Dilated Cardiomyopathy: An Issue of Cardiology Clinics

Dilated Cardiomyopathy: An Issue of Cardiology Clinics

Editor: Cameron Johnson

MURPHY & MOORE
www.murphy-moorepublishing.com

www.murphy-moorepublishing.com

MURPHY & MOORE

Cataloging-in-Publication Data

Dilated cardiomyopathy : an issue of cardiology clinics / edited by Cameron Johnson.
p. cm.
Includes bibliographical references and index.
ISBN 978-1-63987-164-3
1. Myocardium--Diseases. 2. Heart--Dilatation. 3. Congestive heart failure.
4. Cardiology. I. Johnson, Cameron.
RC685.M9 D55 2022
616.124--dc23

Murphy & Moore Publishing,
1 Rockefeller Plaza,
New York City, NY 10020, USA

ISBN 978-1-63987-164-3 (Hardback)

Contents

Preface

The main aim of this book is to educate learners and enhance their research focus by presenting diverse topics covering this vast field. This is an advanced book which compiles significant studies by distinguished experts in the area of analysis. This book addresses successive solutions to the challenges arising in the area of application, along with it; the book provides scope for future developments.

Dilated cardiomyopathy is a disorder of the heart wherein the thinning of the left ventricle of the heart takes place. This leads to the heart not being able to pump blood efficiently. Some of the common symptoms of dilated cardiomyopathy are chest pain, swelling in feet and ankles, and shortness of breath. There are numerous reasons due to which a person might suffer from this disease, such as arrhythmia, hypertension, obesity and diabetes. Dilated cardiomyopathy can lead to severe complications, including heart failure, heart arrest and blood clots. It can be diagnosed through a chest X-ray, echocardiogram or blood tests. This book elucidates the concepts and innovative models around prospective developments with respect to the research on dilated cardiomyopathy. It will also provide interesting topics for research which interested readers can take up. Those in search of information to further their knowledge will be greatly assisted by this book.

It was a great honour to edit this book, though there were challenges, as it involved a lot of communication and networking between me and the editorial team. However, the end result was this all-inclusive book covering diverse themes in the field.

Finally, it is important to acknowledge the efforts of the contributors for their excellent chapters, through which a wide variety of issues have been addressed. I would also like to thank my colleagues for their valuable feedback during the making of this book.

Editor

1

Historical Terminology, Classifications, and Present Definition of DCM

Marco Merlo, Chiara Daneluzzi, Luisa Mestroni, Antonio Cannatà, and Gianfranco Sinagra

Abbreviations and Acronyms

ARVC	Arrhythmogenic right ventricular cardiomyopathy
CMPs	Cardiomyopathies
CMR	Cardiac magnetic resonance
DCM	Dilated cardiomyopathy
EMB	Endomyocardial biopsy
ESC	European Society of Cardiology
HF	Heart failure
HNDC	Hypokinetic non-dilated cardiomyopathy
ICD	Implantable cardioverter defibrillator
LMNA/C	Lamin A/C
LV	Left ventricular
LVRR	Left ventricular reverse remodeling

M. Merlo (✉) · G. Sinagra
Cardiovascular Department, Azienda Sanitaria Universitaria Integrata, Trieste, Italy
e-mail: gianfranco.sinagra@asuits.sanita.fvg.it

C. Daneluzzi · A. Cannatà
Cardiovascular Department, Azienda Sanitaria Universitaria Integrata, University of Trieste (ASUITS), Trieste, Italy

L. Mestroni
Cardiovascular Institute and Adult Medical Genetics Program, University of Colorado Anschutz Medical Campus, Aurora, CO, USA
e-mail: luisa.mestroni@ucdenver.edu

1.1 Dilated Cardiomyopathies: The Classification Pathway

Cardiomyopathies (CMPs) are myocardial disorders in which the heart muscle has structural and functional abnormalities in the absence of other causes sufficient to cause the disease. Until a few decades ago in medical literature, there was uncertainty and confusion about this entity. In the last years, advances in pathophysiology, pathology, biomarkers, genetics and molecular medicine, echocardiography, and cardiac magnetic resonance have brought light in the darkness.

Since 1956 several definitions of CMPs have been adopted using terms as "inflammatory," "non-coronary," "myocardial disorders of unknown etiology" [1]. Classifications tried to make order in the complexity and, historically, were mainly based on phenotype [2, 3] missing multiple other aspects. In 2006 the American Heart Association proposed the definition of CMPs as follows: "cardiomyopathies are a heterogeneous group of diseases of the myocardium associated with mechanical and/or electrical dysfunction that usually (but not invariably) exhibit inappropriate ventricular hypertrophy or dilatation and are due to a variety of causes that frequently are genetic. Cardiomyopathies either are confined to the heart or are part of generalized systemic disorders, often leading to cardiovascular death or progressive heart failure (HF) related disability" [4]. This classification is based on etiology, distinguishing CMP in genetic, acquired, and mixed, and splits CMPs into two groups, primary or secondary, as they involve predominately the heart or as a part of systemic disease. Brugada syndrome, long QT syndromes, short QT syndromes, catecholaminergic ventricular polymorphic tachycardia, and Asian sudden unexplained nocturnal deaths are put separately, but for the first time, channelopathies were mentioned in the classification of genetic cardiomyopathies.

Two years later the European Society of Cardiology (ESC) chose a clinical and morphological classification (Fig. 1.1), reporting CMPs as "myocardial disorders in which structure and function of the myocardium are abnormal, in the absence of coronary artery disease, hypertension, valvular heart disease and congenital heart disease sufficient to cause the observed abnormality". Dilated CMP, hypertrophic CMP, restrictive CMP, and arrhythmogenic right ventricular CMP are the four main specific phenotypes that have to be subsequently subclassified in familial and nonfamilial. Actually the picture is not so simple, with heterogeneity and overlapping forms [5].

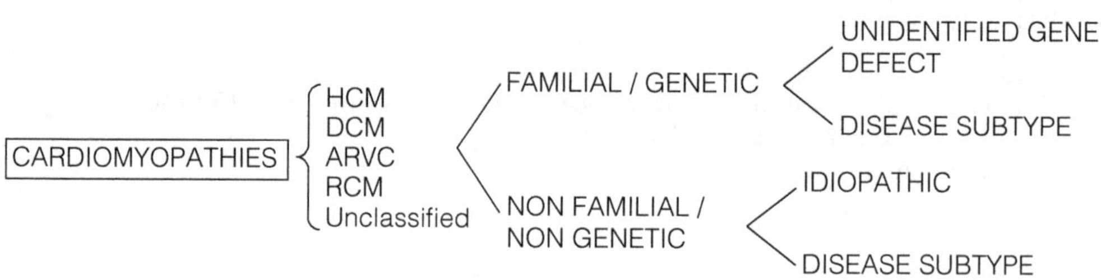

Fig. 1.1 The 2008 ESC classification of cardiomyopathies. From Elliott P. et al. European Heart Journal 2008

The need to integrate the above multiple aspects of CMPs prompts last classification available, proposed by Arbustini et al. in 2013 and endorsed by the World Heart Federation, the MOGE(S), a morphofunctional classification, enriched with extra-cardiac involvement, mode of inheritance with effect of mutation on gene function, and functional status. In details MOGE(S) acronym stands for morphofunctional characteristics (M), organ involvement (O), genetic or familial inheritance pattern (G), etiological information (E), and functional status (S). This system resembles the TNM classification of tumors and provides a genotype-phenotype correlation [6]. It seems to be a challenging way to describe CMPs in everyday life; however, it pushes clinicians to clarify etiology and familiar history and to have a comprehensive approach to the patients, not focusing only on the heart. Actually, even if it represents a translation link between basic science and clinical medicine, However, its use in clinical practice is rare [7].

Although major advances in knowledge as reported above, DCM is the cardiomyopathy that, between all others, still lacks of complete characterization and understanding. The term DCM encloses multiple entities, and, so far, no classification has been able to portrait it adequately.

Anyway, continuous efforts are made by researchers, and in 2016, a new statement has been published. Pinto et al. proposed a revised definition of DCM (Fig. 1.2), which tries to encompass the broad clinical features of the disease and its changes during time. They emphasize the progression of the disease from a preclinical state with no cardiac dilation through isolated ventricular dilation or arrhythmic cardiomyopathy, characterized by arrhythmogenic features as supraventricular/ventricular arrhythmias and/or conduction defects observed in myocarditis, genetic defects, and neuromuscular diseases. Furthermore, they introduce a new entity called “the hypokinetic non-dilated cardiomyopathy (HNDC)” which is the overt phase of systolic dysfunction not associated with ventricular dilation, as it happens in DCM caused by Lamin A/C defects. The final landing remains DCM [8].

Another new concept comes from the recent awareness that DCM overlaps with arrhythmogenic right ventricular cardiomyopathy (ARVC). They may share disease-causing mutations; desmosomal gene defects are known to be mutated in DCM and

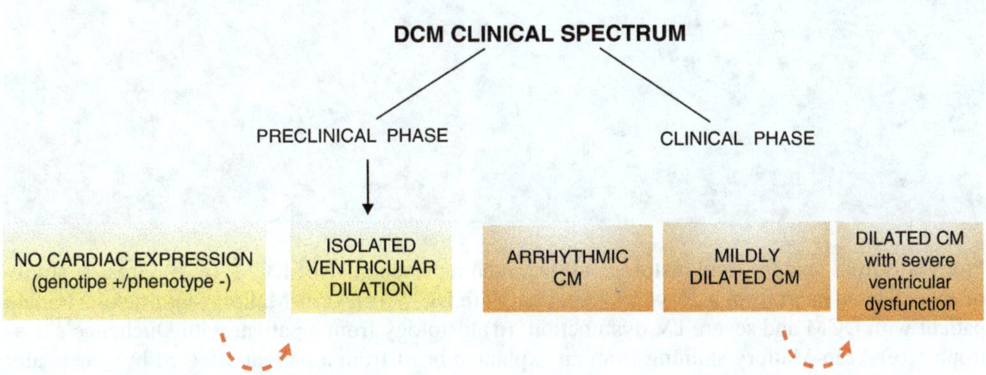

Fig. 1.2 The DCM clinical spectrum. From Pinto Y.M. et al., European Heart Journal 2016

ARVC. Moreover, patients with ARVC can show a left ventricular involvement, and the other way around a DCM relative may demonstrate ventricular ectopy coming from the right ventricle [8].

Maybe in the next classification there will be room for this overlap form with specific gene defects.

Despite major scientific progresses in the last decades, DCM still remains the third cause of HF and the first cause of cardiac transplant worldwide, with high clinical relevance given its mortality-morbidity risk in such a young population with long life expectancy (mean age at diagnosis is 45 years) (Fig. 1.3).

Major advances have been made in DCM since the 1980s when it was considered an end-stage condition, as a cancer, with 50% of mortality at 2 years. Nowadays, the estimated free survival from death and heart transplant is approximately of 85% at 10 years [9]. This is the result of earlier diagnosis with consequent earlier beginning of evidence-based therapy, which has dramatically improved in the last 30 years with introduction of neurohormonal agent (most recent sacubitril-valsartan) and non-pharmacological therapy (implantable cardioverter defibrillator (ICD) and resynchronization therapy). Unfortunately, we are not always able to adequately

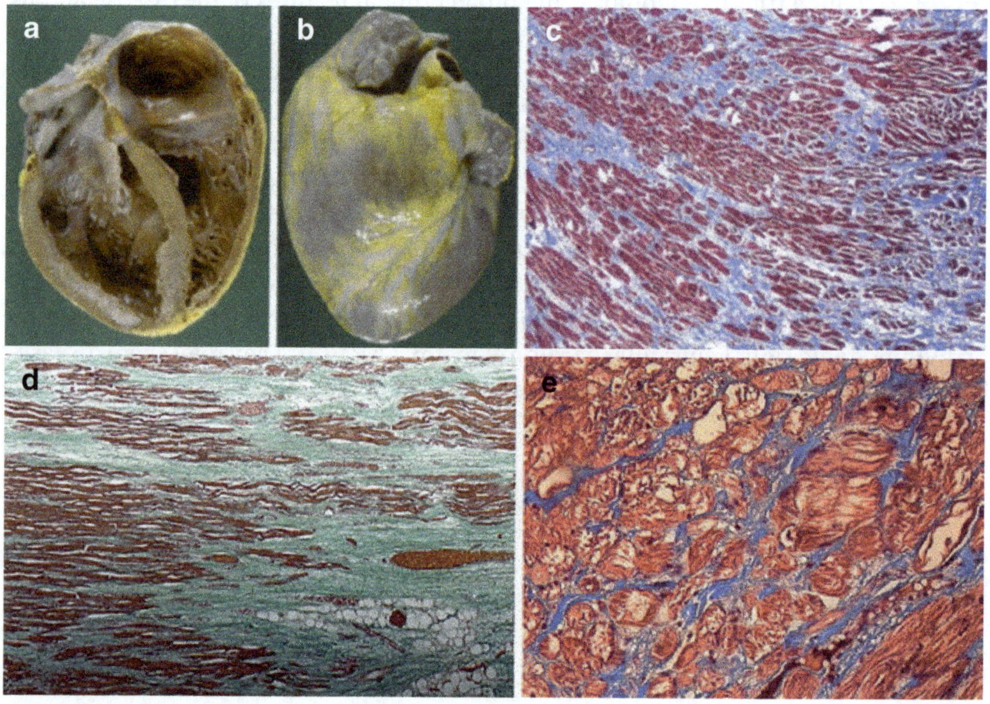

Fig. 1.3 Gross anatomy and histological specimen representative of DCM. (**a**, **b**) Gross anatomy of an explanted heart from a 26-year-old patient with DCM. (**c**) Azan-Mallory staining of a female patient with DCM and severe LV dysfunction; (**d**) histology from a patient with Duchenne's dystrophy; (**e**) Azan-Mallory staining from an explanted heart from a patient affected by genetically determined DCM (double mutation in desmin and potassium channels). Courtesy of Prof. Bussani, University of Trieste

stratify the risk in this population, especially at the beginning of the disease when the adverse left ventricular remodeling is not the only adverse predictor and major arrhythmic events can happen in patients not satisfying criteria for ICD implantation. Anyway, severe mitral regurgitation, right ventricular dysfunction, and restrictive filling pattern have been recognized as predictors of adverse events as expression of advanced disease [10–12]. On the other hand, caution has to be taken to avoid early useless ICD implantation motivated only by low ejection fraction: studies have demonstrated that left ventricular reverse remodeling is a process that lasts 3–9 months after the diagnosis (to be completed in 24 months) [13]. A global evaluation comprehensive of late gadolinium enhancement and peak circumferential strain assessed by cardiac magnetic resonance (CMR) performs better than clinical-echocardiographic evaluation alone in the prediction of left ventricular reverse remodeling (LVRR) in patient recently diagnosed with DCM receiving evidence-based therapy [14].

DCM carries important ethical issues as the identification of asymptomatic carriers of gene mutations in a family, potential risk of pregnancy, and sport participation. These are common situations that the clinical cardiologist has to face with, often without specific guidelines.

Some help in the management of DCM comes from registries enrolling clinical, instrumental, and prognostic data of large cohorts of patients affected and strictly followed in the long term. In our Institution this is a common behavior, since we can extrapolate thousands of data from the Heart Muscle Disease Registry, active from 1978 [15].

1.2 Genetic Dilated Cardiomyopathy and Etiological Classification

Familial forms account for the at least 40% of cases, and thanks to the recent discoveries in the genetic field, clinicians have the opportunity, but also the responsibility, to provide an etiological diagnosis, stratify the risk and treat patients with the best strategy available. So, when acquired causes (e.g. hypertension, coronary artery disease, valvular heart disease, arrhythmias, etc.) have been excluded, there is a family history of DCM and there are clinical clues suggesting the diagnosis (what we used to call "red flags": deafness, blindness, muscular disorders, etc.), we recommend to perform the genetic screening [13]. Anyway, it has to be stressed that de novo mutations exist, so a negative family history doesn't rule out a genetic DCM, and that is mandatory for an appropriate patient selection in order to avoid noise, as will be explained below.

Guidelines and position papers recommend, with level C of evidence, genetic testing in the proband (the first or the most affected in the family, as this gives a high positive predictive value) in order to provide diagnostic/prognostic information, aid therapeutic choices, and prompt cascade screening in relatives [16]. Family screening allows an early diagnosis in a consistent number of patients, facilitating the diagnosis in non-proband DCM patients at an early stage of the disease, giving the chance to start optimal medical therapy earlier [17].

Genetic background of DCM is a wide and complex issue. So far, more than 50 genes encoding for cytoskeleton, sarcomeric proteins, sarcolemma, nuclear envelope ion channels, and intercellular junctions have been found to be implicated in DCM, and several other genes remain to be discovered. There is variable clinical presentation (also in the same family), incomplete penetrance, age-related penetrance, and lack of specific phenotype (meaning that the same gene mutation can cause different cardiomyopathies) [13].

However, unlike few decades ago, when cardiomyopathies were a confused matter, now we are living an historical breakthrough: from a pure phenotype classification, we are moving toward a best understanding of DCM and a more "personal" characterization of the disease, thanks to genetics [18]. In particular, there is growing evidence in the field of genotype-phenotype correlation with remarkable implications in the management of patients.

Although a strong genotype-phenotype relationship is currently accepted only for LMNA/C, recently a body of data is emerging in this field. Some rare sarcomeric variants carry poor prognosis after the age of 50, supporting the role of genetic testing in further risk stratification [19]. Furthermore, cytoskeleton Z-disk mutations are demonstrated as inversely related with LVRR. Moreover, since these proteins are not involved in beta-adrenergic activity, they are not targeted by antineurohormonal drugs limiting the therapeutic effect of the widespread molecules used in HFβ management [20].

Thus, the updated approach to DCM is now comprehensive of genetic evaluation with identification of genes and their corresponding phenotypic expression, accepting that most genotype-phenotype correlation remains unknown and, to date, globally, the genetic background is not able to predict disease evolution and response to therapy.

1.3 Future Perspectives

As frequently happens in medicine, there are unresolved issues, which are outlined below and which will be further explained in the focused chapters of the book.

Our efforts must focus on identifying the underlying DCM cause, in order to further reduce the number of "idiopathic DCM." Progresses have been made in this field; we know that in the 1980s, almost 50% of DCM didn't have a specific cause. Nowadays the etiologic characterization has dramatically improved so that it is possible to understand the etiologic basis of many so-called idiopathic heart muscle disease [3].

Thanks to etiology-directed management, the DCM prognosis has considerably improved and clinicians must persist in this task [21].

In patient with clinically suspected myocarditis as a possible explanation for ventricular dysfunction, there is the need to proceed with endomyocardial biopsy (EMB), with histopathology, immunohistochemistry, and molecular analysis. It has a fundamental role in identifying the underlying etiology (e.g., giant cell, eosinophilic myocarditis, sarcoidosis) which imply different treatments and prognosis. It is also the basis for safe immunosuppressive therapy, after the exclusion of viral infection [22].

Valuable aids in the etiologic characterization of DCM come from the recent advances in echocardiography.

An interesting tool is speckle-tracking strain analysis for assessing cardiac mechanics and segmental and global LV function. This technique allows the evaluation of myocardial deformation in all its components (i.e., longitudinal and circumferential shortening and radial thickening). All parameters may be reduced in DCM, beginning in the preclinical phase and allowing an early identification of disease [23].

Another essential tool is cardiovascular magnetic resonance (CMR). It provides additional prognostic information as it is the gold standard technique for biventricular morphological and functional evaluation and tissue characterization [24].

It is frequently adopted in the setting of myocarditis in stable patients or after EMB in life-threatening presentations, according to Lake Louise criteria [22].

A step toward a comprehensive DCM classification and an attempt to reconcile clinic with genetic in the complexity of the disease is genotype-phenotype correlation, with its prognostic implication in clinical practice. A clear example of this relation is the LMNA/C, but other gene defects are emerging, such as Filamin C [25]. It is possible that in the future genetic cluster classification will be completed studying every gene mutation, thanks to whole-genome sequencing, taking care of the patient instead of the disease.

Our efforts are focused on a personalized medicine approach including technologies at the services of each patient maybe with genic therapy or specific anti-inflammatory therapy targeted to the specific etiology.

References

1. Arbustini E, Narula N, Tavazzi L, et al. The MOGE(S) classification of cardiomyopathy for clinicians. J Am Coll Cardiol. 2014;64:304–18. https://doi.org/10.1016/j.jacc.2014.05.027.
2. Heartjf B. Report of the WHO/ISFC task force on the definition and classification of cardiomyopathies. Br Heart J. 1980;44:672–3. https://doi.org/10.1136/hrt.44.6.672.
3. Richardson P, McKenna W, Bristow M, et al. Report of the 1995 World Health Organization/International Society and Federation of Cardiology Task Force on the definition and classification of cardiomyopathies. Circulation. 1996;93:841–2. https://doi.org/10.1161/01.CIR.93.5.841.
4. Maron BJ, Towbin JA, Thiene G, et al. Contemporary definitions and classification of the cardiomyopathies: an American Heart Association scientific statement from the Council on Clinical Cardiology, Heart Failure and Transplantation Committee. Circulation. 2006;113:1807–16. https://doi.org/10.1161/CIRCULATIONAHA.106.174287.
5. Elliott P, Andersson B, Arbustini E, et al. Classification of the cardiomyopathies: a position statement from the European Society of Cardiology Working Group on Myocardial and Pericardial Diseases. Eur Heart J. 2008;29:270–6. https://doi.org/10.1093/eurheartj/ehm342.
6. Şahan E, Şahan S, Karamanlıoğlu M, et al. The MOGE(S) classification. Herz. 2016;41:503–6. https://doi.org/10.1007/s00059-015-4394-0.
7. Fedele F, Severino P, Calcagno S, Mancone M. Heart failure: TNM-like classification. J Am Coll Cardiol. 2014;63:1959–60.
8. Pinto YM, Elliott PM, Arbustini E, et al. Proposal for a revised definition of dilated cardiomyopathy, hypokinetic non-dilated cardiomyopathy, and its implications for clinical practice:

a position statement of the ESC Working Group on Myocardial and Pericardial Diseases. Eur Heart J. 2016;37:1850–8. https://doi.org/10.1093/eurheartj/ehv727.

9. Merlo M, Gigli M, Poli S, et al. La cardiomiopatia dilatativa come malattia dinamica: storia naturale, rimodellamento inverso e stratificazione prognostica. G Ital Cardiol. 2016;17:15–23.
10. Merlo M, Pyxaras SA, Pinamonti B, et al. Prevalence and prognostic significance of left ventricular reverse remodeling in dilated cardiomyopathy receiving tailored medical treatment. J Am Coll Cardiol. 2011;57:1468–76. https://doi.org/10.1016/j.jacc.2010.11.030.
11. Stolfo D, Merlo M, Pinamonti B, et al. Early improvement of functional mitral regurgitation in patients with idiopathic dilated cardiomyopathy. Am J Cardiol. 2015;115:1137–43. https://doi.org/10.1016/j.amjcard.2015.01.549.
12. Merlo M, Stolfo D, Anzini M, et al. Persistent recovery of normal left ventricular function and dimension in idiopathic dilated cardiomyopathy during long-term follow-up: does real healing exist? J Am Heart Assoc. 2015;4:e001504. https://doi.org/10.1161/JAHA.114.000570.
13. Merlo M, Cannatà A, Gobbo M, et al. Evolving concepts in dilated cardiomyopathy. Eur J Heart Fail. 2017;20(2):228–39. https://doi.org/10.1002/ejhf.1103.
14. Merlo M, Masè M, Vitrella G, et al. Comprehensive structural and functional assessment for prediction of left ventricular reverse remodeling in non-ischemic cardiomyopathy. J Am Coll Cardiol. 2018;71:A877. https://doi.org/10.1016/S0735-1097(18)31418-9.
15. Mestroni L, Rocco C, Gregori D, et al. Familial dilated cardiomyopathy: evidence for genetic and phenotypic heterogeneity. Heart Muscle Disease Study Group. J Am Coll Cardiol. 1999;34:181–90.
16. Hershberger RE, Lindenfeld J, Mestroni L, et al. Genetic evaluation of cardiomyopathy—a Heart Failure Society of America practice guideline. J Card Fail. 2009;15:83–97. https://doi.org/10.1016/j.cardfail.2009.01.006.
17. Moretti M, Merlo M, Barbati G, et al. Prognostic impact of familial screening in dilated cardiomyopathy. Eur J Heart Fail. 2010;12:922–7. https://doi.org/10.1093/eurjhf/hfq093.
18. Sinagra G, Mestroni L, Camerini F, editors. Genetic cardiomyopathies: a clinical approach. Milan: Springer; 2013.
19. Merlo M, Sinagra G, Carniel E, et al. Poor prognosis of rare sarcomeric gene variants in patients with dilated cardiomyopathy. Clin Transl Sci. 2013;6:424–8. https://doi.org/10.1111/cts.12116.
20. Dal Ferro M, Stolfo D, Altinier A, et al. Association between mutation status and left ventricular reverse remodelling in dilated cardiomyopathy. Heart. 2017;103:1704–10. https://doi.org/10.1136/heartjnl-2016-311017.
21. Merlo M, Gentile P, Naso P, Sinagra G. The natural history of dilated cardiomyopathy: how has it changed? J Cardiovasc Med. 2017;18:e161–5. https://doi.org/10.2459/JCM.0000000000000459.
22. Caforio ALP, Pankuweit S, Arbustini E, et al. Current state of knowledge on aetiology, diagnosis, management, and therapy of myocarditis: a position statement of the European Society of Cardiology Working Group on Myocardial and Pericardial Diseases. Eur Heart J. 2013;34:2636–48. https://doi.org/10.1093/eurheartj/eht210.
23. Lang RM, Badano LP, Mor-Avi V, et al. Recommendations for cardiac chamber quantification by echocardiography in adults: an update from the American Society of Echocardiography and the European Association of Cardiovascular Imaging. Eur Heart J Cardiovasc Imaging. 2015;16:233–71. https://doi.org/10.1093/ehjci/jev014.
24. Hombach V, Merkle N, Torzewski J, et al. Electrocardiographic and cardiac magnetic resonance imaging parameters as predictors of a worse outcome in patients with idiopathic dilated cardiomyopathy. Eur Heart J. 2009;30:2011–8. https://doi.org/10.1093/eurheartj/ehp293.
25. Corrado D, Zorzi A. Filamin C: a new arrhythmogenic cardiomyopathy–causing gene? JACC Clin Electrophysiol. 2018;4:515–7.

2

Epidemiology

Paola Naso, Luca Falco, Aldostefano Porcari, Andrea Di Lenarda, and Gerardina Lardieri

Abbreviations and Acronyms

CAD	Coronary artery disease
DCM	Dilated cardiomyopathy
ECG	Electrocardiography
EMB	Endomyocardial biopsy
HCM	Hypertrophic cardiomyopathy
HF	Heart failure
ICD	Implantable cardioverter device
LV	Left ventricular
LVEDD	Left ventricular end-diastolic diameter
LVEF	Left ventricular ejection fraction
NGS	Next-generation sequencing
SCN5A	Sodium channel protein type 5 subunit alpha
WGS	Whole-genome sequencing

Dilated cardiomyopathy (DCM) is a cardiac disease characterized by LV dilatation and impaired systolic function. An acquired dilated phenotype may result from a variety of factors including coronary artery disease (CAD), hypertension, myocarditis, valvular and congenital heart disease, drug toxicity, alcohol abuse and metabolic disease. Indeed, the diagnosis of "primary" DCM is often of exclusion. Among the forms of primitive DCM, familiar forms and idiopathic forms are identified [1–4].

P. Naso (✉) · L. Falco · A. Porcari · A. Di Lenarda · G. Lardieri
Cardiovascular Department, Azienda Sanitaria Universitaria Integrata, University of Trieste (ASUITS), Trieste, Italy
e-mail: andrea.dilenarda@asuits.sanita.fvg.it; gerardina.lardieri@aas2.sanita.fvg.it

Table 2.1 Major epidemiologic studies in dilated cardiomyopathy

Study	Incidence/prevalence
Torp et al. 1978	3/100,000/year [20]
Bagger et al. 1984	0.73/100,000/year [21]
Williams et al. 1985	8.3/100,000 [22]
Codd et al. 1989	36.5/100,000 [6]
Dolara et al. 1989	1.8/100,000/year [23]
Rakar et al. 1997	6.95/100,000/year [5]

The epidemiology of this condition is quite complex, due to misdiagnosis, continuous reclassification and changing definitions. Furthermore, since investigations were performed on small populations in specific geographic areas and were not representative of the general population, epidemiological studies on DCM are affected by many limitations. Another, but substantial, limitation of epidemiological studies conducted on this pathology depends upon the lack of standardized diagnostic criteria [5].

Initial estimations of prevalence data for DCM came from a population-based study by Codd et al. conducted on the Olmsted Country population (Minnesota, USA) between 1975 and 1984. According to this study, the prevalence rates were higher for men, with a male/female ratio of 3:1 [6]. Age- and sex-adjusted prevalence rates reached 36.5/100,000 subjects, and incidence rates were found 6/100,000 person years. Younger patients (<55 years) were more frequently affected (incidence up to 17.9/100,000). Data related to the epidemiology in different ethnicities suggest a 2.7-fold increased risk associated with black race [7]. Death certificates from the National Center for Health Statistics' confirmed a 2.5-fold increased risk in blacks more than in whites, with black men having the highest prevalence (27/100,000 in black men versus 11/100,000 in white men) [8]. In Italy, the first data on the incidence of DCM go back to a prospective post-mortem study on consecutive necropsies performed during a 2-year period (November 1987–November 1989) in the Department of Pathology at Trieste University. Incidence of DCM at autopsy was estimated at 4.5/100,000/year, while clinical incidence in the same period was 2.45/100,000/year. The total incidence was 6.95/100,000/year in accordance with the study by Codd et al. [5, 6]. Table 2.1 shows a summary of major epidemiologic studies.

2.1 Towards Contemporary Clinical Epidemiology in Dilated Cardiomyopathy

The 2008 position statement from the European Working Group on Myocardial and Pericardial Diseases was a definitive turning point and shed new light upon the dark side of cardiomyopathies [9]. Cardiomyopathies were defined as "myocardial disorders in which the heart muscle is structurally and functionally abnormal, in the absence of coronary artery disease, hypertension, valvular disease and congenital heart disease sufficient to cause the observed myocardial abnormality" [10].

They were grouped into specific morphological and functional phenotypes and further divided into familial and nonfamilial forms. Diagnostic criteria have two main objectives: to support and facilitate the recognition of the disease and to allow the early diagnosis in affected asymptomatic family members. The consensus paper combined a clinical mind-set with first- and second-level diagnostic tools (i.e. ECG and echocardiography), placing the emphasis on family history of cardiac and neuromuscular diseases. The diagnostic paradigm shifted from a pathophysiological mechanism to a morphological and functional point of view, and the new awareness of a familial pattern in this disease built the basis of relatives screening [11].

In recent years, the diagnosis of DCM became reliable even in centres of different countries, thus allowing multicentre studies with more numerous and representative populations of well-studied patients. Furthermore, female sex gained attention in scientific literature and gender differences became an important topic to address.

Diagnostic criteria only partially overcame the difficulties faced in epidemiologic studies because of the challenging diagnosis and clinical presentation of the disease. Hershberger and colleagues estimated DCM prevalence on the basis of the known DCM to HCM ratio of ≈2:1. Therefore the surrogate DCM was found to be about 1–250 subjects [12], resulting from the early diagnosis, more effective treatments and a reduced mortality of patient partially linked to the identification of DCM in asymptomatic subjects. Current guidelines report a prevalence of familial DCM ranging from ≈30 to 50% of cases, with 40% having an identifiable genetic cause [13–15].

Table 2.2 shows the frequency of DCM in special categories.

DCM was originally considered a rare disease, and the possibility of a familiar substrate was ignored. Over time, DCM was found to be a major cause of HF affecting especially young patients, with absent or nonsignificant comorbidity and a long life expectancy, thus emerging as a major indication to heart transplantation [1]. The need to improve diagnostic accuracy for this population gave new life to scientific literature. DCM started to be considered a systemic condition rather than an isolated disease, and ventricular dilatation was found a common pathway of several cardiac diseases [3].

The studies carried out more recently were not built upon the solely basis of the phenotype, thus reflecting the epidemiology of the disease with higher accuracy. However, despite major efforts, the true incidence and prevalence of DCM still remains to be determined.

Table 2.2 Frequency of dilated cardiomyopathy in special groups

Categories	Prevalence ratios
Female to male	Between 1:1.3 and 1:1.5 [7, 23]
White (W) to African-Americans (AA)	1:2.45 W 11/100,000 AA 27/100,000 [7]
Familial forms	30–50% [14]

2.2 Genetics and Future Perspectives

As previously discussed, it has been known for decades that familial clinical screening in idiopathic DCM would reveal a significant amount of first-degree affected subjects (20–48%). However, only in the last few years, the role of genetics has become predominant in the approach of DCM patients, and the complexity of genetic mechanisms, genotype and environment interactions and genotype-phenotype correlations have become clearer. A fundamental role for these achievements has been played in recent years by the technological progress with the so-called next-generation sequencing (NGS) techniques, also used to sequence the entire human genome (coding and noncoding regions of DNA), referred to as whole-genome sequencing (WGS), with panels of dozens of genes at reduced cost [16].

In the most recent reports, approximately 40% of DCM cases have an identifiable genetic pathogenic variant. An important issue in this setting is the vast genetic as well as phenotypic heterogeneity in familial DCM, meaning that more than one mutation could be found and sometimes different morphological forms are showed in a single family: this is a major obstacle in clinical practice and in genetic report interpretations, because unreported pathogenic mutations must be validated, a process that needs time and delays the screening of other family members [17].

Thanks to the efforts in this field, a growing number of genes involved in DCM have been identified, and currently most panels cover 30–40 genes. Recently, many European centres have put their data together to create the first "Atlas of the clinical genetics of human Dilated Cardiomyopathy" [18].

Nowadays, the role of genetics is becoming more and more important in clinical practice. In fact, there is an increasing evidence that identifying a disease-causing variant may have important patient management implications in terms of severity of the disease, prognosis and survival rates. For example, McNair et al. reported that 1.7% of DCM families have SCN5A gene mutations linked to a strong arrhythmic pattern [19] and that Lamin A/C mutation carriers have a well-known risk of major ventricular arrhythmias/sudden death and conduction system abnormalities: this evidence may lead clinical cardiologist to consider ICD implantations in a cluster of patients that do not match the usual criteria indicated by the HF guidelines [20].

Epidemiology of DCM is rapidly changing. Furthermore, genetic testing may identify asymptomatic carriers, which lead to redefine prevention strategies, sport recommendations and ICD implantation. Nevertheless, it may guide reproductive decision-making, which could further modify the incidence and prevalence of DCM in the future decades [21].

References

1. Aleksova A, Sabbadini G, Merlo M, Pinamonti B, Barbati G, Zecchin M, et al. Natural history of dilated cardiomyopathy: from asymptomatic left ventricular dysfunction to heart failure—a subgroup analysis from the Trieste Cardiomyopathy Registry. J Cardiovasc Med. 2009;10:699–705.

2. Rapezzi C, Arbustini E, Caforio ALP, Charron P, Gimeno-Blanes J, Helio T, et al. Diagnostic work-up in cardiomyopathies: bridging the gap between clinical phenotypes and final diagnosis. A position statement from the ESC Working Group on Myocardial and Pericardial Diseases. Eur Heart J. 2013;34:1448–58.
3. Pinto YM, Elliott PM, Arbustini E, Adler Y, Anastasakis A, Bohm M, et al. Proposal for a revised definition of dilated cardiomyopathy, hypokinetic non-dilated cardiomyopathy, and its implications for clinical practice: a position statement of the ESC Working Group on Myocardial and Pericardial Diseases. Eur Heart J. 2016;37:1850–8.
4. Caforio ALP, Pankuweit S, Arbustini E, Basso C, Gimeno-Blanes J, Felix SB, et al. Current state of knowledge on aetiology, diagnosis, management, and therapy of myocarditis: a position statement of the European Society of Cardiology Working Group on Myocardial and Pericardial Diseases. Eur Heart J. 2013;34:2636–48, 2648a–2648d.
5. Rakar S, Sinagra G, Di Lenarda A, Poletti A, Bussani R, Silvestri F, et al. Epidemiology of dilated cardiomyopathy. A prospective post-mortem study of 5252 necropsies. The Heart Muscle Disease Study Group. Eur Heart J. 1997;18:117–23.
6. Codd MB, Sugrue DD, Gersh BJ, Melton LJ 3rd. Epidemiology of idiopathic dilated and hypertrophic cardiomyopathy. A population-based study in Olmsted County, Minnesota, 1975–1984. Circulation. 1989;80:564–72.
7. Coughlin SS, Szklo M, Baughman K, Pearson TA. The epidemiology of idiopathic dilated cardiomyopathy in a biracial community. Am J Epidemiol. 1990;131:48–56.
8. Gillum RF. Idiopathic cardiomyopathy in the United States, 1970–1982. Am Heart J. 1986;111:752–5.
9. Elliott P, Andersson B, Arbustini E, Bilinska Z, Cecchi F, Charron P, et al. Classification of the cardiomyopathies: a position statement from the European Society of Cardiology Working Group on Myocardial and Pericardial Diseases. Eur Heart J. 2008;29:270–6.
10. Grunig E, Tasman JA, Kucherer H, Franz W, Kubler W, Katus HA. Frequency and phenotypes of familial dilated cardiomyopathy. J Am Coll Cardiol. 1998;31:186–94.
11. Hershberger RE, Hedges DJ, Morales A. Dilated cardiomyopathy: the complexity of a diverse genetic architecture. Nat Rev Cardiol. 2013;10:531–47.
12. Ganesh SK, Arnett DK, Assimes TL, Basson CT, Chakravarti A, Ellinor PT, et al. Genetics and genomics for the prevention and treatment of cardiovascular disease: update: a scientific statement from the American Heart Association. Circulation. 2013;128:2813–51.
13. Mestroni L, Rocco C, Gregori D, Sinagra G, Di Lenarda A, Miocic S, et al. Familial dilated cardiomyopathy: evidence for genetic and phenotypic heterogeneity. Heart Muscle Disease Study Group. J Am Coll Cardiol. 1999;34:181–90.
14. Hershberger RE, Siegfried JD. Update 2011: clinical and genetic issues in familial dilated cardiomyopathy. J Am Coll Cardiol. 2011;57:1641–9.
15. Sweet M, Taylor MRG, Mestroni L. Diagnosis, prevalence, and screening of familial dilated cardiomyopathy. Expert Opin Orphan Drugs. 2015;3:869–76.
16. Haas J, Frese KS, Peil B, Kloos W, Keller A, Nietsch R, et al. Atlas of the clinical genetics of human dilated cardiomyopathy. Eur Heart J. 2015;36:1123–35a.
17. McNair WP, Sinagra G, Taylor MRG, Di Lenarda A, Ferguson DA, Salcedo EE, et al. SCN5A mutations associate with arrhythmic dilated cardiomyopathy and commonly localize to the voltage-sensing mechanism. J Am Coll Cardiol. 2011;57:2160–8.
18. van Rijsingen IAW, Arbustini E, Elliott PM, Mogensen J, Hermans-van Ast JF, van der Kooi AJ, et al. Risk factors for malignant ventricular arrhythmias in Lamin a/c mutation carriers a European cohort study. J Am Coll Cardiol. 2012;59:493–500.
19. Mestroni L, Taylor MRG. Genetics and genetic testing of dilated cardiomyopathy: a new perspective. Discov Med. 2013;15:43–9.
20. Torp A. Incidence of congestive cardiomyopathy. Postgrad Med J. 1978;54:435–9.
21. Bagger JP, Baandrup U, Rasmussen K, Moller M, Vesterlund T. Cardiomyopathy in western Denmark. Br Heart J. 1984;52:327–31.
22. Williams DG, Olsen EG. Prevalence of overt dilated cardiomyopathy in two regions of England. Br Heart J. 1985;54:153–5.
23. Dolara A, Cecchi F, Ciaccheri M. Cardiomyopathy in Italy today: extent of the problem. G Ital Cardiol. 1989;19:1074–9.

3

Pathophysiology

Valerio De Paris, Federico Biondi, Davide Stolfo, Marco Merlo, and Gianfranco Sinagra

Abbreviations and Acronyms

AD	Alzheimer's disease
ANP	Atrial natriuretic peptide
ARVC	Arrhythmogenic right ventricular Cardiomyopathy
AT1/2R	Angiotensin type 1/2 receptor
ATII	Angiotensin II
BNP	Brain natriuretic peptide
DCM	Dilated cardiomyopathy
ECM	Extracellular matrix
HF	Heart failure
IL1β	Interleukin 1 β
LV	Left ventricular
MCP-1	Monocyte chemoattractant protein-1
MIP 1α	Macrophagic inflammatory protein 1 α
MMP-9	Matrix metalloproteinase-9
PIIINP	N-terminal type III collagen peptide
RAAS	Renin-angiotensin-aldosterone system
RyR2	Ryanodine receptor 2
SERCA	Sarco-/endoplasmic reticulum Ca^{2+}-ATPase
SR	Sarcoplasmic reticulum
TIMP-1	Tissue inhibitor of metalloproteinase-1
TNFα	Tumor necrosis factor

V. De Paris · F. Biondi · D. Stolfo (✉)
Cardiovascular Department, Azienda Sanitaria Universitaria Integrata, University of Trieste (ASUITS), Trieste, Italy
e-mail: Davide.stolfo@asuits.sanita.fvg.it

M. Merlo · G. Sinagra
Cardiovascular Department, Azienda Sanitaria Universitaria Integrata, Trieste, Italy
e-mail: gianfranco.sinagra@asuits.sanita.fvg.it

Dilated cardiomyopathy (DCM) is characterized by dilated left ventricle with systolic dysfunction that is not caused by ischemic or valvular heart disease.

The hallmark pathophysiologic feature of DCM is systolic dysfunction of the left or both ventricles. Reduced sarcomere contractility increases ventricular volumes to maintain cardiac output through the Frank-Starling mechanism, producing the thin-walled dilated LV appearance that is observed in overt DCM.

Frank and Starling demonstrated that increased ventricular preload augments contractility, but excessive pressure and volume induces a plateau and then a reduction in myocardial contraction [1]. Abnormal hemodynamics leads further to left ventricular (LV) remodeling.

Cardiac remodeling in response to an inciting myocardial insult or an underlying genetic abnormality has been classically considered the pathognomonic aspect of DCM.

3.1 Ventricular Remodeling in DCM

The term ventricular remodeling refers to alteration in ventricular architecture, with associated increased volume and altered chamber configuration, driven on a histologic level by a combination of pathologic myocyte hypertrophy, myocyte apoptosis, myofibroblast proliferation, and interstitial fibrosis.

Pathologic LV remodeling is closely linked to activation of a series of neuroendocrine, paracrine, and autocrine factors, which are upregulated after myocardial injury and in the setting of increased LV wall stress and hemodynamic derangement. Contributing factors include the renin-angiotensin-aldosterone (RAA) axis, the adrenergic nervous system, increased oxidative stress, pro-inflammatory cytokines, and endothelin. Both RAA system inhibition and beta-adrenergic blockade have shown to markedly attenuate or reverse LV remodeling in patients with heart failure and LV dilation.

Left ventricular remodeling results in characteristic alterations of left ventricular function that can be described in terms of altered left ventricular pressure-volume relationship. Left ventricular dilatation and reduced systolic function induce a rightward displacement of the pressure-volume curve with increased left ventricular end-diastolic volumes and pressures. Despite increased preload, stroke volume may be reduced, and end-systolic pressure to volume ratio (index of contractility) is depressed. In addition to this, diastolic dysfunction due to incomplete relaxation after disturbed excitation-contraction coupling processes and increased stiffness due to altered extracellular matrix composition cause an additional upward shift of the pressure-volume relation.

When the preload reserve is exhausted, the stroke volume becomes sensitive to alterations in the afterload. It depends on blood viscosity, vascular resistance, vascular distensibility, and mainly myocardial wall tension.

Calculations of myocardial wall tension are defined by the Laplace equation and are expressed in terms of tension, T, per unit of cross-sectional area (dynes per centimeter [dyn/cm]).

Within a cylinder, the law of Laplace states that wall tension is equal to the pressure within a thick-walled cylinder times the radius of curvature of the wall:

$$T = P \times R / h$$

where T is wall tension (dyn/cm), P is pressure (dyn/cm^2), R is the radius (cm), and h is wall thickness.

Two fundamental principles stem from the relationship between the geometry of the ventricular cavity and the tension on its muscular walls: (1) dilatation of the ventricles leads directly to an increase in tension and (2) an increase in wall thickness reduces the tension on any individual muscle fiber. Therefore, ventricular hypertrophy reduces afterload by distributing tension among more muscle fibers.

Dilatation of the heart decreases cardiac efficiency as measured by myocardial oxygen consumption unless hypertrophy is sufficient to normalize wall stress. In HF, wall tension (or stress) is high, and thus, afterload is increased. The energetic consequences of the law of Laplace can have some role in progressive deterioration of energy-starved cardiac myocytes in the failing heart.

3.2 Genetic Pathophysiology and New Possible Proteins Involved in DCM [2]

A great diversity of pathogenetic pathways has been hypothesized to explain the development of DCM, depending on the affected genes and the dislodged intracellular structures or pathways.

The wide variety of genes involved in the pathophysiology of DCM gives an insight to think of DCM as a group of diseases, instead of a single form of cardiomyopathy (Fig. 3.1).

Genetic mutations suggest several mechanisms of ventricular dysfunction in DCM as follows:

- *Deficit in force generation* (*sarcomere DCM*): Mutations within genes encoding titin, myosin, actin, troponin, and tropomyosin result in the expression of abnormally functioning proteins, thus leading to myocardial dysfunction and DCM. Sarcomere gene mutations are the most frequent causes of DCM with truncating mutations in titin (TTNtvs) occur in 25% of end-stage disease and in 15% of ambulatory DCM patients [3, 4].
- *Defects in nuclear envelope* (*laminopathies*): These diseases are characterized by variable degrees of heart and skeletal muscle involvement. Mutations involve Lamin-A/C and emerin coding genes. Dominant Lamin A/C mutations occur in approximately 6% of DCM cases and are far more common in DCM with conduction system disease [5]. Electrophysiological abnormalities (conduction system block and atrial fibrillation) often precede DCM that relentlessly progresses to HF [6, 7]. The severity of the associated skeletal myopathy is variable. Most Lamin A/C mutations cause haploinsufficiency, and mouse models of these mutations demonstrate inadequate response to mechanical strain, which may promote premature cardiomyocyte death.

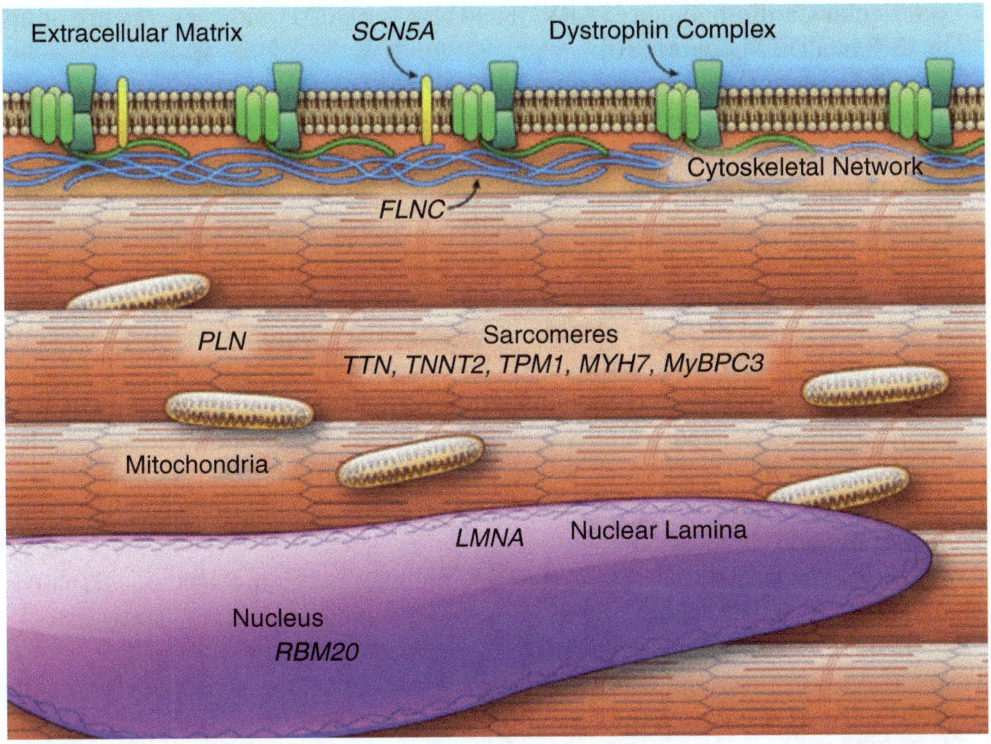

Fig. 3.1 Cardiomyocyte compartments contributing to genetically mediated dilated cardiomyopathy. See Legend for abbreviations and acronyms. (Adapted from McNally EM, Mestroni L, Dilated Cardiomyopathy Genetic Determinants and Mechanisms *CircRes*. 2017;121:731–748. DOI: https://doi.org/10.1161/CIRCRESAHA.116.309396)

- *Deficit in force transmission* (*cytoskeletal cardiomyopathies*): Mutations involving protein members of the cytoskeletal apparatus, like filamins, dystrophin, desmin, d-sarcoglycan, and vinculin, are responsible for muscular dystrophies, which are often associated with DCM.
- Filamins are large cytoskeletal actin cross-linking proteins that stabilize the actin filament networks and link them to the cell membrane by binding transmembrane proteins and ion channels [8]. Filamin C encodes a large protein (2725 amino acids) primarily expressed in the cardiac and skeletal muscle that interacts with sarcomeric proteins in the Z-disc and the sarcolemma. Filamin C truncation variants are associated with a severe arrhythmogenic DCM phenotype in the absence of overt skeletal muscle disease.
- *Deficit in protein post-translational modifications* (*glycosylation processes-cardiomyopathies*): An example comes from dolichol kinase gene mutations, resulting in impairment of protein glycosylation processes inside the cell organelles, thus manifesting as syndromic conditions with hypertrophic phenotype and as non-syndromic DCM phenotype [9].
- *Impaired cell-to-cell adhesion* (*desmosomal cardiomyopathies*): Mutations in genes encoding desmosomal proteins are responsible for arrhythmogenic right

ventricular Cardiomyopahty (ARVC) and also for DCM, with a prevalence of up to 13% in a DCM cohort [10].

- *Deficit in energy production* (*mitochondrial cardiomyopathies*): They are characterized by defects in the oxidative phosphorylation that result in deficient energy production in the form of ATP. They include hypertrophic, dilated, and LV non-compaction phenotypes.
- *Calcium-cycling abnormalities*: A DCM mutation has been described in the phospholamban gene. Phospholamban is responsible for inhibition of sarco-/endoplasmic reticulum $Ca2^+$ –ATPase (SERCA) function. Mutations in the gene result in increased SERCA inhibition with defective calcium reuptake, with consequent reduction in contractility and heart dilation.
- *Ion channel abnormalities*: Mutations in ion channel genes (SCN5A, ABCC9) are typically associated with a variety of arrhythmic disorders. The ventricular dilation and DCM pattern is less common and almost always preceded by arrhythmias and/or conduction system defects [11, 12]. The pathogenetic mechanisms are poorly understood.
- *Spliceosomal defects*: RBM20 is an RNA binding protein involved in alternative splicing process. DCM associated with RBM20 mutations is frequently associated with early onset, severe heart failure, and high arrhythmic potential.
- *Epigenetic perturbation*: Missense mutation in GATAD1 gene is associated with DCM. GATAD1 encodes for a protein that is thought to bind to a histone modification site that regulates gene expression.
- *Protein misfolding disease*: Mutations in presenilin genes have been recently identified in patients with DCM [13]. Presenilins are also expressed in the heart and play a role in heart development. Aβ amyloid is a possible novel cause of myocardial dysfunction. Echocardiographic measurements of myocardial function suggest that patients with Alzheimer's disease (AD) present with an anticipated diastolic dysfunction. As in the brain, A β40 and A β42 are present in the heart, and their expression is increased in AD [14].
- *RAS-MAPK pathway disruption*: Mutations in RAF-1 gene are responsible for rare variants of childhood-onset, non-syndromic DCM.

3.3 Molecular Mechanisms of Cardiac Remodeling in HF [15]

DCM is histologically characterized by diffuse fibrosis, compensatory hypertrophy of the other myocytes, and myocyte dropout. Myocyte hypertrophy is promoted by catecholaminergic stimulation, stretch activation of integrins by myocyte and fibroblast, G protein-mediated intracellular signaling, and micro-RNA networks. A new gene expression toward a fetal pattern results in profound morphological rearrangements. The rate of myocyte apoptosis and consequently progressive cells lost is increased in DCM. This process is partly favored by the elevated expression of fetal genes.

Neurohormonal systems. Acutely reduced cardiac output or vascular underfilling leads to baroreceptor-mediated sympathetic nervous activity with elevation of heart rate, blood pressure, and vasoconstriction. Although these changes maintain an adequate cardiac output, at the end they lead to vicious circle. Catecholamines promote arrhythmias, myocardial ischemia, myocyte hypertrophy, and apoptosis and cause different signal-transduction abnormalities (e.g., beta-1 receptor downregulation) [16].

HF results from increased sympathetic nervous activity, but the renin-angiotensin-aldosterone system (RAAS) is also pathologically activated.

Angiotensin II (ATII) is the most powerful mediator of the RAAS. Its activity is mediated by two major G protein receptor associated receptors: angiotensin type-1 and type-2 receptor (AT1R and AT2R). AT1R is expressed mainly in the vasculature, kidney, adrenal cortex, lungs, and brain, and its activation promotes vasoconstriction; AT2R is mainly expressed in the myocardium and promotes vasodilatation and antiproliferative, anti-oxidative, and anti-inflammation effects.

ATII contributes to the increased activity of the sympathetic nervous system by stimulating the adrenal glands and the juxtaglomerular apparatus of the kidney with resulting elevation of plasma renin levels.

Furthermore, ATII stimulates adrenal secretion of aldosterone which, together with vasopressin, reduces renal excretion of water and sodium [17], configuring an inappropriate ADH secretion syndrome.

Finally, ATII contributes to cardiac remodeling promoting myocyte hypertrophy and apoptosis and structural and biochemical alterations in the ECM [18, 19].

Natriuretic peptides. Natriuretic peptides are hormones produced by the heart. The most important ones are atrial natriuretic peptide (ANP), mainly produced in the atria, and B-type natriuretic peptide (BNP) which is mainly released by ventricular myocardium. They are released in response to myocardial stretch and act as counter-regulatory hormones promoting natriuresis, diuresis, and vasodilation. Their plasma concentrations raise in proportion to HF severity and are consolidated markers of poor prognosis in overt HF.

Inflammation. Inflammation may also play a role in pathophysiology of DCM. Many studies have shown an increase in different inflammatory mediators (e.g., tumor necrosis factor α (TNFα), interleukin (IL) 1beta). IL-2, IL-6, Fas ligand, monocyte chemoattractant protein-1 (MCP-1), and macrophage inflammatory protein α (MIP-1α) in HF have also been renamed as an inflammatory disease.

TNFα, for example, has a negative inotropic toxic effect on the myocardium that is connected to adverse ventricular remodeling in DCM.

Extracellular matrix. The extracellular matrix in the heart provides the scaffolding within which contractile cardiomyocytes are housed; it contains a basement membrane, collagen network, proteoglycans, and glycosaminoglycans. Of the different types of collagens, type I and III collagens are the predominant forms found in fibrils deposited in scar tissue after myocardial injury, more specifically demonstrated in myocardial infarction models. These collagens are initially synthesized by cardiac fibroblasts as procollagen precursors before both the N-terminal and the C-terminal are cleaved by proteinases, and then the resulting tropocollagen is assembled into mature fibrils. Markers of collagen turnover such as serum N-terminal type III collagen peptide (PIIINP) have been associated with increased mortality and hospitalization rates, and procollagen type I and PIIINP levels appeared to decrease following aldosterone antagonist therapy in chronic HF patients [20]. In the 967 Framingham subjects without HF, PIIINP levels were not independently associated with LV mass, fractional shortening, end-diastolic dimensions, or left atrial size [21].

The extracellular matrix is a rather dynamic system that is constantly turned over. In the setting of cardiac or extracardiac injury, regulation of extracellular matrix likely plays an important role in ventricular remodeling and fibrosis. For example, bone morphogenetic protein 1, a C-proteinase, plays a crucial role in the processing of extracellular matrix proteins and collagen deposition and regulation of excessive collagen deposition in fibrosis after tissue injury [22]. Recent studies have found that gene expression of tissue inhibitor of metalloproteinases-1 (TIMP-1) and matrix metallopeptidase-9 (MMP-9) was significantly increased in the border zone of myocardial infarct models as well as ischemic HF models in rats and that treatment with antifibrotic therapy can prevent the upregulation of MMP-9, ultimately leading to suppression of collagen deposition [23, 24]. Interestingly, concentrations of TIMP-1 appeared to correlate with diastolic LV dysfunction [25]. In a multimarker analysis of HF patients, a panel that included TIMP-1 as well as NT-proBNP, hs-TnT, growth differentiation factor 15, and insulin-like growth factor-binding protein 4 had the best performance in predicting all-cause mortality at 3-year follow-up.

Calcium. Cytoplasmic Ca^{2+} has a key role in cardiac contraction triggering the interaction of the myosin-thick and actin-thin myofilament. During the depolarization of the myocyte, Ca^{2+} enters the myocyte through L-type Ca^{2+} channels known as transverse tubules, which are close to the sarcoplasmic reticulum (SR) and stimulates the release of much greater quantities of Ca^{2+} from the SR into the cytoplasm through the Ca^{2+} release channels, the ryanodine receptors (RyR2). After reaching a critical concentration, the cytoplasmic Ca^{2+} activates the contractile system of the myocyte. The sarco-/endoplasmic reticular adenosine triphosphate-driven [Ca^{2+}] (SERCA2a) pump returns cytoplasmic Ca^{2+} to the SR against a concentration gradient, and this ends contraction and initiates myocyte relaxation.

Several abnormal Ca^{2+} cycling may be observed in HF. A first condition is a diastolic leak of Ca^{2+} through altered RyR2 with the reduction of the Ca^{2+} content of the SR and then a reduction of Ca^{2+} that can be released during activation [26]. Some have attributed this mechanism to the hyper-phosphorylation of RyR2 at serine 2808 by phosphokinase A [27], others to the phosphorylation at serine 2814 by another enzyme, Ca^{2+}/calmodulin-dependent protein kinase II [28].

Another alteration of calcium metabolism is due to a loss of function of the SERCA2a pump with a reduction of Ca^{2+} content of cardiac SR. Phospholamban is SERCA2a-protein regulator. In the dephosphorylated state, phospholamban inhibits SERCA2a. Stimulation of b-adrenergic receptors normally causes the phosphorylation of phospholamban and thereby disinhibits SERCA2a, enhancing both cardiac contraction and relaxation. For the desensitization of myocardial b-receptors that occurs in HF, this mechanism provided by adrenergic stimulation may be reduced in this condition [29].

References

1. Sarnoff SJ, Berglund E. Ventricular function: I. Starling's law of the heart studied by means of simultaneous right and left ventricular function curves in the dog. Circulation. 1954;9(5):706–18. https://doi.org/10.1161/01.CIR.9.5.706.
2. Araco M, Merlo M, Carr-White G, Sinagra G. Genetic bases of dilated cardiomyopathy. J Cardiovasc Med. 2017;18:123–30. https://doi.org/10.2459/JCM.0000000000000432.
3. Herman DS, Lam L, Taylor MR, et al. Truncations of titin causing dilated cardiomyopathy. N Engl J Med. 2012;366(7):619–28. https://doi.org/10.1056/NEJMoa1110186.
4. Roberts AM, Ware JS, Herman DS, Schafer S, Baksi J, Bick AJ, et al. Integrated allelic, transcriptional, and phenomic dissection of the cardiac effects of titin truncations in health and disease. Sci Transl Med. 2015;7(270):270ra6. https://doi.org/10.1126/scitranslmed.3010134.
5. McNally EM, Golbus JR, Puckelwartz MJ. Genetic mutations and mechanisms in dilated cardiomyopathy. J Clin Invest. 2013;123:19–26. https://doi.org/10.1172/JCI62862.
6. Fatkin D, MacRae C, Sasaki T, Wolff MR, Porcu M, Frenneaux M, et al. Missense mutations in the rod domain of the Lamin A/C gene as causes of dilated cardiomyopathy and conduction-system disease. N Engl J Med. 1999;341:1715–24. https://doi.org/10.1056/NEJM199912023412302.
7. Taylor MRG, Fain PR, Sinagra G, Robinson ML, Robertson AD, Carniel E, et al., Familial Dilated Cardiomyopathy Registry Research Group. Natural history of dilated cardiomyopathy due to Lamin A/C gene mutations. J Am Coll Cardiol. 2003;41:771–80. https://doi.org/10.1016/S0735-1097(02)02954-6.
8. Zhou AX, Hartwig JH, Akyurek LM. Filamins in cell signaling, transcription and organ development. Trends Cell Biol. 2010;20:113–23. https://doi.org/10.1016/j.tcb.2009.12.001.
9. Garcia-Pavia P, Syrris P, Salas C, Evans A, Mirelis JG, Cobo-Marcos M, et al. Desmosomal protein gene mutations in patients with idiopathic dilated cardiomyopathy undergoing cardiac transplantation: a clinicopathological study. Heart. 2011;97:1744–52. https://doi.org/10.1136/hrt.2011.227967.
10. Brun F, Barnes CV, Sinagra G, Slavov D, Barbati G, Zhu X, et al., Familial Cardiomyopathy Registry. Titin and desmosomal genes in the natural history of arrhythmogenic right ventricular cardiomyopathy. J Med Genet. 2014;51:669–76. https://doi.org/10.1136/jmedgenet-2014-102591.
11. McNair WP, Sinagra G, Taylor MRG, Di Lenarda A, Ferguson DA, Salcedo EE, et al., Familial Cardiomyopathy Registry Research Group. SCN5A mutations associate with arrhythmic dilated cardiomyopathy and commonly localize to the voltage-sensing mechanism. J Am Coll Cardiol. 2011;57:2160–68. https://doi.org/10.1016/j.jacc.2010.09.084.
12. Zaklyazminskaya E, Dzemeshkevich S. The role of mutations in the SCN5A gene in cardiomyopathies. Biochim Biophys Acta. 2016;1863(7 Pt B):1799–805. https://doi.org/10.1016/j.bbamcr.2016.02.014.
13. Li D, Parks SB, Kushner JD, Nauman D, Burgess D, Ludwigsen S, et al. Mutations of presenilin genes in dilated cardiomyopathy and heart failure. Am J Hum Genet. 2006;79:1030–9. https://doi.org/10.1086/509900.
14. Troncone L, Luciani M, Coggins M, Wilker EH, Ho C-Y, Codispoti KE, et al. Ab amyloid pathology affects the hearts of patients with Alzheimer's disease. J Am Coll Cardiol. 2016;68:2395–407. https://doi.org/10.1016/j.jacc.2016.08.073.
15. Johnson FL. Pathophysiology and etiology of heart failure. Cardiol Clin. 2014;32(1):9–19. https://doi.org/10.1016/j.ccl.2013.09.015.
16. Bristow MR, Ginsburg R, Minobe W, Cubicciotti RS, Sageman WS, Lurie K, et al. Decreased catecholamine sensitivity and β-adrenergic-receptor density in failing human hearts. N Engl J Med. 1982;307:205–11. https://doi.org/10.1056/NEJM198207223070401.
17. Schrier RW, Abraham WT. Hormones and hemodynamics in heart failure. N Engl J Med. 1999;341(8):577–85. https://doi.org/10.1056/NEJM199908193410806.

18. McEwan PE, Gray GA, Sherry L, Webb DJ, Kenyon CJ. Differential effects of angiotensin II on cardiac cell proliferation and intramyocardial perivascular fibrosis in vivo. Circulation. 1998;98:2765–73. https://doi.org/10.1161/01.CIR.98.24.2765.
19. Liu Y, Leri A, Li B, Wang X, Cheng W, Kajstura J, et al. Angiotensin II stimulation in vitro induces hypertrophy of normal and postinfarcted ventricular myocytes. Circ Res. 1998;82:1145–59. https://doi.org/10.1161/01.RES.82.11.1145.
20. Zannad F, Dousset B, Alla F. Treatment of congestive heart failure: interfering the aldosterone-cardiac extracellular matrix relationship. Hypertension. 2001;38:1227–32. https://doi.org/10.1161/hy1101.099484.
21. Wang TJ, Larson MG, Benjamin EJ, Siwik DA, Safa R, Guo C-Y, et al. Clinical and echocardiographic correlates of plasma procollagen type III amino-terminal peptide levels in the community. Am Heart J. 2007;154:291–7. https://doi.org/10.1016/j.ahj.2007.04.006.
22. Shalitin N, Schlesinger H, Levy MJ, Kessler E, Kessler-Icekson G. Expression of procollagen C-proteinase enhancer in cultured rat heart fibroblasts: evidence for co-regulation with type I collagen. J Cell Biochem. 2003;90:397–407. https://doi.org/10.1002/jcb.10646.
23. Shi J, Dai W, Hale SL, Brown DA, Wang M, Han X, et al. Bendavia restores mitochondrial energy metabolism gene expression and suppresses cardiac fibrosis in the border zone of the infarcted heart. Life Sci. 2015;141:170–8. https://doi.org/10.1016/j.lfs.2015.09.022.
24. Nural-Guvener H, Zakharova L, Feehery L, Sljukic S, Gaballa M. Anti-fibrotic effects of class I HDAC inhibitor, mocetinostat is associated with IL-6/Stat3 signaling in ischemic heart failure. Int J Mol Sci. 2015;16:11482–99. https://doi.org/10.3390/ijms160511482.
25. Sanchis L, Andrea R, Falces C, Llopis J, Morales-Ruiz M, Lopez-Sobrino T, et al. Prognosis of new-onset heart failure outpatients and collagen biomarkers. Eur J Clin Investig. 2015;45:842–9. https://doi.org/10.1111/eci.12479.
26. Belevych AE, Terentyev D, Terentyeva R, Nishijima Y, Sridhar A, Hamlin RL, et al. The relationship between arrhythmogenesis and impaired contractility in heart failure: role of altered ryanodine receptor function. Cardiovasc Res. 2011;90:493–502. https://doi.org/10.1093/cvr/cvr025.
27. Shan J, Betzenhauser MJ, Kushnir A, Reiken S, Meli AC, Wronska A, et al. Role of chronic ryanodine receptor phosphorylation in heart failure and beta-adrenergic receptor blockade in mice. J Clin Invest. 2010;120:4375–87. https://doi.org/10.1172/JCI37649.
28. Respress JL, van Oort RJ, Li N, Rolim N, Dixit SS, DeAlmeida A, et al. Role of RyR2 phosphorylation at S2814 during heart failure progression. Circ Res. 2012;110:1474–83. https://doi.org/10.1161/CIRCRESAHA.112.268094.
29. El-Armouche A, Eschenhagen T. β-adrenergic stimulation and myocardial function in the failing heart. Heart Fail Rev. 2009;14:225–41. https://doi.org/10.1007/s10741-008-9132-8.

4

Etiological Definition and Diagnostic Work-Up

Marco Merlo, Marco Gobbo, Jessica Artico, Elena Abate, and Stefania Franco

Abbreviations and Acronyms

AL	Amyloid light chain
ATTR	Amyloid transthyretin
BNP	Brain natriuretic peptide
CMR	Cardiovascular magnetic resonance
CS	Cardiac sarcoidosis
DCM	Dilated cardiomyopathy
EF	Ejection fraction
EMB	Endomyocardial biopsy
FDG	Fluorodeoxyglucose
HF	Heart failure
HRS	Heart Rhythm Society
ICD	Implantable cardioverter defibrillator
LGE	Late gadolinium enhancement
LV	Left ventricle
LVRR	Left ventricular reverse remodeling
RV	Right ventricle

M. Merlo (✉)
Cardiovascular Department, Azienda Sanitaria Universitaria Integrata, Trieste, Italy

M. Gobbo · J. Artico · S. Franco
Cardiovascular Department, Azienda Sanitaria Universitaria Integrata, University of Trieste (ASUITS), Trieste, Italy

E. Abate
Cardiovascular Department, Azienda Sanitaria Universitaria Integrata, University of Trieste (ASUITS), Trieste, Italy

Klinik für Innere Medizin 3, Universitätsklinikum Halle (Saale), Halle (Saale), Germany
e-mail: Elena.Abate@uk-halle.de

4.1 Clinical Presentation

Most patients affected by dilated cardiomyopathy (DCM) present between the ages of 20 and 60, but the disease can occur also in children and older adults. They are most commonly Caucasian males. Furthermore, with respect to other heart failure etiologies, the comorbidity profile of DCM patients is very low. Finally, due to the frequent long-standing asymptomatic left ventricular dysfunction, these patients are often scarcely symptomatic for heart failure (HF) at diagnosis in spite of importantly remodeled left ventricle. Useful patterns in diagnosing DCM are:

1. Heart failure symptoms (progressive dyspnea with exertion, impaired exercise capacity, orthopnea, paroxysmal nocturnal dyspnea, and peripheral edema)
2. Incidental detection of asymptomatic cardiomegaly
3. Incidental detection of left bundle branch block (e.g., sport screening in countries with ECG sport screening)
4. Symptoms related to coexisting arrhythmia, conduction disturbance, thromboembolic complications
5. Sudden death
6. Familial screening

4.2 Etiological Classification: A Critical Issue in Clinical Management of DCM

DCM prognoses have changed dramatically in the last decades [1]. This aspect is due to an improvement in HF therapy, both pharmacologic and non-pharmacologic (e.g., devices and MitraClip©), promoting left ventricular reverse remodeling (LVRR). However, the diagnostic effort facing a newly discovered DCM phenotype is critical to address a tailored therapy and to improve the LVRR amount and long-term survival [2]. In fact, DCM is a generic term that encases several different diseases. Timing is also a crucial aspect since delaying an accurate etiological definition of nonischemic DCM could mean to increase the event rate. In this sense a red flags approach appears important, and advanced diagnostic tools should be used not in every patient but in whom red flags suggest utility rather than futility [3].

4.2.1 Need of Reclassification of the Disease During Follow-Up

The overall improvement of prognosis in DCM makes quite frequent to see in clinical practice patients with >10 years of disease. In these patients an eventual worsening of systolic function or arrhythmias could be explained by a progression of the disease but also by a developed superimposed coronary artery disease, valvulopathy, or active myocarditis. In this sense repeated etiological classification of disease is advocated and appears crucial periodically during follow-up [4].

4.3 Exclusion of Reversible Causes of Left Ventricular Dysfunction/Dilation

It is pivotal to exclude possible removable causes of left ventricular dysfunction [4]. First and by far most important is to exclude an ischemic cardiomyopathy that is conventionally distinguished from DCM by the presence of >50% stenosis in the left main stem, proximal left anterior descending artery, or two or more epicardial coronary arteries on invasive or computed tomography coronary angiography (2). Late gadolinium enhancement (LGE) at cardiovascular magnetic resonance (CMR) provides an alternative approach and may identify prior myocardial infarction (subendocardial or transmural LGE) in as many as 13% of patients with suspected DCM and unobstructed coronary arteries [5]. In addition to ischemic cardiomyopathy, DCM must also be distinguished from other nonischemic cardiomyopathies and physiological adaptations that may generate similar patterns of left ventricle (LV) remodeling [6]. One example is represented by valvular heart disease associated with left ventricular systolic dysfunction.

Hypertensive dilated cardiomyopathy is a challenging entity from diagnostic standpoint. These patients usually are older and with more comorbidities, tolerating higher doses of drugs, or with high pressure in spite of LV dysfunction and a septal thickness of more than 12 mm [7]. However, it is still unknown why only few hypertensive patients develop LV systolic dysfunction in the absence of concomitant coronary artery disease. A genetic background favorable to develop DCM is likely, but future focused studies are advocated to elucidate this issue.

The term "idiopathic DCM" is often used in clinical practice and in some series accounts for 20–30% of nonischemic HF. However, the approach to a patient with nonischemic DCM rarely seeks reversible factors other than hypertension, valve disease, and congenital heart disease. Other examples of commonly overlooked or underappreciated reversible environmental triggers for LV dysfunction include sustained supraventricular arrhythmias or very frequent ventricular ectopic beats, which can lead to tachycardia-induced cardiomyopathy; substance abuse (e.g., alcohol, cocaine); acute emotional stress or chemotherapies that cause catecholamine (i.e., Takotsubo) or toxin-induced cardiomyopathies; and systemic autoimmune disorders (e.g., Churg–Strauss syndrome and sarcoidosis). New-onset HF with LV dysfunction occurring during pregnancy or the postpartum period could identify a peripartum cardiomyopathy. Confirmation of active myocarditis as the cause of recent onset severe HF is particularly important as it may require investigations (e.g., endomyocardial biopsy) [8].

Accordingly, a comprehensive integrated approach, including third-level diagnostic tools, should be systematically implemented in clinical practice to remove every possible reversible cause through specific therapeutic interventions. This issue appears essential to promote left ventricular reverse remodeling and subsequent outcome improvement [2] (Fig. 4.1).

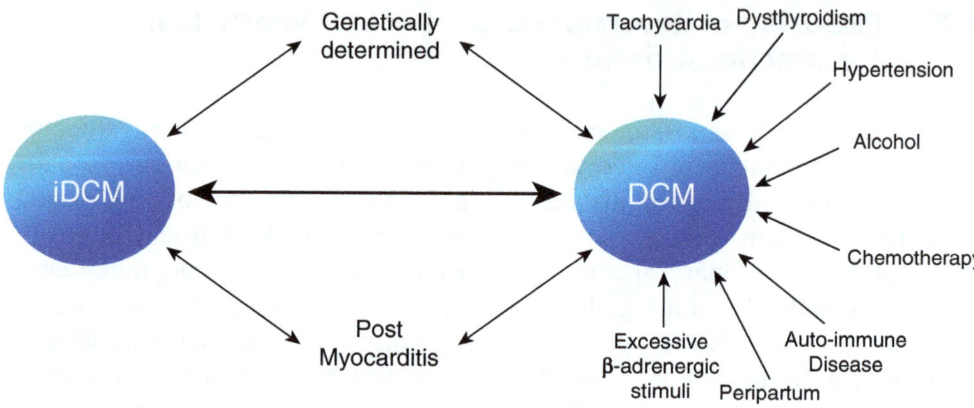

Fig. 4.1 Etiological characterization of DCM. *DCM* dilated cardiomyopathy, *IDCM* idiopathic dilated cardiomyopathy. From Merlo et al. Evolving Concepts in Dilated Cardiomyopathy, EJHF.2018. 20(2):228–239

4.4 Diagnostic Work-Up in New-Onset LV Dysfunction/ Dilation: A "Red Flags" Approach

As previously stated, DCM may present with multiple clinical scenarios. However, the clinical approach to a suspected DCM requires a step-by-step work-up. It is crucial to start from the family and personal history, to perform a comprehensive physical examination and to interpret all the available diagnostic tools. Rapezzi and colleagues first described the so-called red flags approach in cardiomyopathies to guide the selection of the appropriate diagnostic techniques [3]. The easily missed boxes (see below) provide some important examples of this approach and of difficulties of differential diagnosis in approaching a newly diagnosed nonischemic DCM.

4.4.1 Personal and Family History

In the adulthood, the onset of the disease is generally observed during the third or fourth decade of life. This is "unusual" in classic genetic diseases. Since genetic forms account for 20–50% of DCM cases, the first clinical examination should include a very careful assessment of the patient's family history [9]. The recording of a complete family pedigree is helpful in determining the possible mode of genetic transmission (autosomal dominant, autosomal recessive, X-linked, matrilinear) and in detecting other cardiac and non-cardiac traits associated with DCM. The pedigree is by far the most important genetic tool in the systematic approach to DCM [9]. Importantly, a negative family history does not rule out a genetic form of DCM as de novo genetic mutations can be responsible for sporadic DCM. Systematic familial screening is an important way of diagnosis shedding light on early phases of disease with favorable prognosis [10].

A distinct clinical entity is the DCM formed in pediatric patients. The prognosis in this specific population is poorer than in adulthood, carrying more HF and arrhythmic events. This translates in a need of more aggressive treatments and follow-up in pediatric DCMs [11], implicating difficult clinical choices due to the age of the patients. The reasons of this particularly aggressive form in children are largely unknown. Other forms of LV dysfunction, such as active myocarditis, appear to carry an ominous prognosis in children [12]. It is possible that specific immunologic pathways could be involved, but this represents an important field for future research.

4.4.2 Symptoms and Physical Examination

Clinically, signs and symptoms of heart failure often characterize the onset of the disease, but young individuals can remain asymptomatic for a long time despite having LV dysfunction. A history of palpitations and syncope should be carefully investigated, as they can be the clinical expressions of serious ventricular arrhythmias. Neurologic examination is of paramount importance. A search for multisystem involvement should be part of the clinical examination, in particular looking for signs of skeletal myopathy or neurosensory disorders [3]. For example, cases of DCM associated with learning difficulties, blindness, and deafness should be recognized.

4.4.3 12 Lead Electrocardiogram

Historically, electrocardiogram in DCM has been considered non-specific. However, in some cases it can provide clues to specific forms of DCM. For example, posterolateral pseudonecrosis (that requires exclusion of true necrosis with coronary angiogram) is typical of dystrophin-related DCM. Atrioventricular blocks (of various degrees) can suggest a mutation in *LMNA* and are usually related to an important arrhythmic burden [13]. Sinus bradycardia and atrial standstill have been associated to myotonic dystrophy and Emery–Dreifuss muscular dystrophy [3]. Other important red flags include low QRS voltages, right bundle branch conduction abnormalities, and anterolateral/inferior negative T waves which can lead to a diagnosis of biventricular or left-dominant arrhythmogenic cardiomyopathy [14]. Left bundle branch block and left atrial enlargement are usually markers of long-standing disease, the former also having prognostic and therapeutic implications (i.e., resynchronization therapy) [15]. Finally, in contrast to other cardiomyopathies, there is a lack of studies on a systematic evaluation of ECG in a large cohort of DCM. These studies could provide in the future possible diagnostic and prognostic tools derived by a simple and often neglected tool as ECG.

4.4.4 Laboratory Tests

In HF with reduced ejection fraction, natriuretic peptides have clinical utility for the diagnosis and prognostic stratification. In fact, guidelines recommend dosage of brain natriuretic peptide (BNP) or N-terminal pro-BNP at the time of the first evaluation and systematically during follow-up [16]. However, BNP rises irrespective of HF etiology. Instead, elevations in serum creatine phosphokinase can suggest specific genetic disorders such as dystrophinopathy, laminopathy, or desminopathy [3]. Whether clinical evidence of neuromuscular involvement is found or not, in these patients a complete neurological work-up is generally warranted. Other important laboratory markers suggesting specific etiologies are high transferrin saturation and hyperferritinemia in hemochromatosis, or lactic acidosis and leucopoenia in rare forms of mitochondrial diseases [3].

4.4.4.1 Genetic Testing

While there is a general appreciation that DCM can be caused by many different disease processes, in everyday clinical practice it is often considered under the catch-all heading of "nonischemic HF" with reduced ejection fraction. However, the concept that DCM represents a family of diseases characterized by complex interactions between environment and genetic predispositions is gaining prominence as the clinical impact of a precise diagnosis is better appreciated [17]. Nowadays, after the exclusion of possible removable causes of LV dysfunction, in both familial and sporadic cases, particularly in the presence of "red flags" suggesting possible genetic forms of DCM, a genetic testing with a next-generation sequencing approach is indicated. Despite current guidelines recognize a genotype–phenotype correlation only in LMNA carriers, there is a growing amount of data that supports genotype–phenotype correlations also for other genes (i.e., desmosomal, FLNC [18], TTN [19], sarcomere) (see Chap. 5). In this sense, it is emerging a new, widely unexplored, and important overlap syndrome between DCM and right ventricular cardiomyopathy called arrhythmogenic cardiomyopathy, often determined by mutations of LMNA, FLNC, or desmosomal genes. Therefore, it exists the next future perspective of an extensive use of genetic testing in DCM, even if the current knowledge on genotype–phenotype correlation and application of precision medicine in DCM is still embryonic [20].

4.4.5 Echocardiography

Two-dimensional Doppler echocardiography has an important role in the diagnostic and prognostic assessment of DCM [21]. Echocardiography has the main advantage of being very practical and quite affordable making it the perfect tool for first-line diagnosis and follow-up of DCM patients. In fact, evaluation of LV ejection fraction and LV dimensions represents the first-line approach to a DCM patient and should be periodically repeated during the follow-up. Different patterns of DCM have been described according to the grade of LV dilation. Hypokinetic non-dilated cardiomyopathy (or mildly dilated cardiomyopathy) has been recently introduced as a distinct clinical entity [6, 22]. Specific genetic forms, such as *LMNA* mutations, can cause isolated LV systolic dysfunction without dilatation and have a much higher arrhythmic burden [23]. A reduced LV ejection fraction with preserved LV size can be also observed in the early (preclinical) stages of disease and is generally associated with a good prognosis [22]. The presence of some particular features such as a restrictive LV filling pattern and non-sustained ventricular arrhythmia carries a higher risk of an adverse outcome [24, 25]. Similar clues may suggest involvement of specific genes. Alternatively, active myocarditis can also present with depressed ejection fraction but not extensive LV remodeling, frequently in association with a high arrhythmic burden [8, 12].

Myocardial deformation imaging techniques (e.g., speckle tracking) offer greater sensitivity than LV ejection fraction for identifying subtle abnormalities of systolic function and may assist in the early detection of disease [26].

In addition to the examination of LV systolic function and size, the presence and the severity of functional mitral regurgitation [27] have important implications for therapeutic and prognostic strategies. Left ventricular diastolic function should be systematically assessed for the estimation of left ventricular filling pressures and the identification of restrictive filling pattern [24]. The right ventricle along with the estimation of pulmonary arterial pressure is also essential in the stratification of the disease [28].

Box 4.1 Easily Missed: Cardiac Amyloidosis

Amyloidosis is a disease complex caused by extracellular deposition of insoluble abnormal fibrils composed of misfolded proteins, which can alter tissue structure and impair function of multiple organs including the heart. Types of amyloidosis which commonly affect the heart include primary systemic amyloidosis (amyloid light chain (AL)) and transthyretin amyloidosis (amyloid transthyretin), the latter of which may be acquired in older individuals (wild type) or inherited in younger patients (hereditary).

Cardiac amyloidosis usually starts as restrictive cardiomyopathy with normal or mildly depressed LV systolic dysfunction and significant diastolic HF and can progress to severe systolic dysfunction in advanced stages. Once amyloid infiltration involves the heart, prognosis significantly worsens. In fact, median survival in AL amyloidosis is ≈13 months but decreases drastically to 4 months with the onset of HF symptoms [29].

Reduced QRS voltage amplitude on ECG is noted in the limb leads in ≈50% of cases, but the true electrocardiographic hallmark of cardiac amyloidosis is the disproportion between left ventricular wall thickness and QRS voltages [29]. A pseudoinfarct pattern in the precordial leads is another electrocardiographic feature.

In some cases, echocardiography could suggest the diagnosis and hence enhance the sensitivity of physical examination. Typical echocardiographic features of amyloidosis include thickened ventricular walls (right and left) in the setting of normal ventricular size, biatrial dilatation, the presence of a pericardial effusion, and valvular thickening without significant dysfunction [30]. Increased echogenicity of the myocardium, termed *granular sparkling*, is not very sensitive or specific when evaluated in isolation. Even if the global LV function is usually impaired only in advanced cardiac amyloidosis, longitudinal dysfunction precedes the onset of heart failure. This is best detected by strain imaging, which typically shows impairment of longitudinal strain at the base of the left ventricle, with relatively well-preserved apical strain. When strain is color coded, a "bull's eye" with an apical sparing pattern is found; it is both sensitive and specific for the diagnosis of cardiac amyloidosis [31]. In contrast CMR findings in cardiac amyloidosis are aspecific. In fact late gadolinium enhancement is simply an expression of interstitial expansion that can be frequently found in storage diseases (e.g., Anderson–Fabry and Danon disease) [30].

Scintigraphy with bone-seeking tracers (DPD Tc in Europe and PYP Tc in the USA) is an important technique in the diagnosis of amyloidosis. Myocardial uptake is strictly dependent on etiology: absent or mild in AL, present in ATTR, and variable in other rarer genetic forms [32]. A strong myocardial tracer uptake is highly sensitive for ATTR cardiac amyloidosis (both hereditary and wild type). Furthermore, specificity in relation to sarcomeric hypertrophic cardiomyopathy has also been shown to be high [30]. There are potential pitfalls since a negative scintigraphy does not rule out a diagnosis of cardiac amyloidosis and mild myocardial tracer uptake does not allow a differential diagnosis between ATTR and AL [30].

4.4.6 Cardiovascular Magnetic Resonance

Cardiovascular magnetic resonance (CMR) imaging is considered the gold standard for assessment of ventricular volumes and ejection fraction, enabling confident diagnosis of DCM in borderline cases and improving the characterization of disease severity in patients with known LV dysfunction.

Another crucial aspect of CMR is tissue characterization that can be useful in diagnosis of specific forms of DCM [5, 33]. The identification of myocardial edema (in T2-weighted images) suggests active myocarditis and late gadolinium enhancement (LGE) representing replacement fibrosis and is detectable in approximately one-third of cases of DCM with a distinctive mid-wall distribution, more frequently within the septal wall [5]. The presence of LGE in DCM carries important prognostic implications in terms of low probability of LV reverse remodeling and increased risk of sudden cardiac death [5, 34]. Moreover, the distribution of LGE may be suggestive of some DCM phenotypes; for instance, an inferolateral or posterolateral location is typical of muscular dystrophy, whereas subepicardial or transmural patchy distribution of LGE is suggestive of myocarditis or sarcoidosis [35].

Emerging CMR techniques, specifically T1 mapping, provide assessment of the interstitial fibrosis and could represent in the future a tool for early diagnosis and risk stratification of DCM [36].

CMR T2* imaging is the preferred technique for the detection and quantification of iron deposits within the myocardium in patients with hemochromatosis.

Box 4.2 Easily Missed: Cardiac Sarcoidosis

Sarcoidosis is a multisystemic inflammatory disease of unknown origin characterized by noncaseating granuloma formation in multiple organ systems. The disease affects more frequently the lung (more than 90% of patients), but it can also involve the heart, liver, spleen, skin, eyes, parotid gland, and other organs and tissues. A certain diagnosis requires histopathologic demonstration of noncaseating granulomas at lung biopsy. Clinically cardiac involvement occurs in about 5% of patients with sarcoidosis, but autopsy findings and, more recently, data based on CMR studies showed that 25–50% of patients with sarcoidosis have some degree of cardiac involvement. The principal manifestations are conduction abnormalities, ventricular arrhythmias (including sudden death), and heart failure [37, 38].

Diagnosis of cardiac sarcoidosis is challenging, and diagnostic criteria rely on the presence of noncaseating granuloma on histological examination of myocardial tissue. Among patients with extra-cardiac sarcoidosis, diagnosis of cardiac sarcoidosis is probable in the presence of reduced LVEF, unexplained ventricular tachycardia, conduction block (Mobitz type II or 3° heart blocks), patchy uptake at cardiac FDG–PET or a LGE on CMR, or gallium uptake in a pattern consistent with cardiac sarcoidosis [39].

Preliminary tests, such as ECG, chest radiography, and echocardiography, are non-specific for cardiac sarcoidosis (CS).

Abnormal electrocardiographic findings include various degrees of conduction block, such as bundle branch block (right bundle branch block more common than left bundle branch block) and fascicular block, QRS complex fragmentation, pathological Q waves, and ST–T changes. Notably, only a small proportion (3–9%) of patient with asymptomatic cardiac sarcoidosis have an abnormal ECG [38, 39].

Echocardiographic abnormalities are variable and non-specific and are present in about 77% of patients with systemic sarcoidosis [40]. The most common features are interventricular thinning, especially basal focal areas of akinesia or dyskinesia or aneurysm, and other common findings are cardiac chambers enlargement, left and/or right ventricular systolic dysfunction, and/or and diastolic dysfunction [40]. Granulomatous inflammation can be rarely seen as macroscopic areas of bright echoes, with a "speckled" or "snowstorm" pattern at two-dimensional echocardiography [39].

In the recent years, CMR has emerged as a valuable imaging tool for early diagnosis of cardiac sarcoidosis [41]. Thanks to its accuracy and resolution, it is able to detect both structural and functional abnormalities and to differentiate them from ischemic lesions. CMR has a specificity of about 78% for cardiac sarcoidosis making it the diagnostic tool of choice [41]. CMR abnormalities include not only granulomatous infiltration but also inflammation, edema, and fibrosis [41]. Different patterns of LGE can be found in patients with cardiac sarcoidosis. Early enhancement of granulomas in T2-weighted images is suggestive of the presence of inflammation and edema [41, 42]. The most common patterns of LGE distribution are subepicardial and mid-myocardial, with preferential involvement of the basal septum or inferolateral wall [43]. Right ventricular involvement has been described, too [43].

Another important imaging technique for CS diagnosis is FDG–PET. Focal or focal-on-diffuse FDG uptake, which represents active inflammation, can suggest CS. These findings have a low specificity, since these patterns are seen in other inflammatory myocardial diseases, too.

EMB is still considered an important tool for certain diagnosis of cardiac sarcoidosis. However, it has low sensitivity (25%) due to the focal localization of lesions. Moreover, EMB is most commonly performed from the right ventricle, while disease involvement is more common in the basal septum and inferolateral LV wall, regions that are more difficult to biopsy [39]. Current consensus guidelines now suggest electrophysiological (electroanatomic mapping) or image-guided (PET or CMR) biopsy procedures to increase its sensitivity [39].

The arrhythmic risk in cardiac sarcoidosis patients raises the issue of the risk stratification of sudden death and when to consider ICD implantation. Several studies demonstrated that the only consistent association with ICD intervention in these patients was with reduced LVEF. However, a significant rate of ICD intervention occurred also in patients with low to moderate LVEF reduction, while none of those with normal LV and RV ejection fraction had appropriate ICD therapy [44]. Current consensus guidelines recommend ICD implantation in patients with known cardiac sarcoidosis and spontaneous sustained ventricular arrhythmias or prior cardiac arrest and/or if LVEF <35% (despite optimal medical therapy and trial of immunosuppression). ICD implantation can also be useful in patients with unexplained syncope and inducible ventricular arrhythmias. ICD implantation has also been considered at the time of pacemaker implantation (when indicated) and may be considered in patients with LVEF in the range of 36–49%, despite optimal medical therapy for heart failure and a period of immunosuppression [39].

Interestingly, these guidelines, enhancing the role of CMR, stated that ICD implantation may be considered if patients have evidence of late gadolinium enhancement on CMR [40].

4.4.7 Cardiac Catheterizations and Procedures

4.4.7.1 Coronary Angiogram

In the diagnostic assessment of a depressed LV ejection fraction of unknown origin, coronary angiography is required to rule out coronary artery disease, particularly in patients above 35 years, males, and those carrying cardiovascular risk factors. Computed tomography angiography can be considered as an alternative, particularly if the pretest probability of ischemic disease is low to moderate.

4.4.7.2 Cardiac Catheterization

Right heart catheterization should be limited to selected cases, such as in patients with advanced disease who are candidates for cardiac transplantation, due to its limited importance in the diagnostic work-up. However it is pivotal for prognostic stratification.

4.4.7.3 Endomyocardial Biopsy

The role of endomyocardial biopsy in the diagnosis of DCM remains controversial. Modern immunohistochemical methods improve sensitivity compared with the traditional histopathological Dallas criteria [45], but endomyocardial biopsy should generally be reserved for selected cases such as patients with severe heart failure, refractory hemodynamic impairment or life-threatening arrhythmias that are potentially caused by myocarditis and might be responsive to immunosuppression or antiviral therapy [8, 46, 47]. Endomyocardial biopsy can also be useful when specific diseases with targeted treatment strategies are suspected (i.e., sarcoidosis and hemochromatosis).

Box 4.3 Easily Missed: Active Myocarditis

Myocarditis represents an underdiagnosed cause of DCM. Myocarditis is an inflammatory disease of the myocardium characterized by a great heterogeneity of presentation and evolution. Common clinical scenarios associated with myocarditis may range from subclinical asymptomatic myocarditis to perimyocarditis resembling an acute coronary syndrome, to syncope from ventricular arrhythmias or heart block, to heart failure associated with progressive or chronic DCM, to severe acute heart failure in some cases requiring intensive hemodynamic support [48].

Myocarditis can be caused by a broad range of infectious agents, including viruses, bacteria, fungi, and protozoa, as well as noninfectious triggers, such as toxins and hypersensitive reactions. Among these triggers, viral infection has been documented to constitute the most prevalent cause of myocarditis.

Clinical suspicion of inflammatory heart disease is crucial in the clinical scenarios presented above, especially in newly diagnosed DCM or in the presence of life-threatening arrhythmias: history of recent flu-like symptoms (present in 35–65% of cases) or viral gastroenteritis may raise this suspicion. A previous insect bite, suspicious of *Borrelia* or rickettsiae, should always be investigated [8].

In patients with clinically suspected acute myocarditis, confirmatory testing usually begins with serum biomarkers. However, Troponin I may be raised in only 34% of patients with acute myocarditis [49]. Non-specific serum markers of inflammation, such as C-reactive protein, erythrocyte sedimentation rate, and leucocyte count, are frequently increased in patients with suspected myocarditis, but low specificity limits their diagnostic value.

Patients with myocarditis might mostly have non-specific changes on ECG. These include sinus tachycardia, ST wave and T wave abnormalities, and, sometimes, PR depression and diffuse ST segment elevation (if there is concomitant peri-epicardial inflammation). Electrocardiographic changes that are associated with poor prognosis in acute myocarditis include widened QRS and Q waves [50].

Echocardiography is mandatory in patients with suspected myocarditis. The entity of left ventricular dysfunction and wall motion abnormalities not associated with a coronary distribution are useful tool to suggest an acute myocarditis. In fulminant cases, there might be wall thickening due to edema [51].

Cardiac MRI sensitivity varies with clinical presentation and extent of cell necrosis [52]. In high- and intermediate-risk forms (i.e., myocarditis presenting with heart failure or arrhythmias associated with LV dysfunctions), cardiac MRI has modest diagnostic accuracy, in fact the edema may be absent in T2-weighted images since its presence highly depends by the timing of MRI performance. In patients with biopsy-proven viral myocarditis, the presence of myocardial scar, indicated by LGE, is an independent predictor of all-cause mortality and cardiac mortality, but no data are available about the prognostic value of additional cardiac MRI-related parameters, such as the pattern of distribution and the extension of LGE [53].

Endomyocardial biopsy (EMB) is the gold standard for the diagnosis of myocarditis, although its role is still controversial. Indeed, it is associated with a non-negligible rate of major complications, even in specialized centers (around 1% of the cases) [54], and its diagnostic accuracy is still debated, highly depending on the operator experience, on the number and the location of tissue samples, and on the timing of the EMB. Therefore, EMB should be performed only in selected life-threatening scenarios, such as heart failure with severe ventricular dysfunction and/or life-threatening arrhythmias refractory to optimized medical therapy in the short term (usually 3 weeks) [8, 55].

Recently, practical and clinically oriented classification of myocarditis and its clinical management has been proposed based on event risk derived by clinical and laboratory presentation and short-term evolution, as seen in Fig. 4.2 [8].

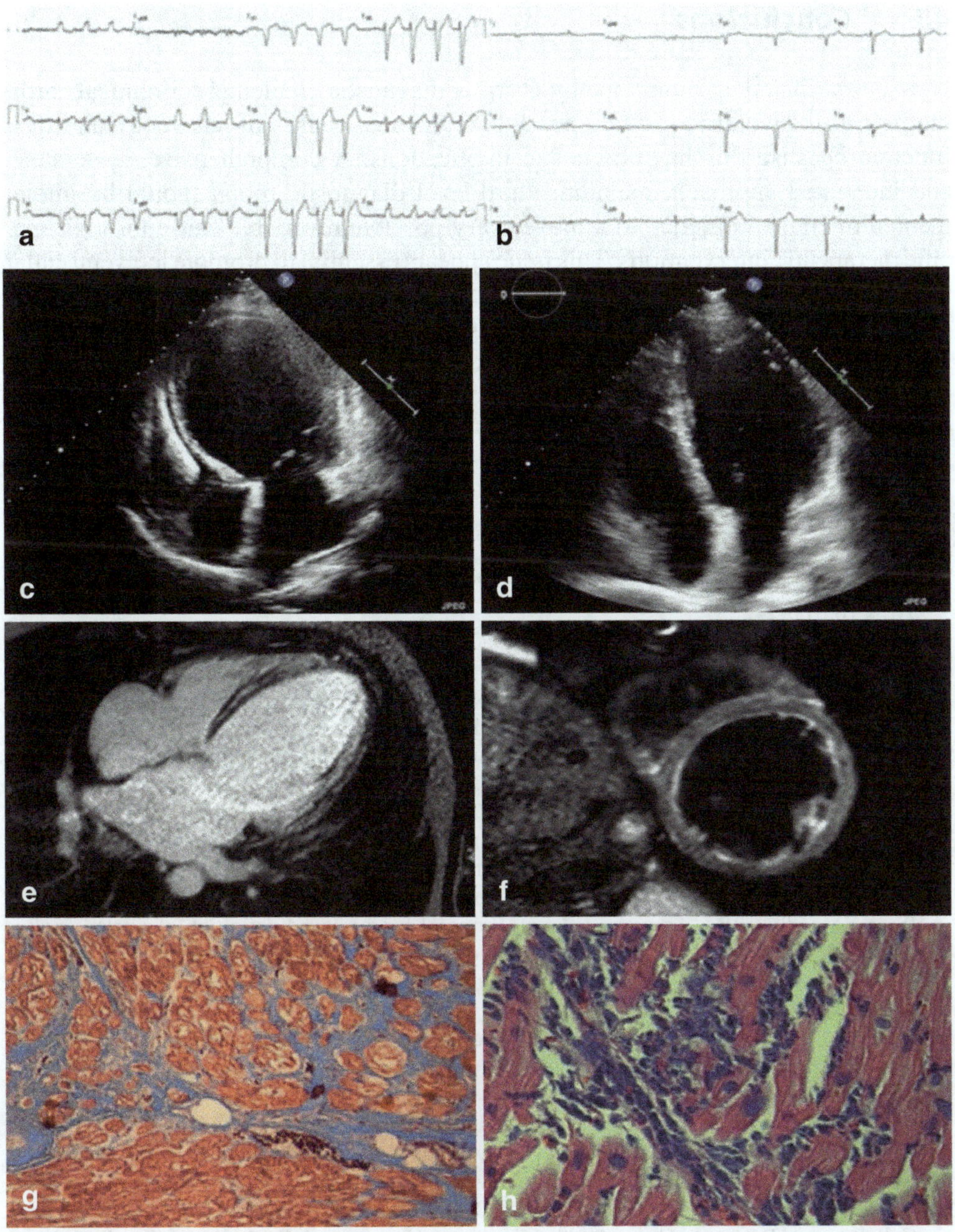

Fig. 4.2 Characterization of DCM vs. active myocarditis at diagnosis. The role of ECG (panels (**a**) vs. (**b**): note the left bundle branch block vs. low QRS voltages), echocardiography (panels (**c**) vs. (**d**): note the huge vs. mild left ventricular/atrial dilation), cardiac magnetic resonance (panels (**e**) vs. (**f**): note the mid-wall distribution pattern of late gadolinium enhancement vs. myocardial edema at T2-weighted imaging), endomyocardial biopsy (panels (**g**) vs. (**h**): note the cardiomyocyte damage and the myocardial fibrosis [in blue] vs. active lymphocytic inflammation). Reproduced with permission from Merlo et al. Evolving Concepts in Dilated Cardiomyopathy, EJHF.2018. 20(2):228–239

4.5 Conclusions

New-onset dilated cardiomyopathy is still a diagnostic challenge for clinical cardiologists. It is pivotal to exclude possible removable causes of left ventricular dysfunction because this has prognostic implications. A comprehensive, systematic, and integrated approach, including third-level diagnostic tools, should be implemented in clinical practice to remove every possible reversible cause through specific therapeutic interventions. This issue appears essential to promote left ventricular reverse remodeling and subsequent outcome improvement. Excluding treatable causes is by far the most important issue. Cardiac sarcoidosis, cardiac amyloidosis, and acute myocarditis are paradigmatic examples and should be carefully excluded.

References

1. Merlo M, Pivetta A, Pinamonti B, Stolfo D, Zecchin M, Barbati G, Di Lenarda A, Sinagra G. Long-term prognostic impact of therapeutic strategies in patients with idiopathic dilated cardiomyopathy: changing mortality over the last 30 years. Eur J Heart Fail. 2014;16:317–24.
2. Merlo M, Pyxaras SA, Pinamonti B, Barbati G, Di Lenarda A, Sinagra G. Prevalence and prognostic significance of left ventricular reverse remodeling in dilated cardiomyopathy receiving tailored medical treatment. J Am Coll Cardiol. 2011;57:1468–76.
3. Rapezzi C, Arbustini E, Caforio ALP, et al. Diagnostic work-up in cardiomyopathies: bridging the gap between clinical phenotypes and final diagnosis. A position statement from the ESC Working Group on Myocardial and Pericardial Diseases. Eur Heart J. 2013;34:1448–58.
4. Merlo M, Cannatà A, Gobbo M, Stolfo D, Elliott P, Sinagra G. Evolving concepts in dilated cardiomyopathy. Eur J Heart Fail. 2018;20(2):228–39.
5. Gulati A, Jabbour A, Ismail TF, et al. Association of fibrosis with mortality and sudden cardiac death in patients with nonischemic dilated cardiomyopathy. JAMA. 2013;309:896–908.
6. Pinto YM, Elliott PM, Arbustini E, et al. Proposal for a revised definition of dilated cardiomyopathy, hypokinetic non-dilated cardiomyopathy, and its implications for clinical practice: a position statement of the ESC working group on myocardial and pericardial diseases. Eur Heart J. 2016;37:1850–8.
7. Bobbo M, Pinamonti B, Merlo M, et al. Comparison of patient characteristics and course of hypertensive hypokinetic cardiomyopathy versus idiopathic dilated cardiomyopathy. Am J Cardiol. 2017;119:483–9.
8. Sinagra G, Anzini M, Pereira LN, Bussani R, Finocchiaro G, Bartunek J, Merlo M. Myocarditis in clinical practice. A clinical approach to myocarditis. Mayo Clin Proc. 2016.
9. Mestroni L, Maisch B, McKenna WJ, Schwartz K, Charron P, Rocco C, Tesson F, Richter A, Wilke A, Komajda M. Guidelines for the study of familial dilated cardiomyopathies. Collaborative Research Group of the European Human and Capital Mobility Project on Familial Dilated Cardiomyopathy. Eur Heart J. 1999;20:93–102.
10. Moretti M, Merlo M, Barbati G, Di Lenarda A, Brun F, Pinamonti B, Gregori D, Mestroni L, Sinagra G. Prognostic impact of familial screening in dilated cardiomyopathy. Eur J Heart Fail. 2010;12:922–7.
11. Puggia I, Merlo M, Barbati G, Rowland TJ, Stolfo D, Gigli M, Ramani F, Di Lenarda A, Mestroni L, Sinagra G. Natural history of dilated cardiomyopathy in children. J Am Heart Assoc. 2016; https://doi.org/10.1161/JAHA.116.003450.
12. Anzini M, Merlo M, Sabbadini G, et al. Long-term evolution and prognostic stratification of biopsy-proven active myocarditis. Circulation. 2013;128:2384–94.

13. Taylor MRG, Fain PR, Sinagra G, et al. Natural history of dilated cardiomyopathy due to lamin A/C gene mutations. J Am Coll Cardiol. 2003;41:771–80.
14. Sen-Chowdhry S, Syrris P, Prasad SK, Hughes SE, Merrifield R, Ward D, Pennell DJ, McKenna WJ. Left-dominant arrhythmogenic cardiomyopathy: an under-recognized clinical entity. J Am Coll Cardiol. 2008;52:2175–87.
15. Aleksova A, Carriere C, Zecchin M, Barbati G, Vitrella G, Di Lenarda A, Sinagra G. New-onset left bundle branch block independently predicts long-term mortality in patients with idiopathic dilated cardiomyopathy: data from the Trieste Heart Muscle Disease Registry. Europace. 2014;16:1450–9.
16. Ponikowski P, Voors AA, Anker SD, et al. 2016 ESC Guidelines for the diagnosis and treatment of acute and chronic heart failure. Eur Heart J. 2016;37:2129–200.
17. Hazebroek MR, Moors S, Dennert R, et al. Prognostic relevance of gene-environment interactions in patients with dilated cardiomyopathy: applying the MOGE(S) classification. J Am Coll Cardiol. 2015;66:1313–23.
18. Ortiz-Genga MF, Cuenca S, Dal Ferro M, et al. Truncating FLNC mutations are associated with high-risk dilated and arrhythmogenic cardiomyopathies. J Am Coll Cardiol. 2016;68:2440–51.
19. Herman DS, Lam L, Taylor MRG, et al. Truncations of titin causing dilated cardiomyopathy. N Engl J Med. 2012;366:619–28.
20. Haas J, Frese KS, Peil B, et al. Atlas of the clinical genetics of human dilated cardiomyopathy. Eur Heart J. 2015;36:1123–35a.
21. Lang RM, Bierig M, Devereux RB, et al. Recommendations for chamber quantification: a report from the American Society of Echocardiography's Guidelines and Standards Committee and the Chamber Quantification Writing Group, developed in conjunction with the European Association of Echocardiograph. J Am Soc Echocardiogr. 2005;18:1440–63.
22. Gigli M, Stolfo D, Merlo M, Barbati G, Ramani F, Brun F, Pinamonti B, Sinagra G. Insights into mildly dilated cardiomyopathy: temporal evolution and long-term prognosis. Eur J Heart Fail. 2017;19:531–9.
23. van Rijsingen IAW, Arbustini E, Elliott PM, et al. Risk factors for malignant ventricular arrhythmias in lamin a/c mutation carriers a European cohort study. J Am Coll Cardiol. 2012;59:493–500.
24. Pinamonti B, Zecchin M, Di Lenarda A, Gregori D, Sinagra G, Camerini F. Persistence of restrictive left ventricular filling pattern in dilated cardiomyopathy: an ominous prognostic sign. J Am Coll Cardiol. 1997;29:604–12.
25. Spezzacatene A, Sinagra G, Merlo M, et al. Arrhythmogenic phenotype in dilated cardiomyopathy: natural history and predictors of life-threatening arrhythmias. J Am Heart Assoc. 2015;4:e002149.
26. Japp AG, Gulati A, Cook SA, Cowie MR, Prasad SK. The diagnosis and evaluation of dilated cardiomyopathy. J Am Coll Cardiol. 2016;67:2996–3010.
27. Stolfo D, Merlo M, Pinamonti B, Poli S, Gigli M, Barbati G, Fabris E, Di Lenarda A, Sinagra G. Early improvement of functional mitral regurgitation in patients with idiopathic dilated cardiomyopathy. Am J Cardiol. 2015;115:1137–43.
28. Merlo M, Gobbo M, Stolfo D, et al. The prognostic impact of the evolution of RV function in idiopathic DCM. JACC Cardiovasc Imaging. 2016; https://doi.org/10.1016/j.jcmg.2016.01.027.
29. Bozkurt B, Colvin M, Cook J, et al. Current diagnostic and treatment strategies for specific dilated cardiomyopathies: a scientific statement from the American Heart Association. Circulation. 2016;134:e579–646.
30. Rapezzi C, Lorenzini M, Longhi S, Milandri A, Gagliardi C, Bartolomei I, Salvi F, Maurer MS. Cardiac amyloidosis: the great pretender. Heart Fail Rev. 2015;20:117–24.
31. Phelan D, Collier P, Thavendiranathan P, Popovic ZB, Hanna M, Plana JC, Marwick TH, Thomas JD. Relative apical sparing of longitudinal strain using two-dimensional speckle-tracking echocardiography is both sensitive and specific for the diagnosis of cardiac amyloidosis. Heart. 2012;98:1442–8.

32. Hutt DF, Quigley A-M, Page J, et al. Utility and limitations of 3,3-diphosphono-1,2-propanodicarboxylic acid scintigraphy in systemic amyloidosis. Eur Heart J Cardiovasc Imaging. 2014;15:1289–98.
33. Assomull RG, Prasad SK, Lyne J, Smith G, Burman ED, Khan M, Sheppard MN, Poole-Wilson PA, Pennell DJ. Cardiovascular magnetic resonance, fibrosis, and prognosis in dilated cardiomyopathy. J Am Coll Cardiol. 2006;48:1977–85.
34. Masci PG, Doulaptsis C, Bertella E, et al. Incremental prognostic value of myocardial fibrosis in patients with non-ischemic cardiomyopathy without congestive heart failure. Circ Heart Fail. 2014;7:448–56.
35. Satoh H, Sano M, Suwa K, Saitoh T, Nobuhara M, Saotome M, Urushida T, Katoh H, Hayashi H. Distribution of late gadolinium enhancement in various types of cardiomyopathies: Significance in differential diagnosis, clinical features and prognosis. World J Cardiol. 2014;6:585–601.
36. Puntmann VO, Carr-White G, Jabbour A, et al. T1-mapping and outcome in nonischemic cardiomyopathy: all-cause mortality and heart failure. JACC Cardiovasc Imaging. 2016;9:40–50.
37. Sekhri V, Sanal S, DeLorenzo LJ, Aronow WS, Maguire GP. Cardiac sarcoidosis: a comprehensive review. Arch Med Sci. 2011;7:546–54.
38. Mehta D, Lubitz SA, Frankel Z, Wisnivesky JP, Einstein AJ, Goldman M, Machac J, Teirstein A. Cardiac involvement in patients with sarcoidosis: diagnostic and prognostic value of outpatient testing. Chest. 2008;133:1426–35.
39. Birnie DH, Nery PB, Ha AC, Beanlands RSB. Cardiac Sarcoidosis. J Am Coll Cardiol. 2016;68:411–21.
40. Houston BA, Mukherjee M. Cardiac sarcoidosis: clinical manifestations, imaging characteristics, and therapeutic approach. Clin Med Insights Cardiol. 2014;8(Suppl 1):31–7. https://doi.org/10.4137/CMC.S15713.
41. Greulich S, Deluigi CC, Gloekler S, et al. CMR imaging predicts death and other adverse events in suspected cardiac sarcoidosis. JACC Cardiovasc Imaging. 2013;6:501–11.
42. Patel MR, Cawley PJ, Heitner JF, et al. Detection of myocardial damage in patients with sarcoidosis. Circulation. 2009;120:1969–77.
43. Hulten E, Aslam S, Osborne M, Abbasi S, Bittencourt MS, Blankstein R. Cardiac sarcoidosis—state of the art review. Cardiovasc Diagn Ther. 2016;6:50–63.
44. Betensky BP, Tschabrunn CM, Zado ES, Goldberg LR, Marchlinski FE, Garcia FC, Cooper JM. Long-term follow-up of patients with cardiac sarcoidosis and implantable cardioverter-defibrillators. Heart Rhythm. 2012;9:884–91.
45. Caforio ALP, Pankuweit S, Arbustini E, et al. Current state of knowledge on aetiology, diagnosis, management, and therapy of myocarditis: a position statement of the European Society of Cardiology Working Group on Myocardial and Pericardial Diseases. Eur Heart J. 2013;34:2636–48, 2648a–2648d
46. Cooper LT, Baughman KL, Feldman AM, et al. The role of endomyocardial biopsy in the management of cardiovascular disease: a scientific statement from the American Heart Association, the American College of Cardiology, and the European Society of Cardiology Endorsed by the Heart Failure Society of America and the Heart Failure Association of the European Society of Cardiology. Eur Heart J. 2007;28:3076–93.
47. Pollack A, Kontorovich AR, Fuster V, Dec GW. Viral myocarditis: diagnosis, treatment options, and current controversies. Nat Rev Cardiol. 2015;12:670–80.
48. Sagar S, Liu PP, Cooper LTJ. Myocarditis. Lancet (London, England). 2012;379:738–47.
49. Smith SC, Ladenson JH, Mason JW, Jaffe AS. Elevations of cardiac troponin I associated with myocarditis. Experimental and clinical correlates. Circulation. 1997;95:163–8.
50. Ukena C, Mahfoud F, Kindermann I, Kandolf R, Kindermann M, Bohm M. Prognostic electrocardiographic parameters in patients with suspected myocarditis. Eur J Heart Fail. 2011;13:398–405.
51. Mendes LA, Dec GW, Picard MH, Palacios IF, Newell J, Davidoff R. Right ventricular dysfunction: an independent predictor of adverse outcome in patients with myocarditis. Am Heart J. 1994;128:301–7.

52. Francone M, Chimenti C, Galea N, Scopelliti F, Verardo R, Galea R, Carbone I, Catalano C, Fedele F, Frustaci A. CMR sensitivity varies with clinical presentation and extent of cell necrosis in biopsy-proven acute myocarditis. JACC Cardiovasc Imaging. 2014;7:254–63.
53. Grun S, Schumm J, Greulich S, et al. Long-term follow-up of biopsy-proven viral myocarditis: predictors of mortality and incomplete recovery. J Am Coll Cardiol. 2012;59:1604–15.
54. Chimenti C, Verardo R, Scopelliti F, Grande C, Petrosillo N, Piselli P, De Paulis R, Frustaci A. Myocardial expression of Toll-like receptor 4 predicts the response to immunosuppressive therapy in patients with virus-negative chronic inflammatory cardiomyopathy. Eur J Heart Fail. 2017;19:915–25.
55. Heymans S, Eriksson U, Lehtonen J, Cooper LTJ. The quest for new approaches in myocarditis and inflammatory cardiomyopathy. J Am Coll Cardiol. 2016;68:2348–64.

5

Genetics of Dilated Cardiomyopathy: Current Knowledge and Future Perspectives

Matteo Dal Ferro, Giovanni Maria Severini, Marta Gigli, Luisa Mestroni, and Gianfranco Sinagra

Abbreviations and Acronyms

ACMG	American College of Medical Genetics and Genomics
DCM	Dilated cardiomyopathy
HCM	Hypertrophic cardiomyopathy
HF	Heart failure
HMDR	Heart Muscle Disease Registry of Trieste
LV	Left ventricular
LVEF	Left ventricular ejection fraction
LVNC	LV non-compaction
LVRR	Left ventricular reverse remodeling
RV	Right ventricular
MAF	Major allele frequency
NGS	Next-generation sequencing
PPCM	Peripartum cardiomyopathy
PSI	Proportion or percentage (of exons) spliced in
RCM	Restrictive cardiomyopathy

M. Dal Ferro (✉) · M. Gigli
Cardiovascular Department, Azienda Sanitaria Universitaria Integrata, University of Trieste (ASUITS), Trieste, Italy
e-mail: matteo.dalferro@asuits.sanita.fvg.it; marta.gigli@asuits.sanota.fvg.it

G. M. Severini
Medical Genetics Laboratory, Institute of Maternal and Child Health IRCCS Burlo Garofolo, Trieste, Italy
e-mail: gianmaria.severini@burlo.trieste.it

L. Mestroni
Cardiovascular Institute and Adult Medical Genetics Program, University of Colorado Anschutz Medical Campus, Aurora, CO, USA
e-mail: Luisa.Mestroni@ucdenver.edu

G. Sinagra
Cardiovascular Department, Azienda Sanitaria Universitaria Integrata, Trieste, Italy
e-mail: gianfranco.sinagra@asuits.sanita.fvg.it

5.1 DCM-Associated Genes

Nowadays, genetic laboratories from the USA and Europe offer different panels of genes related to DCM, ranging from 30 to more than 150 genes, with a great part of them only anecdotally associated with the disease or with a putative link on the basis of biological relationship with known genes. A detailed analysis of each different gene is far beyond the aim of this chapter, which will be focused in the complexity of the interpretation of "evidence-based" DCM genetic background. Here below is presented a brief list of the most investigated and evidence-based genes, grouped according to functional intracellular similarity. Cardiac sarcomeric and cytoskeletal genes (*TTN* overall) are the most frequently encountered. Other involved genes spread all over cardiomyocyte biological pathways and cell compartments, encoding components of desmosome, structural cytoskeleton, nuclear lamina, mitochondria, and ion flux-handling proteins [1] (Fig. 5.1).

We must premise that in these years times are rapidly changing, and this list may be no more representative of the entire genetic landscape of the disease in the next years.

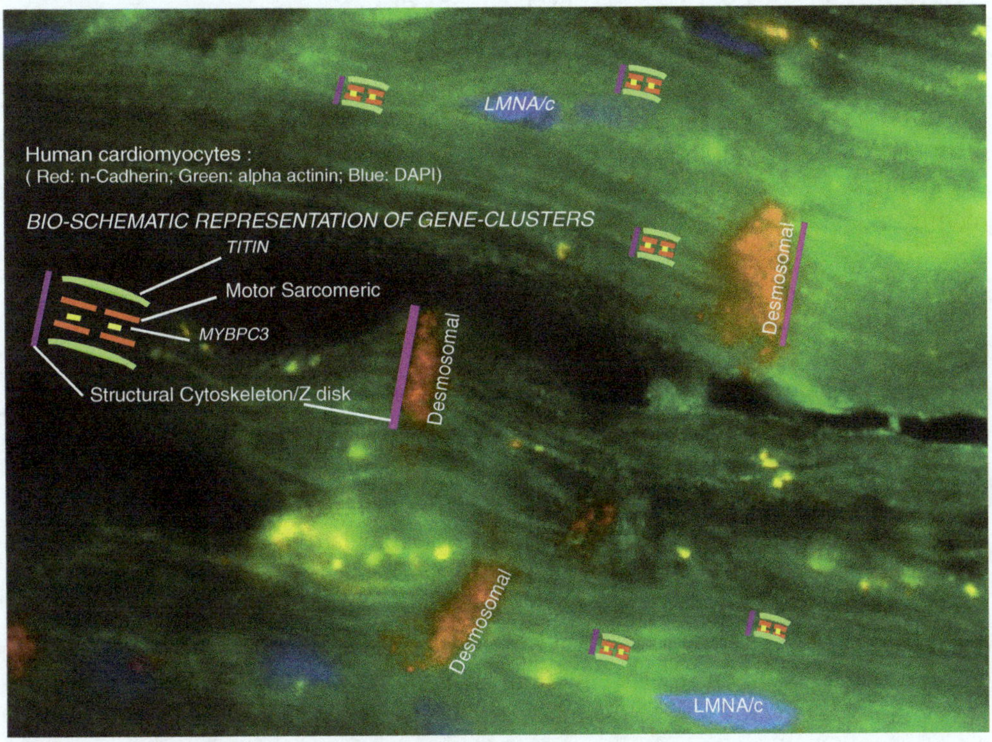

Fig. 5.1 Cardiomyocytes' immunofluorescence, with schematic representation of gene clusters involved in DCM pathogenesis (courtesy of the authors)

5.1.1 Titin

(See Sect. 5.5.1)

5.1.2 Lamin A/C

(See Sect. 5.5.2)

5.1.3 Structural Cytoskeleton Z-Disk Genes

Cardiomyocyte's structural integrity, sarcomeric orientation and contraction, and mechano-sensing transductions depend on cytoskeleton and Z-disk correct function. *DES*, *DMD*, *FLNC*, *NEXN*, *NEBL*, *LDB3*, and *VCL* encode for component of both sarcolemmal and sarcoplasmatic intermediate filaments, co-localizing to sarcolemmal membrane, sarcoplasmic membrane, and Z-disk structure. Notably, no or only a mild ATPase activity is known for these genes; thus all belongs to non-motor actin-binding protein group inside Z-disk structure. Mutations in these genes accounted for 5–10% of familial DCM, but this prevalence could increase after the inclusion of the recently discovered Filamin C (*FLNC*) gene.

Desmin (*DES*): Desmin is a cytoskeletal protein which forms muscle-specific intermediate filaments.

Mutations in the gene encoding Desmin cause a wide spectrum of phenotypes of different cardiomyopathies, skeletal myopathies, and mixed skeletal and cardiac myopathies. Desmin mutations account for 1–2% of all cases of DCM. Cardiac manifestations include restrictive cardiomyopathy (RCM), DCM, conduction system diseases, arrhythmias, and sudden death. Isolate cardiac phenotype is reported, or it can precede skeletal muscle involvement [2–4]. Truncating *DES* variants are associated with anticipated and more severe forms of DCM with diffuse LV fibrosis (unpublished data from Heart Muscle Disease Registry of Trieste, HMDR).

Dystrophin (*DMD*): The Dystrophin gene is located on the short arm of the X chromosome and consequently shows an x-linked pattern of inheritance. The dystrophin protein, in conjunction with the dystrophin glycoprotein complex, has an important role in force transmission, being integral to the mechanical link between the intracellular cytoskeleton and the extracellular matrix. Cardiac involvement is present in approximately 90% of the cases of Duchenne's muscular dystrophy and 70% of Becker's muscular dystrophy. Abnormal Q waves ("pseudonecrosis") in lead I, aVL, and V6 or in lead II, III, and aVF have been described. Right bundle branch block, atrioventricular block, and supraventricular arrhythmias can be present. About 10% of female carriers of *DMD* mutations (Duchenne or Becker type) may develop a DCM in the absence of clinical involvement of skeletal muscle and, although in anecdotal forms, missense and truncating variants of *DMD* may present with isolated cardiac involvement in males, with DCM, and no signs of muscular dystrophy [5–8].

Filamin C (See Sect. 5.5.3)

Vinculin (*VCL*): This gene encodes a cytoskeletal protein (Vinculin) involved in cell-matrix and cell-cell adhesion. Specifically, Vinculin is involved in the linkage of integrin adhesion molecules to the actin cytoskeleton. Mutations in this gene, especially in cardiac-specific isoform metavinculin, are very rarely found (less than ten variants described so far) and have been mainly related to DCM but also to hypertrophic cardiomyopathy (HCM). Nowadays, only a limited number of cases sustain these associations, and segregation studies were no or only marginally in support of it. Moreover, some of the described families harbored a second mutation that explained the phenotype [9, 10].

Lim Domain Binding 3 (*LDB3*, or Cypher Zasp): LDB3 interact with alpha-actinin-2 and to protein kinase C, maintaining the structure of the Z-disk during muscle contraction and contributing to signal transduction cascades including cardiac hypertrophy and ventricular remodeling pathways. Mutations in this gene have been associated with left ventricular non-compaction (LVNC), DCM, HCM, skeletal myopathy, and peripheral neuropathy. The evidence on the pathogenicity of many of the first described variants is actually weak, as some of them have been found with similar frequency in patients and controls [11]. Those variants that are more likely pathogenic are mainly located in some of the zinc-binding LIM domains of the protein [12].

5.1.4 Desmosomal Genes

Desmosome is a symmetric myocyte structure in which each part resides in the cytoplasm of one of a pair of adjacent cells, anchoring intermediate filaments in the cytoskeleton to the cell surface. In combination with the adherents and gap junctions, it connects myocardial cells maintaining both the mechanical and electrical integrity of the heart. Several desmosome genes have been identified in patients with DCM, usually inherited with an autosomal dominant pattern. Interestingly, desmosome genes (Plakophilin-2 (*PKP2*), Desmoplakin (*DSP*), Desmocollin-2 (*DSC2*), Desmoglein-2 (*DSG2*), and Plakoglobin (*JUP*)) were initially described as causing arrhythmogenic right ventricular cardiomyopathy (ARVC), but in 2010, Elliott et al. demonstrated a prevalence of 5% of desmosomal protein coding genes mutations among 100 unrelated DCM patients [13]: in relation to this aspect, it is now useful to introduce the concept of "overlapping, gene-driven phenotype" between different forms of cardiomyopathies (which turns out to be a recurrent feature in many genotypes)—even if originally described as linked to a peculiar phenotype (in the case of *JUP* and *DSP* genes with Naxos and Carvajal diseases and with ARVC), a specific genotype can manifest itself in different ways according to others, also non-genetic, modifiers.

Furthermore, the genetic overlap between ARVC and DCM has also been shown in most of non-desmosomal ARVC-related genes (e.g., *LMNA*, *TMEM43*), increasing the possibility of a clinical overlap between different forms of cardiomyopathy.

It is worth mentioning the similarity between specific cardiac and cutaneous desmosomal protein isoforms: Desmoplakin, plakoglobin, and plakophilin-2 are, in fact, constitutively expressed in desmosomes of both cardiomyocytes and keratinocytes, and a radical mutation in one of these two proteins often may result in cardio-cutaneous syndromes. Cadherins, conversely (*DSC* and *DSG*), have different isoforms preferentially expressed in the heart (isoform 2) or in the cutis (isoforms 1 and 3) [14, 15].

Desmoplakin (*DSP*): *DSP* codes for the protein desmoplakin, an intracellular obligate component of desmosomes that anchors intermediate filaments, such as desmin and filamins, to the inner desmosomal plaques, while the N terminus of the protein (extracellular domains) interacts with plakophilin and plakoglobin. *DSP*-related DCM is associated with increased ventricular arrhythmic burden and left ventricular fibrosis, with or without right ventricular involvement (arrhythmogenic cardiomyopathy). In general, frameshift and nonsense mutations in *DSP* are considered as disease causing, even when they have not been previously described, while missense variants must be evaluated case by case. As previously mentioned, *DSP* mutations, if present in homozygosity and with autosomal recessive inheritance pattern, have also been associated with a series of diseases characterized by cardiac and cutaneous involvement, such as Carvajal syndrome (woolly hair, keratoderma, DCM), keratosis palmoplantaris striata II, woolly hair, and lethal acantholytic epidermolysis bullosa. To date, large observational studies investigating the prognosis and the clinical manifestation related to *DSP*-DCM in respect to other genotypes are still lacking, but preliminary data from single-family studies and from HMDR of Trieste seems to confirm the increased risk of malignant ventricular arrhythmias.

5.1.5 Sarcomeric (Motor) Genes

Mutations in genes encoding for proteins that form sarcomeric thick and thin filaments have been largely recognized as DCM causing. These proteins (Myosin-heavy chain alpha and beta (*MYH6* and *MYH7*, respectively), myosin-binding protein C*3 (MYBPC3)*, troponins *(TNNT2, TNNI3, TNNC1)*, tropomyosin 1 (*TPM1*), cardiac actinin 1 *(ACTN1)*, myopalladin *(MYPN)*) share catalytic activity and are involved in sarcomeric contraction (*MYPN* shares also structural properties with Z-disk genes); comprehensively, these genes are involved in about 10% of cases of genetic DCM. Also this group of genes is characterized by a large overlapping of phenotypes: this is due to increased allelic heterogeneity, where different mutations resulting in different phenotypes are scattered and intercalated through the entire nucleotide sequence of a given gene, and, more interestingly, a single variant may express itself in different phenotypes inside the same family [16, 17]. Here below a brief list of most frequently encountered sarcomeric genes in DCM genotyping:

Myosin-heavy chain alpha (*MYH7*): *MYH6* codes for the alpha subunit of cardiac myosin heavy chain. It is the predominant isoform of myosin heavy chain at the embryonic myocardium. The ATPase activity and the shortening velocity of this isoform are higher than those of the adult beta-myosin isoforms. After birth, *MYH6* expression decreases and represents on average 7% of ventricular myosin in the adult heart. Despite its low expression, the presence of alpha-myosin is important for ventricular function, and its expression in adult atrial myocardium remains elevated, being the main isoform in this tissue (*MYH6* variants are also strongly associated with atrial septal defects). The characterization of this gene in DCM is representative of the evolving knowledge in cardiac genetics: previous studies have highlighted the importance of *MYH6* mutations in DCM patients, elucidating also a possible negative prognostic effect [18]. These *MYH6* mutations were distributed in highly conserved residues and were predicted to negatively affect protein function, but, nevertheless, the progression of knowledge of genetic databases has cast some doubts about the real contribute of this gene in DCM, since there seems to be no significant mutation excess in DCM patients in respect to controls. Variant is this gene should be evaluated carefully case by case [11].

Myosin-heavy chain beta (*MYH7*): β myosin heavy chain was the first sarcomeric protein to be linked with cardiomyopathy, and mutations in *MYH7* are now common causes of HCM and are also associated with DCM, LVNC, and RCM. In respect to DCM, they are responsible for about 4–6% of cases of familial DCM. Truncating variants should generally be considered pathogenic. The converter region of the protein (amino acid: 700–790) represents a mutation hotspot which have been shown to correlate with possible overlapping phenotypes and severe prognosis [16, 17].

Troponin T type 2 (*TNNT2*):The protein troponin T type 2 is the tropomyosin-binding subunit of the troponin complex, which is located on the thin filament of striated muscles and regulates muscle contraction in response to alterations in intracellular calcium ion concentration. Mutations in *TNNT2* have also been associated with HCM, DCM, RCM, and LVNC. Patients with *TNNT2* mutations generally exhibit a high frequency of premature sudden cardiac death. It accounts for 2–3% of DCM familial forms. Variant Arg173Trp has been clearly associated almost exclusively with dilated phenotype [19].

Myosin-binding protein C3 (*MYBPC3*): This gene *3* encodes for a member of myosin-associated proteins, which localized in the cross-bridge-bearing zone (C region) of A bands in cardiac muscle. It is the most common mutated gene in HCM, and, as others sarcomeric genes, it has been associated also with dilated or non-compaction phenotype. The more recent evidences raise questions about its contribution to DCM phenotype, given the relatively similar prevalence of *MYBPC3* rare variants in healthy and affected individuals of explored populations [11]. However, it must be underlined that some HCM that develop "burnout" physiology may turn in dilated phenotype: particular attention should be paid to this aspect when facing a DCM patient with a rare variant in *MYBPC3*.

5.1.6 Ion Channel-Related Genes

Genes encoding for ion-channel proteins are strongly associated with channelopaties, but, in the last years, a growing amount of studies extended the phenotypical spectrum of clinical entities related to a defect in one of these genes to also to structural (dilated or non-compaction) phenotypes. The mechanistic links behind these associations is still poorly understood, but it is potentially related to altered membrane stability (i.e., syntrophin-mediated interaction between *SCN5A* and *DMD*) or altered calcium handling leading to sarcomeric inefficiency (phospholamban (*PLN*) and *RYR2* variants). *HCN4* (hyperpolarization-activated cyclic nucleotide-gated potassium channel 4) mutations have also been recently shown to be associated with LVNC, with or without DCM overlap (NB: the association between *HCN4* and DCM needs still to be demonstrated) [20–23].

SCN5A: This gene encodes the voltage-gated sodium channel known as tetrodotoxin-resistant Nav1.5 dependent. The protein expression is predominant at heart. It is responsible for the fast sodium current that causes phase 0 of the action potential. Mutations in this gene, with marked allelic heterogeneity, have been strongly associated with Brugada syndrome in case of loss of function effect and long QT type 3 in case of gain of function effect, both diseases with autosomal dominant transmission. The association with DCM has been, in proportion, very rarely reported; it is generally accepted that these mutations are located in two specific regions of the channel: in the voltage-sensitive domain (VSD) and intracellular loops. One of the best characterized mutations is Arg222Gln [20], which affects the VSD. This mutation is also associated with frequent ventricular arrhythmias, cardiac conduction disease, and, in some cases, atrial fibrillation. None of the carriers presented a prolonged QTc. Recently, especially for truncating variants, the association with DCM has been further confirmed [11].

Ryanodine Receptor 2 (*RYR2*): This gene encodes a ryanodine receptor found in cardiac muscle sarcoplasmic reticulum. The encoded protein is one of the components of calcium channel, mediating the release of Ca^{2+} from the sarcoplasmic reticulum into the cytoplasm and thereby playing a key role in triggering cardiac muscle contraction. Mutations (>95% missense) in this gene are known to result in catecholaminergic polymorphic ventricular tachycardia (CPVT), typically in the absence of structural heart disease. Some missense mutations have also been originally associated with the development of ARVC; however, it is now accepted that these carriers had not fulfilled current diagnostic criteria for the disease. Among missense variants, only one has been clearly associated with the development of structural (hypertrophic) heart disease in patients diagnosed with CPVT. A different variant (exon 3 deletion) has been demonstrated, in two families, to segregate with CPVT and progressive left ventricular dysfunction and/or cavity enlargement in some members [20]. Thus, the presence of DCM without CPVT phenotype related to RYR2 (radical) mutations is yet to be demonstrated.

5.1.7 Other Genes

BCL2-Associated Athanogene 3, *BAG3*: Members of the *BAG* family, including *BAG3*, are cytoprotective proteins that bind to and regulate Hsp70 family molecular chaperones. Heterozygous mutations in *BAG3* have been associated with DCM. Mechanism of disease may, at least in part, depends on a decreased capability to compensate external stressors. The severity of DCM, in fact, has been shown to vary considerably between carriers. By the age of 70, the disease penetrance is apparently 100%. Both non-truncating and truncating *BAG3* mutations are reported, with variable penetrance. A specific variant (Pro209Leu), typically a spontaneous de novo variant, is linked to pediatric myofibrillar myopathy [24, 25].

RNA-Binding Motif Protein 20, *RBM20*: This gene encodes a RNA-binding protein that acts as a regulator of mRNA splicing of a subset of genes involved in cardiac development, mainly sarcomeric genes (*TTN*, but also *MYH7*, *TNNT2*, and others). The association of this gene with DCM was firstly established in 2009 by genome-wide linkage analysis and progressively confirmed by subsequent studies. Remarkably, these mutations were located in exon 9, which appears to be a mutational hotspot. Nowadays, also mutations out of exon 9 are reported to be DCM causative, with similar penetrance and clinical manifestations. In respect to prevalence in DCM families, *RBM 20* represents a rare genotype, accounting for 2–3% of cases. For this reason, so far, we should underline that evidence-based genotype-phenotype correlations are still lacking: only a small number of studies, in fact, with small numbers of index-patients or families, and short follow-up, reported a phenotype characterized by "severe heart failure, arrhythmia, and the need for cardiac transplantation" [26, 27], which still need to be confirmed in further studies.

5.2 Technical Issues in Genetic Sequencing

Over the last three decades, different approaches and technologies have been used to obtain genetic information in families or sporadic patients with hereditary diseases. Linkage analysis was the first method used to identify new disease genes, but this technique requires very large families or a large number of sporadic cases. The advent of "old" sequencing technology (Sanger method) has made genetic analysis much more effective, but with timing analysis and high costs, especially for pathologies with high genetic heterogeneity such as cardiomyopathies.

More recently we are witnessing a revolution in medical genetics and scientific research applied both to the identification of new disease genes and to the massive parallel study of a large number of genes. This is due to the discovery of high-efficiency instruments (NGS) that allowed the entry into what is called the era of the precision medicine; speed, reliability, and limited costs are the advantages peculiar of these techniques that allow the parallel analysis of a large number of genes.

NGS technologies can be applied in various formats, with the aim of sequencing the entire genome (including non-coding parts), or the exome, which includes only the coding regions of the genome, or a group (panel) of selected genes. Currently (but technologies are continuously improving), the latter application seems to offer the best compromise between costs, execution speed, and accuracy for certified diagnostic purposes, as it usually guarantees greater coverage of the analyzed genes [28, 29].

Different next-generation platforms have been proposed, differing from each other mainly in their methods of clonal amplification of short DNA fragments (50–400 bases) as a genomic library template and how these fragment libraries are subsequently sequenced through repetitive cycles to provide a nucleotide readout (see Table 5.1) [30].

Table 5.1 Comparison between the most common NGS platforms

	NGS whole genome platforms			Compact NGS sequencers	
Sequencer	SOLID 5500 XL W (Applied Biosystems®, Thermo Fisher®)	454 GS FLX Titanium XL (Roche®)	HiSeq 4000 (Illumina®)	MiSeq (Illumina)	PGM Ion torrent (Thermo Fisher)
Methods	Sequencing by ligation	Pyrosequencing	Sequencing by synthesis	Sequencing by synthesis	Semiconductor sequencing
Most used sequencing application	Whole exome/ genome	Whole exome/ genome	Whole exome/ genome	Target	Target
Read length (bp)	35–50	700	150	300	400
Reads per run	1.2–1.4 billion	1 million	2.5–5 billion	15 million	80 million
Run time	2–7 days	24 h	1–3 days	24 h	3 h
Advantage	Low error rate	Read length, fast	Low error rate High throughput	Low error rate	Short time Less expensive
Disadvantage	Short read length, long run time	Homopolymer errors	Short read length	Higher cost	Homopolymer errors

However, the discovery of new single nucleotide variants (SNVs) using NGS still requires validation with Sanger sequencing methods because of the possible loss of precision in obtaining a really high number of short DNA fragments using the polymerase chain reaction (PCR) during library building. NGS platforms have in fact error rates of approximately ten times higher (1 in 1000 bases with 20× coverage) than Sanger sequencing (1 in 10,000 bases). Although the reading depth cutoff for NGS platforms is conventionally set at 20×, many studies indicate that average reading depths greater than 100× are required for the use of these platforms as independent tool for newly discovered variants, even under optimal conditions [31].

5.3 The Complexity in Variant Classification Process

Traditionally, a mutation is defined as a permanent change in the nucleotide sequence, whereas a polymorphism is defined as a variant with a frequency above 1%. These terms, however, which have been used widely, actually seem no longer suitable to describe the complexity of interindividual genetic variability. The Human Genome Project, culminating in 2001 with the determination of the complete sequence of human DNA [32], provided a first quantitative assessment of the interindividual genetic variability and the possible impact that this variability has on human health. Subsequent multiple international projects (like ESP and 1000 genomes, recently merged with other projects in the most comprehensive exome and genome database: gnomAD; http://gnomad.broadinstitute.org) led to the conclusion that about 1 in 1000 nucleotides in the human genome (three million in total) differs between people, and this variation is largely responsible for the physical, behavioral, and medical unique characteristics of each individual. In this line, the term "mutation" is no more strictly associated with the concept of pathogenicity, as the term polymorphism with the concept of benignity.

Taking into account the higher complexity of genetic information, the American College of Medical Genetics and Genomics (ACMG) 2015 guidelines defined a new standard [33]; both terms, mutation and polymorphism, should now be replaced by the term "variant," followed by one of these modifiers: (I) pathogenic, (II) likely pathogenic, (III) uncertain significance, (IV) likely benign, or (V) benign. Several stringent criteria are required to reach one of these different modifiers, which are defined by crosschecking the evidence that derives from different categories of evaluation: (a) population and disease-specific genetic databases, (b) in silico predictive algorithms, (c) biochemical characteristics, (d) literature evidences. A free access website, http://wintervar.wglab.org/results.php, released from ACMG, allows a guideline-based, point-by-point analysis of each—missense—variant of interest.

This classification approach is more stringent than the previous ones and may result in a larger proportion of variants being categorized as uncertain significance. It is hoped that this approach will reduce the substantial number of variants being reported as "causative" of disease without having sufficient supporting evidence for that classification. It is important to keep in mind that when a variant is classified as pathogenic, healthcare providers are highly likely to take that as "actionable," i.e., to alter the treatment or surveillance of a patient or remove such management in a genotype-negative family member, based on that determination [11].

In recent years, in fact, genetic laboratories often showed a lack of uniformity in the definition of variants, especially for variants originally described in the past literature, which are still reported as pathogenic in older databases but were subsequently found to be too common in general population, so unlikely to be disease causing. This dis-homogeneity potentially led to different clinical management of similar variants.

A similar argument is related to new candidate genes: these genes are included in offered extended panel tests on the basis of a putative biological relationship with known disease-causing genes, but—still—in the absence of solid population or scientific supporting data. The actual net effect of extended gene panels is an increase in the amount of variants of unknown significance and a relative decrease in actionable variants.

It is important now to provide a brief mention to the mostly used of these "clinically oriented variant classification" databases: ClinVar and HGMD [34, 35]. The ClinVar database (https://www.ncbi.nlm.nih.gov/clinvar/) is a public database that better represents the "historical" process that characterizes the classification of each variant: quoting, "ClinVar is a freely accessible, public archive of reports 'coming from research and diagnostic laboratories' of the relationships among human variations and phenotypes, with supporting evidence. ClinVar thus facilitates access to (…) the history of that interpretation." The Human Gene Mutation Database (HGMD®, https://portal.biobase-international.com/hgmd/pro/start.php), available under subscription in the most updated version (last 3 years), is the other most reliable source of information about "known (published) gene lesions responsible for human inherited disease." Since nowadays not all laboratories are active submitters to ClinVar or HGMD®, clinicians should still be careful in referring to them as a gold standard for variant classification: when a potentially disease related rare variant is found in a patient, these databases should be intended as a valuable source of informations to crosscheck with, but representing only a part of the multi-parametric approach that finally lead to definite variant classification.

In respect to variants in DCM-related genes, a recent report [11] shed some light in this topic, helping the clinicians to reassess the classification of variants and genes offered by clinical laboratories according to the new guideline standards, in order to elucidate the common characteristics of true actionable variants. The authors found that in some genes, previously strongly associated with a given cardiomyopathy, a rare variant was not clinically informative because there is an unacceptably high likelihood of false positive interpretation, while, by contrast, in other genes, diagnostic laboratories may have been overly conservative when assessing variant pathogenicity. Interestingly, some genes proposed on the basis of several (but dated) studies as among the most common causes of DCM (e.g., *MYBPC3*, *MYH6*, and missense variants in *SCN5A*) showed no excess variation among affected cases, raising an important question about their contribution to DCM phenotype development. Identifying the frequency of the most common HCM pathogenic variant in the available population databases (c.1504C>T in *MYBPC3*: 2.5×10^{-5}) as the conservative upper bound, this study clearly elucidated what is the major allele frequency (MAF) threshold for a rare variant to be considered pathogenic: 0.0001 in ExAC (ExAC is the first release version of gnomAD, composed by exome data).

The emerging concept is the odds ratio (OR) of a given variant, to be disease causing (e.g., *LMNA*-truncating variants (tv) reached an OR of ~99 to develop DCM, *TTN*-truncating variant an OR ~20 to ~50, *FLNC* not tested): the higher OR corresponds to higher actionability.

To summarize, clinicians should be aware that the "pathogenicity" of a variant is a fluid and evolving definition that should be periodically re-evaluated with the evidence coming from database and scientific progress, in order to be continuously customized to the patient.

5.4 The External Modulation of Genotype: Environmental Triggers

In DCM, both in sporadic and in familial cases, the pathogenicity of a gene variant is modulated by interfering, non-genetic environmental factors: this interaction could be largely responsible for variability in disease phenotype and prognosis. It is important to keep in mind how the actual knowledge in this field (contribution of interfering factors) may still be invalidated by a different accuracy in underlying genetic characterization, with the oldest reports being published before the release of 2015 ACMG standard. Below is reported a brief summary of known interfering environmental factors: inflammation, toxic exposure, hormones, and metabolic profile. Notably, in this field the research is currently very active, and all the following statements are susceptible to possible modifications in the next future (Table 5.2).

To conclude, we may say that the phenotypically normal heart with a pathogenic variant (definition that should be constantly re-evaluated) represents a model of failing but compensated heart, which is no or less able to sustain a second, environmental, failing hit [48]: all these potential "second hits" must be taken into account in DCM treatment and prognosis stratification.

5.5 Evidence-Based Genotype-Phenotype Correlations

As previously mentioned, the key factor for a correct genotype-phenotype analysis is the accuracy of the underlying variant classification: reliable genotype-dependent phenotypic informations are in fact achievable only if driven by a solid pathogenicity assessment.

Then, as patient's phenotype represents the final results of a long-lasting process of interactions between genetic background and environment, clinicians are aware that discovering the net effect of the pathogenic variant requires a careful "pruning" of "confounding" factors. Furthermore, some correlations could also be outlined "a posteriori", i.e., by the type of response to the medical therapy.

Finally, in assessing this correlation, it is important to focus on what is the best starting point: specific mutation versus specific gene versus specific clusters of genes with similar function inside the cardiomyocyte.

In this line, in respect to truly personalized medicine, the most correct approach should be the correlation between a specific pathogenic variant in a gene and its "private" phenotype, but, in order to achieve a more clinically meaningful classification, gene clustering attempts have been made and were shown to allow a rough, but functional, orientation, especially in therapeutic management [49]. At the current state of knowledge, a good compromise could be represented by the correlation between a specific gene and its phenotype, just preceded by a brief general distinction on the two main categories of variant (in respect to structural protein effect): missense and truncating (or radical). Generally speaking, the former is expected to affect protein morphology and/or function by changing a single amino acid in the protein sequence, while the latter is expected to cause a premature truncation of the amino acid sequence, leading to a decrease of total protein amount or effectiveness at the cellular level, mainly through nonsense-mediated decay (NMD). Consequently, truncating variants are generally considered less tolerated and linked to haploinsufficiency. Among all the human genes, the ones that are most conserved, expressed in early development, and highly tissue specific usually do not tolerate to be expressed in a single copy and are called haploinsufficient genes [50]. All

Table 5.2 Known DCM predisposing background in respect to external modifiers

Environmental modifier	Known DCM-predisposing genetic background		References	Recommendation
	Trigger-specific	Cardiomyopathy-specific		
Inflammation (myocarditis)	Innate immune system-related genes? (not demonstrated)	*BAG3*, *DSP*, *PKP2*, *RYR2*, *SCN5A*, *TNNI3*, *TTN*	[36–38] HMDR (unpublished data)	Genetic predisposition to DCM should be ruled out in some cases of myocarditis, especially (1) in the setting of known familial DCM, (2) in the presence of LV dysfunction and remodeling associated with only mild histological inflammation, or, finally, (3) in cases of persistent LV dysfunction despite immunosuppressive therapy
Toxic (alcohol, chemotherapeutics)	SNPs in genes involved in ethanol metabolisms (such as ADH1B, A/A; ALDH2, A/G or A/A; and CYP2E1-T/C or T/T) or in pathways modulating anthracycline cardiotoxicity (as topoisomerase 2-beta, carbonyl reductases, ROS generation, and intrinsic antioxidant species)	*TTN*	[39–42]	Only anecdotal reports investigate the prevalence of variants in cardiomyopathy-related genes across patients with toxic exposure and cardiac dysfunction; however, the effect of toxics is likely supposed to be even more deleterious in the presence of a gene defect that predisposes to DCM

(continued)

Table 5.2 continued

Environmental modifier	Known DCM-predisposing genetic background		References	Recommendation
	Trigger-specific	Cardiomyopathy-specific		
Hormones (peripartum cardiomyopathy (PPCM))	Poorly elucidated: basic research and animal studies linked PPCM to prolactin hormones, in which oxidative stress turns prolactin into an angiostatic fragment that plays a role in the progression of the disease (Broad trial-44). Strong ethnic predisposition: Nigeria (PPCM incidence: 1 in 100 to 1 in 1000 pregnancies) or Haiti (1 in 299 pregnancies)	*TTN, MYBPC3, MYH6, MYH7, PSEN2, SCN5A, TNNC1, and TNNT2:* pregnancy-related effect on the manifestation of the disease is supposed to be due not only to hormonal changes but more comprehensively to a different hemodynamic state in which the "mutation-harboring" heart is required to sustain an high output state for a long time (usually without associated hypertension)	[43, 44]	Only anecdotal reports investigate the prevalence of variants in cardiomyopathy-related genes across patients with toxic exposure and cardiac dysfunction; however, the effect of toxics is likely supposed to be even more deleterious in the presence of a gene defect that predisposes to DCM
Sport, lifestyle	Not investigated	Desmosomal genes: The combination of neurohormonal, mechanical, and oxidative stressors that characterize competitive sport activities may modulate disease penetrance in the presence of a predisposing genetic background, exacerbating or accelerating it: this potential deleterious role, if present, is still poorly investigated in DCM and needs further studies		

Metabolic profile and cardiovascular risk factors	Not specifically investigated: There is compelling evidence that diabetes has a direct negative effect on the heart, being an independent risk factor for heart failure, with multiple mechanisms including mitochondrial dysfunction, oxidative stress, and shift in energetic substrate utilization. In respect to hypertension, unpublished data from HMDR of Trieste highlight the role of untreated elevated arterial hypertension in the first manifestation of heart failure in a minor proportion of patients harboring a pathogenic variant, and, from the other side, the presence of arterial hypertension is a positive predictor of LV reverse remodeling (LVRR) in DCM patients	All known DCM-associated genes (*TTN* overall, HMDR unpublished data). Furthermore, recent evidence binds a specific LMNA variant—p.G602S—and type 2 diabetes	[45–47]	In HMDR registry, few families are enrolled in which DCM and diabetes co-segregate in the absence of a pathogenic identified variants: the suggestions are that (1) in DCM families, diabetic patients may be at risk of a worse disease prognosis, and (2) in some cases diabetes and dilated cardiomyopathy seem to be genetically correlated. Both these hypotheses need to be deeply elucidated

cardiomyopathy-causing genes are included in this category, but they are not mutated with similar proportions of truncating and missense variants: for example, truncating variants on *TTN* have been discovered as the most frequent mutations in all DCM, whereas, in other DCM disease-causing genes, missense variants are the most frequently encountered (with, interestingly, similar actionability). With these principles in mind, among the several papers published on this topic, only few of them demonstrate evidence-based genotype-phenotype correlations that are helpful in the clinical management of patients with genetic DCM. To date, the best characterized correlations regard *LMNA* and *TTN* genes. Filamin C and other genes, in the next future, may reach a similar level of evidence (Fig. 5.2).

5.5.1 Lamin A/C

LMNA represent the more investigated gene in DCM, and the natural history of *LMNA*-DCM has been outlined in several papers [52–54]. Comprehensively, with a confirmed mortality rate around 12% at 4 years (up to 30% at 12 years of follow-up), it could be considered the more aggressive genotype in DCM. Its phenotypic expression is characterized by a relatively high incidence of sudden cardiac death or major ventricular arrhythmias, even before the development of systolic left ventricular dysfunction. The median age at disease onset is between 30 and 40 years, and penetrance is almost complete at the age of 70 [52].

It is associated also to a primary disease of the conduction system, with supraventricular arrhythmias and atrioventricular block, by some authors called *LMNA* "atriopathy." To date, *LMNA* pathogenic variants represent the only genetic background in DCM that is included in current guidelines, as it may change clinical choices such as the implantable cardioverter-defibrillator (ICD) therapy in primary prevention regardless of left ventricular ejection fraction values (Class IIa, level of evidence B, for ICD implantation in the presence of risk factors [55]: NSVT during ambulatory electrocardiogram monitoring, LVEF < 45% at first evaluation, male sex, and non-missense mutations).

The type of variant (missense versus truncating) and its site (before or after the nuclear lamina interacting domain) have also been addressed in respect to prognosis: actual evidence shows that mortality rates are similar, but truncating variants are related to anticipated penetrance of the disease. No clear effect is still demonstrated in respect to the site of variants [56].

5.5.2 Titin

Titin (*TTN*) is known as the largest sarcomeric protein that resides within the heart muscle. Due to alternative splicing of *TTN*, the heart expresses two major isoforms (N2B and N2BA) that incorporate four distinct regions termed the Z-line, I-band, A-band, and M-line. The amino terminus of Titin is embedded in the sarcomere Z-disk and participates in myofibril assembly, stabilization, and maintenance. The

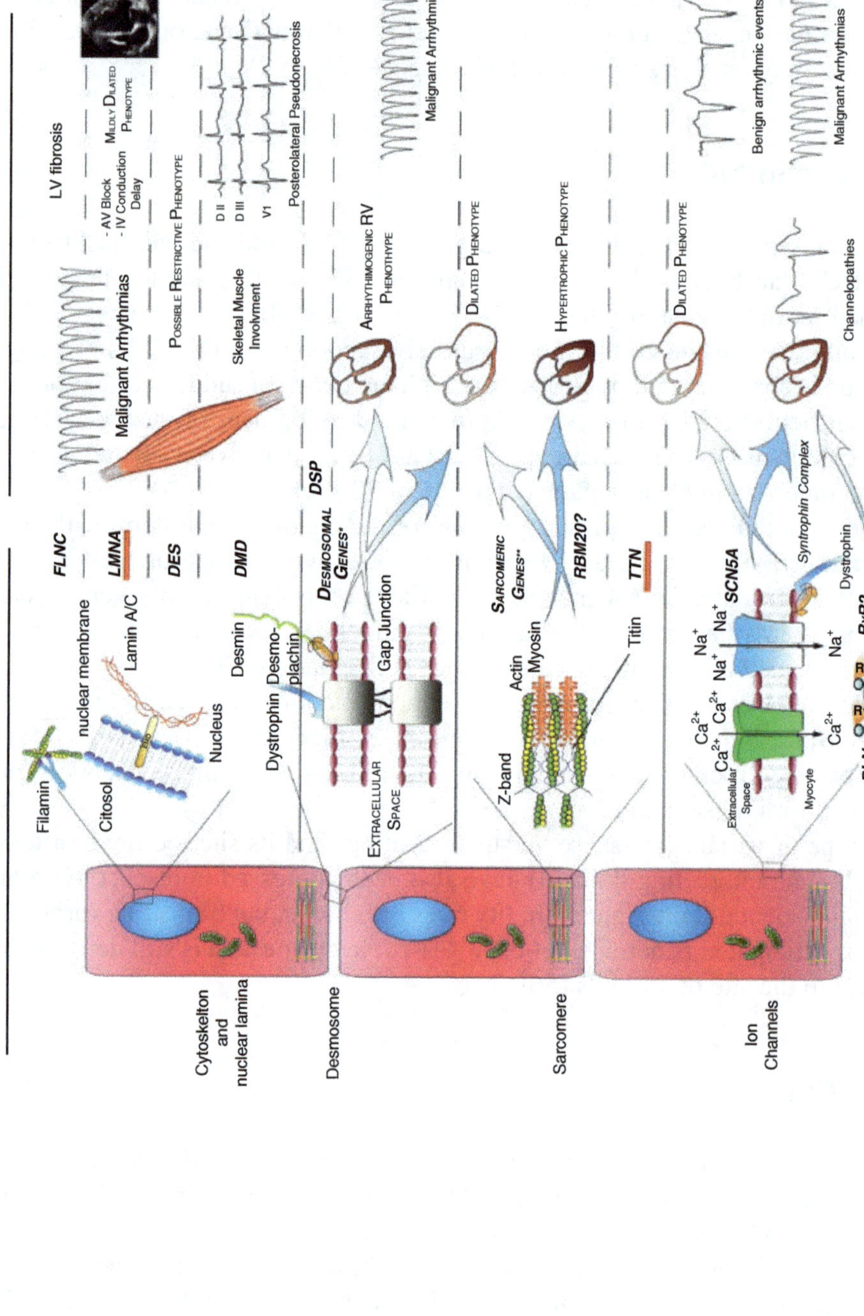

Fig. 5.2 Schematic representation of genotype-phenotype correlations (*adapted from* [51])

elastic I-band behaves as a bidirectional spring, restoring sarcomeres to their resting length after systole and limiting their stretch in early diastole. The inextensible A-band binds myosin and myosin-binding protein and is thought to be critical for biomechanical sensing and signaling. The M-band contains a kinase that may participate in strain-sensitive signaling and affect gene expression and cardiac remodeling in DCM.

Due to its higher prevalence in DCM population in respect to Lamin A/c (*TTN* 12–18% of whole DCM population, versus *LMNA* 4–6%), Titin is becoming the more broadly assessed genotype, despite its relatively recent discovery as a DCM-related gene [57]. To date, the evidence of pathogenicity is related almost exclusively to truncating variants. Since Titin-truncating variants (*TTN*tv) were reported also in 2–3% of general population without overt cardiomyopathy, many efforts have been made, firstly, to outline the characteristics that distinguish the disease-related truncating variants from the benign ones.

An important study by Roberts et al. elucidated the importance of the specific site of truncating variants: of the 364 exons of the entire gene, only a part of them is translated in cardiac isoforms N2B and N2BA [58]: Proportion (or percentage) of exons spliced in (PSI) is the concept that allows to correlate the exon site of the truncating variant with the molecular—and clinical—consequences of this truncation, with a PSI > 15% set as a lowest threshold to be penetrant and PSI > 90% describing exons sites with higher cardiac expression and higher association with fully penetrant DCM phenotype. The entire A-band and the proximal or terminal part of I-band contain exons with PSI proximal to 100%. Tv in M-band exons and Z-band exons should be evaluated case by case. This is the reason why the OR of a TTNtv varies between 20 and 50 according to the site involved by the mutation.

A second paper by the same group further demonstrates this concept, showing that also in general population without overt cardiomyopathy, the presence of *TTN*tv in sites with PSI > 15% mildly, but significantly, affects cardiac dimensions and function when assessed with 3D cardiac magnetic resonance [48].

Lower ventricular mass values, with lower ventricular wall thickness, have been recently outlined as a peculiar phenotypic manifestation of TTNtv [49, 59].

In respect to other clinical manifestations of *TTN*-related DCM, evidences are in favor of a relatively mild and treatable form of the disease in respect to *LMNA*-related one, with lower mortality rates, in line with the general DCM population. This could be true, especially in relatives that are diagnosed in a preclinical state [49, 59].

Clinicians must be aware that *TTN*tv, even if in small proportion of cases, could be linked to malignant ventricular arrhythmias especially in the presence of external modifiers: comprehensively, the sum of the actual evidences recommends a complete and continuous clinical follow-up of patients with *TTN*tv-related DCM and their relatives, even in the absence of overt cardiomyopathy [60].

Titin missense variants, on the contrary, nowadays are considered mostly as benign. This assumption has been tested in a recent multicenter study that sequenced

TTN gene in a cohort of 147 DCM patients in which the outcome was not affected by the presence of Titin missense variants, confirming that most of these variants could be in fact benign (despite a highly conservative and accurate selection of variants: lowest population frequency, familial segregation, software predictions of pathogenicity) [61]. Recently, however, this "simple" classification has been questioned: a report in fact elucidated the pathogenicity of a specific *TTN* missense variant in DCM phenotype with non-compaction aspects, raising the threshold of complexity in *TTN* variant evaluation [62].

5.5.3 Filamin C

FLNC encodes filamin C, an intermediate filament that cross-links polymerized actin, contributing in anchoring cellular membrane proteins to cytoskeleton and in maintaining sarcomeric and Z-disk stability. It directly interacts with two protein complexes that link the subsarcolemmal actin cytoskeleton to the extracellular matrix: (1) the dystrophin-associated glycoprotein and (2) the integrin complexes, while, at intercalated disks, filamin C is located in the fascia adherens [63].

The association with DCM was initially reported by two separate studies [63, 64]. Ortiz et al. evaluated with NGS panels a cohort of 2877 patients referred for various cardiac diseases (including channelopathies and HCM, the latter representing almost one half of the cases) and identified 28 unrelated probands with *FLNC*-truncating variants, previously diagnosed mainly with DCM or, in minor part, with arrhythmogenic or RCM. Truncating variants in *FLNC* came out to cause an overlapping phenotype of dilated and left dominant arrhythmogenic cardiomyopathy complicated by frequent premature sudden death, with the phenotypic hallmark represented by subepicardial-transmural fibrosis in inferolateral LV wall. Interestingly, a small portion of probands (<5%) had prominent right ventricular involvement or restrictive phenotype.

The cumulative incidence of MVA or SD was found to be between 15 and 20% in a median follow-up of 5 years, and the mortality rate was about 6% for the same follow-up. We should underline that these data refer to a limited cohort of probands referred for genetic testing due to aggressive familial disease, representing a potential selection bias. Data on large cohorts of *FLNC*tv-related DCM patients are still lacking to confirm or modulate this aggressive phenotype.

Furthermore, it is worth mentioning that *FLNC missense* variants have been identified in a previous study also in families with HCM, although with a mild degree of LV hypertrophy. As for other cytoskeletal or sarcomeric genotypes with allelic heterogeneity, this fact suggests that filaminopathies can generate a spectrum of different cardiac disorders that at least in part may be related to the type of variant [65].

FLNC has only recently been included in the genetic screening of patients with inherited cardiomyopathies and sudden death, and its real prevalence in DCM has still to be elucidated. Figure 5.3 shows familial pedigrees of three families carrying *FLNC*tv.

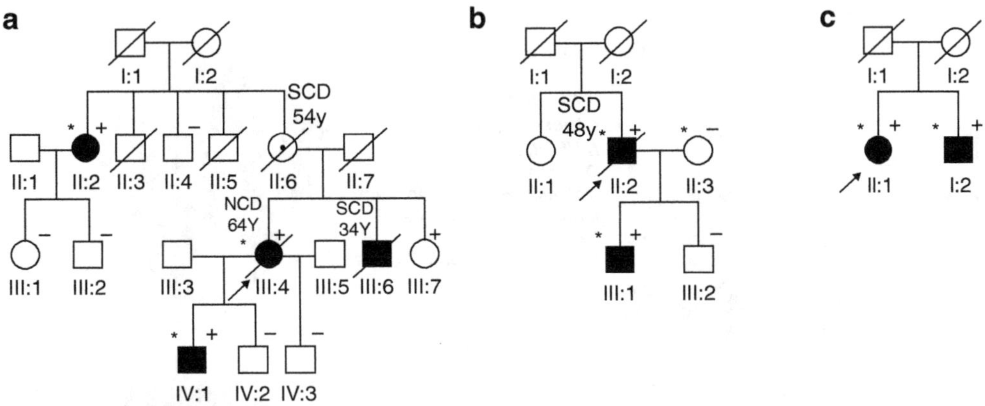

Fig. 5.3 Familial pedigrees of three families carrying *FLNC*tv

5.5.4 Insights from Clinical Presentation and Left Ventricular Reverse Remodeling (LVRR)

In clinical practice, especially in newly diagnosed DCM patients without familial history of cardiac disease, cardiologists may find useful to know peculiar findings that are representative of a specific genotype and, hopefully, able to guide disease treatment and prognostic assessment, at least in the short time.

A recent report from HMDR of Trieste tried to shed some light in this sense, differentiating genotypes on the basis of response to therapy: a different response, in fact, can be interpreted as the indirect evidence of different, mutation-driven, underlying pathogenic processes [49]. These mutation-dependent processes may not, or only marginally, be detectable otherwise.

Despite several limitations (possible selection bias in single referral center, limited number of patients partially grouped in gene clusters, thus introducing a possible heterogenic genetic background), this study allowed some interesting observations both in clinical presentation and LVRR rate in different genetic-based DCM, especially in relatively less investigated genotypes.

In respect to clinical presentation, most of the clinical and instrumental characteristics did not differ between the different genotypes. Except for a lower rate of left bundle-brunch block in both *TTN* and structural cytoskeleton Z-disk group and a trend toward a mild degree of LV dilation and dysfunction in *LMNA* mutation carriers (part of these findings have been subsequently confirmed in other studies) [59, 60], symptoms, electrocardiographic, and echocardiographic findings were grossly similar across different genotypes, being consistent with the hypothesis that DCM represents the final common phenotype of multiple genetic-based cardiac diseases and their relationship with environmental modifiers.

The most interesting finding was related to LVRR: a significant association was in fact demonstrated between lack of LVRR and specific genotypes (*FLNC*, *DES*, *DMD*, and other cytoskeletal Z-disk genes overall, followed by *LMNAc*). Conversely, *TTN* genotypes were most frequently associated with positive LVRR on optimal medical therapy (Fig. 5.4).

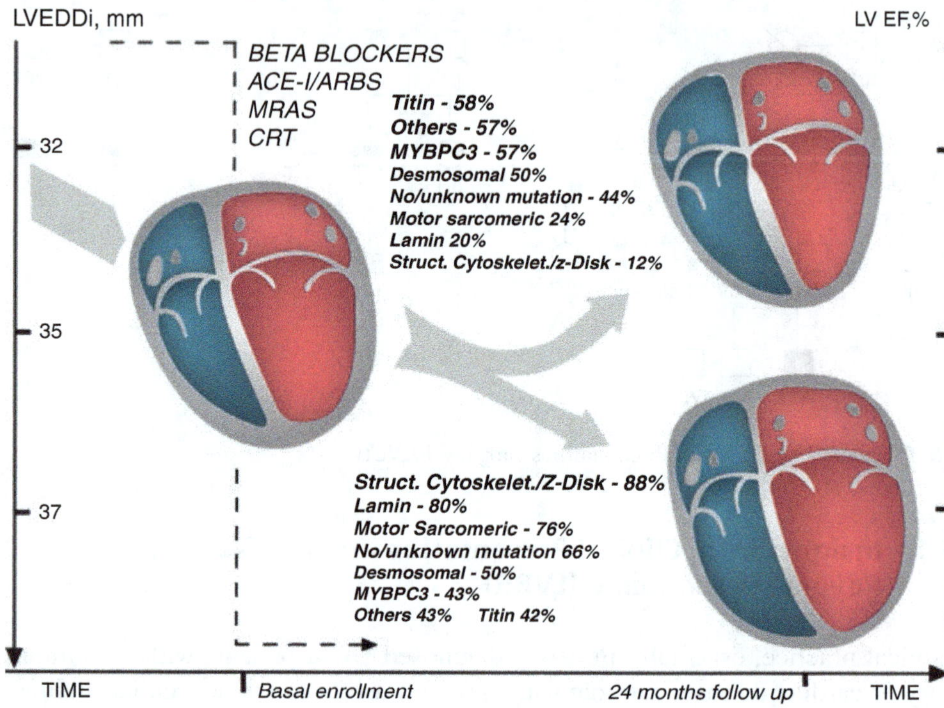

Fig. 5.4 Association between LVRR and absence of LVRR according to different genotypes (data from HMDR) [49]

This kind of approach showed how phenotype correlations can be inferred also in this way, as an "ongoing" process, once more related to the interactions with external modifiers, in these cases represented by medications.

To conclude, the emerging concept elucidated in this chapter is that disease manifestation and prognosis are the results of the interaction between genotype and environment: the contribution of each factor to the patient's clinical status is modulated by (1) genetic variant's actionability and (2) type and severity of environmental factor(s). Summarizing, high actionable genotypes (with higher OR, as *LMNA*tv, or double pathogenic variants) may be per se the major determinants of disease manifestation/prognosis, while strong interfering environmental factors (e.g., chemotherapy) play a major role especially in cases with less actionable genotype.

Future perspectives in genetics will further investigate these aspects.

References

1. McNally EM, Mestroni L. Dilated cardiomyopathy: genetic determinants and mechanisms. Circ Res. 2017;121(7):731–48.
2. Dalakas MC, Park KY, Semino-Mora C, Lee HS, Sivakumar K, Goldfarb LG. Desmin myopathy, a skeletal myopathy with cardiomyopathy caused by mutations in the desmin gene. N Engl J Med. 2000;342(11):770–80.

3. Li D, Tapscoft T, Gonzalez O, Burch PE, Quinones MA, Zoghbi WA, et al. Desmin mutation responsible for idiopathic dilated cardiomyopathy. Circulation. 1999;100(5):461–4.
4. Taylor MR, Slavov D, Ku L, Di Lenarda A, Sinagra G, Carniel E, et al. Prevalence of desmin mutations in dilated cardiomyopathy. Circulation. 2007;115(10):1244–51.
5. Jefferies JL, Eidem BW, Belmont JW, Craigen WJ, Ware SM, Fernbach SD, et al. Genetic predictors and remodeling of dilated cardiomyopathy in muscular dystrophy. Circulation. 2005;112(18):2799–804.
6. Lapidos KA, Kakkar R, McNally EM. The dystrophin glycoprotein complex: signaling strength and integrity for the sarcolemma. Circ Res. 2004;94(8):1023–31.
7. Melacini P, Fanin M, Danieli GA, Villanova C, Martinello F, Miorin M, et al. Myocardial involvement is very frequent among patients affected with subclinical Becker's muscular dystrophy. Circulation. 1996;94(12):3168–75.
8. Politano L, Nigro V, Nigro G, Petretta VR, Passamano L, Papparella S, et al. Development of cardiomyopathy in female carriers of Duchenne and Becker muscular dystrophies. JAMA. 1996;275(17):1335–8.
9. Olson TM, Illenberger S, Kishimoto NY, Huttelmaier S, Keating MT, Jockusch BM. Metavinculin mutations alter actin interaction in dilated cardiomyopathy. Circulation. 2002;105(4):431–7.
10. Wells QS, Ausborn NL, Funke BH, Pfotenhauer JP, Fredi JL, Baxter S, et al. Familial dilated cardiomyopathy associated with congenital defects in the setting of a novel VCL mutation (Lys815Arg) in conjunction with a known MYPBC3 variant. Cardiogenetics. 2011;1(1). pii: e10.
11. Walsh R, Thomson KL, Ware JS, Funke BH, Woodley J, McGuire KJ, et al. Reassessment of Mendelian gene pathogenicity using 7,855 cardiomyopathy cases and 60,706 reference samples. Genet Med. 2017;19(2):192–203.
12. Vatta M, Mohapatra B, Jimenez S, Sanchez X, Faulkner G, Perles Z, et al. Mutations in Cypher/ZASP in patients with dilated cardiomyopathy and left ventricular non-compaction. J Am Coll Cardiol. 2003;42(11):2014–27.
13. Elliott P, O'Mahony C, Syrris P, Evans A, Rivera Sorensen C, Sheppard MN, et al. Prevalence of desmosomal protein gene mutations in patients with dilated cardiomyopathy. Circ Cardiovasc Genet. 2010;3(4):314–22.
14. Delmar M, McKenna WJ. The cardiac desmosome and arrhythmogenic cardiomyopathies: from gene to disease. Circ Res. 2010;107(6):700–14.
15. Corrado D, Basso C, Pilichou K, Thiene G. Molecular biology and clinical management of arrhythmogenic right ventricular cardiomyopathy/dysplasia. Heart. 2011;97(7):530–9.
16. Hershberger RE, Hedges DJ, Morales A. Dilated cardiomyopathy: the complexity of a diverse genetic architecture. Nat Rev Cardiol. 2013;10(9):531–47.
17. Garcia-Giustiniani D, Arad M, Ortiz-Genga M, Barriales-Villa R, Fernandez X, Rodriguez-Garcia I, et al. Phenotype and prognostic correlations of the converter region mutations affecting the beta myosin heavy chain. Heart. 2015;101(13):1047–53.
18. Merlo M, Sinagra G, Carniel E, Slavov D, Zhu X, Barbati G, et al. Poor prognosis of rare sarcomeric gene variants in patients with dilated cardiomyopathy. Clin Transl Sci. 2013;6(6):424–8.
19. Campbell N, Sinagra G, Jones KL, Slavov D, Gowan K, Merlo M, et al. Whole exome sequencing identifies a troponin T mutation hot spot in familial dilated cardiomyopathy. PLoS One. 2013;8(10):e78104.
20. Marjamaa A, Laitinen-Forsblom P, Lahtinen AM, Viitasalo M, Toivonen L, Kontula K, et al. Search for cardiac calcium cycling gene mutations in familial ventricular arrhythmias resembling catecholaminergic polymorphic ventricular tachycardia. BMC Med Genet. 2009;10:12.
21. McNair WP, Sinagra G, Taylor MR, Di Lenarda A, Ferguson DA, Salcedo EE, et al. SCN5A mutations associate with arrhythmic dilated cardiomyopathy and commonly localize to the voltage-sensing mechanism. J Am Coll Cardiol. 2011;57(21):2160–8.
22. Schweizer PA, Koenen M, Katus HA, Thomas D. A distinct cardiomyopathy: HCN4 syndrome comprising myocardial noncompaction, bradycardia, mitral valve defects, and aortic dilation. J Am Coll Cardiol. 2017;69(9):1209–10.

23. van der Zwaag PA, van Rijsingen IA, Asimaki A, Jongbloed JD, van Veldhuisen DJ, Wiesfeld AC, et al. Phospholamban R14del mutation in patients diagnosed with dilated cardiomyopathy or arrhythmogenic right ventricular cardiomyopathy: evidence supporting the concept of arrhythmogenic cardiomyopathy. Eur J Heart Fail. 2012;14(11):1199–207.
24. Knezevic T, Myers VD, Gordon J, Tilley DG, Sharp TE III, Wang J, et al. BAG3: a new player in the heart failure paradigm. Heart Fail Rev. 2015;20(4):423–34.
25. Norton N, Li D, Rieder MJ, Siegfried JD, Rampersaud E, Zuchner S, et al. Genome-wide studies of copy number variation and exome sequencing identify rare variants in BAG3 as a cause of dilated cardiomyopathy. Am J Hum Genet. 2011;88(3):273–82.
26. Brauch KM, Karst ML, Herron KJ, de Andrade M, Pellikka PA, Rodeheffer RJ, et al. Mutations in ribonucleic acid binding protein gene cause familial dilated cardiomyopathy. J Am Coll Cardiol. 2009;54(10):930–41.
27. Maatz H, Jens M, Liss M, Schafer S, Heinig M, Kirchner M, et al. RNA-binding protein RBM20 represses splicing to orchestrate cardiac pre-mRNA processing. J Clin Invest. 2014;124(8):3419–30.
28. Djemie T, Weckhuysen S, von Spiczak S, Carvill GL, Jaehn J, Anttonen AK, et al. Pitfalls in genetic testing: the story of missed SCN1A mutations. Mol Genet Genomic Med. 2016;4(4):457–64.
29. Consugar MB, Navarro-Gomez D, Place EM, Bujakowska KM, Sousa ME, Fonseca-Kelly ZD, et al. Panel-based genetic diagnostic testing for inherited eye diseases is highly accurate and reproducible, and more sensitive for variant detection, than exome sequencing. Genet Med. 2015;17(4):253–61.
30. Rothberg JM, Hinz W, Rearick TM, Schultz J, Mileski W, Davey M, et al. An integrated semiconductor device enabling non-optical genome sequencing. Nature. 2011;475(7356):348–52.
31. Gullapalli RR, Desai KV, Santana-Santos L, Kant JA, Becich MJ. Next generation sequencing in clinical medicine: challenges and lessons for pathology and biomedical informatics. J Pathol Inform. 2012;3:40.
32. McPherson JD, Marra M, Hillier L, Waterston RH, Chinwalla A, Wallis J, et al. A physical map of the human genome. Nature. 2001;409(6822):934–41.
33. Richards S, Aziz N, Bale S, Bick D, Das S, Gastier-Foster J, et al. Standards and guidelines for the interpretation of sequence variants: a joint consensus recommendation of the American College of Medical Genetics and Genomics and the Association for Molecular Pathology. Genet Med. 2015;17(5):405–24.
34. Landrum MJ, Lee JM, Benson M, Brown G, Chao C, Chitipiralla S, et al. ClinVar: public archive of interpretations of clinically relevant variants. Nucleic Acids Res. 2016;44(D1):D862–8.
35. Stenson PD, Ball EV, Mort M, Phillips AD, Shiel JA, Thomas NS, et al. Human Gene Mutation Database (HGMD): 2003 update. Hum Mutat. 2003;21(6):577–81.
36. Merlo M, Anzini M, Bussani R, Artico J, Barbati G, Stolfo D, et al. Characterization and long-term prognosis of postmyocarditic dilated cardiomyopathy compared with idiopathic dilated cardiomyopathy. Am J Cardiol. 2016;118(6):895–900.
37. Belkaya S, Kontorovich AR, Byun M, Mulero-Navarro S, Bajolle F, Cobat A, et al. Autosomal recessive cardiomyopathy presenting as acute myocarditis. J Am Coll Cardiol. 2017;69(13):1653–65.
38. Frantz S, Falcao-Pires I, Balligand JL, Bauersachs J, Brutsaert D, Ciccarelli M, et al. The innate immune system in chronic cardiomyopathy: a European Society of Cardiology (ESC) scientific statement from the Working Group on Myocardial Function of the ESC. Eur J Heart Fail. 2018;20(3):445–59.
39. Guzzo-Merello G, Cobo-Marcos M, Gallego-Delgado M, Garcia-Pavia P. Alcoholic cardiomyopathy. World J Cardiol. 2014;6(8):771–81.
40. Marichalar-Mendia X, Rodriguez-Tojo MJ, Acha-Sagredo A, Rey-Barja N, Aguirre-Urizar JM. Oral cancer and polymorphism of ethanol metabolising genes. Oral Oncol. 2010;46(1):9–13.
41. Renu K, V GA PBT, Arunachalam S. Molecular mechanism of doxorubicin-induced cardiomyopathy - An update. Eur J Pharmacol. 2018;818:241–53.

42. Ware JS, Amor-Salamanca A, Tayal U, Govind R, Serrano I, Salazar-Mendiguchia J, et al. Genetic etiology for alcohol-induced cardiac toxicity. J Am Coll Cardiol. 2018;71(20):2293–302.
43. European Society of Gynecology, Association for European Paediatric Cardiology, German Society for Gender Medicine, Regitz-Zagrosek V, Blomstrom Lundqvist C, Borghi C, et al. ESC Guidelines on the management of cardiovascular diseases during pregnancy: the Task Force on the Management of Cardiovascular Diseases during Pregnancy of the European Society of Cardiology (ESC). Eur Heart J. 2011;32(24):3147–97.
44. Hilfiker-Kleiner D, Haghikia A, Berliner D, Vogel-Claussen J, Schwab J, Franke A, et al. Bromocriptine for the treatment of peripartum cardiomyopathy: a multicentre randomized study. Eur Heart J. 2017;38(35):2671–9.
45. Merlo M, Pyxaras SA, Pinamonti B, Barbati G, Di Lenarda A, Sinagra G. Prevalence and prognostic significance of left ventricular reverse remodeling in dilated cardiomyopathy receiving tailored medical treatment. J Am Coll Cardiol. 2011;57(13):1468–76.
46. Ernande L, Derumeaux G. Diabetic cardiomyopathy: myth or reality? Arch Cardiovasc Dis. 2012;105(4):218–25.
47. Florwick A, Dharmaraj T, Jurgens J, Valle D, Wilson KL. LMNA sequences of 60,706 unrelated individuals reveal 132 novel missense variants in A-type lamins and suggest a link between variant p.G602S and type 2 diabetes. Front Genet. 2017;8:79.
48. Schafer S, de Marvao A, Adami E, Fiedler LR, Ng B, Khin E, et al. Titin-truncating variants affect heart function in disease cohorts and the general population. Nat Genet. 2017;49(1):46–53.
49. Dal Ferro M, Stolfo D, Altinier A, Gigli M, Perrieri M, Ramani F, et al. Association between mutation status and left ventricular reverse remodelling in dilated cardiomyopathy. Heart. 2017;103(21):1704–10.
50. Rivas MA, Pirinen M, Conrad DF, Lek M, Tsang EK, Karczewski KJ, et al. Human genomics. Effect of predicted protein-truncating genetic variants on the human transcriptome. Science. 2015;348(6235):666–9.
51. Merlo M, Cannata A, Gobbo M, Stolfo D, Elliott PM, Sinagra G. Evolving concepts in dilated cardiomyopathy. Eur J Heart Fail. 2018;20(2):228–39.
52. van Rijsingen IA, Nannenberg EA, Arbustini E, Elliott PM, Mogensen J, Hermans-van Ast JF, et al. Gender-specific differences in major cardiac events and mortality in lamin A/C mutation carriers. Eur J Heart Fail. 2013;15(4):376–84.
53. Kumar S, Baldinger SH, Gandjbakhch E, Maury P, Sellal JM, Androulakis AF, et al. Long-term arrhythmic and nonarrhythmic outcomes of lamin A/C mutation carriers. J Am Coll Cardiol. 2016;68(21):2299–307.
54. Taylor MR, Fain PR, Sinagra G, Robinson ML, Robertson AD, Carniel E, et al. Natural history of dilated cardiomyopathy due to lamin A/C gene mutations. J Am Coll Cardiol. 2003;41(5):771–80.
55. Priori SG, Blomstrom-Lundqvist C, Mazzanti A, Blom N, Borggrefe M, Camm J, et al. 2015 ESC Guidelines for the management of patients with ventricular arrhythmias and the prevention of sudden cardiac death: The Task Force for the Management of Patients with Ventricular Arrhythmias and the Prevention of Sudden Cardiac Death of the European Society of Cardiology (ESC). Endorsed by: Association for European Paediatric and Congenital Cardiology (AEPC). Eur Heart J. 2015;36(41):2793–867.
56. Nishiuchi S, Makiyama T, Aiba T, Nakajima K, Hirose S, Kohjitani H, et al. Gene-based risk stratification for cardiac disorders in LMNA mutation carriers. Circ Cardiovasc Genet. 2017;10(6). pii: e001603.
57. Herman DS, Lam L, Taylor MR, Wang L, Teekakirikul P, Christodoulou D, et al. Truncations of titin causing dilated cardiomyopathy. N Engl J Med. 2012;366(7):619–28.
58. Roberts AM, Ware JS, Herman DS, Schafer S, Baksi J, Bick AG, et al. Integrated allelic, transcriptional, and phenomic dissection of the cardiac effects of titin truncations in health and disease. Sci Transl Med. 2015;7(270):270ra6.

59. Jansweijer JA, Nieuwhof K, Russo F, Hoorntje ET, Jongbloed JD, Lekanne Deprez RH, et al. Truncating titin mutations are associated with a mild and treatable form of dilated cardiomyopathy. Eur J Heart Fail. 2017;19(4):512–21.
60. Verdonschot JAJ, Hazebroek MR, Derks KWJ, Barandiaran Aizpurua A, Merken JJ, Wang P, et al. Titin cardiomyopathy leads to altered mitochondrial energetics, increased fibrosis and long-term life-threatening arrhythmias. Eur Heart J. 2018;39(10):864–73.
61. Begay RL, Graw S, Sinagra G, Merlo M, Slavov D, Gowan K, et al. Role of titin missense variants in dilated cardiomyopathy. J Am Heart Assoc. 2015;4(11). pii: e002645.
62. Hastings R, de Villiers CP, Hooper C, Ormondroyd L, Pagnamenta A, Lise S, et al. Combination of whole genome sequencing, linkage, and functional studies implicates a missense mutation in titin as a cause of autosomal dominant cardiomyopathy with features of left ventricular noncompaction. Circ Cardiovasc Genet. 2016;9(5):426–35.
63. Begay RL, Tharp CA, Martin A, Graw SL, Sinagra G, Miani D, et al. FLNC gene splice mutations cause dilated cardiomyopathy. JACC Basic Transl Sci. 2016;1(5):344–59.
64. Ortiz-Genga MF, Cuenca S, Dal Ferro M, Zorio E, Salgado-Aranda R, Climent V, et al. Truncating FLNC mutations are associated with high-risk dilated and arrhythmogenic cardiomyopathies. J Am Coll Cardiol. 2016;68(22):2440–51.
65. Valdes-Mas R, Gutierrez-Fernandez A, Gomez J, Coto E, Astudillo A, Puente DA, et al. Mutations in filamin C cause a new form of familial hypertrophic cardiomyopathy. Nat Commun. 2014;5:5326.

6

Clinical Presentation, Spectrum of Disease, and Natural History

Marco Merlo, Davide Stolfo, Thomas Caiffa, Alberto Pivetta, and Gianfranco Sinagra

Abbreviations and Acronyms

CMR	Cardiac magnetic resonance
CRT	Cardiac resynchronization therapy
DCM	Dilated cardiomyopathy
EMB	Endomyocardial biopsy
HF	Heart failure
KM	Kaplan-Meier
LBBB	Left bundle branch block
LGE	Late gadolinium enhancement
LV	Left ventricular
LVEF	Left ventricular ejection fraction
LVRR	Left ventricular reverse remodeling
RV	Right ventricular
SCD	Sudden cardiac death

M. Merlo (✉) · G. Sinagra
Cardiovascular Department, Azienda Sanitaria Universitaria Integrata, Trieste, Italy
e-mail: gianfranco.sinagra@asuits.sanita.fvg.it

D. Stolfo · T. Caiffa · A. Pivetta
Cardiovascular Department, Azienda Sanitaria Universitaria Integrata, University of Trieste (ASUITS), Trieste, Italy
e-mail: Davide.stolfo@asuits.sanita.fvg.it

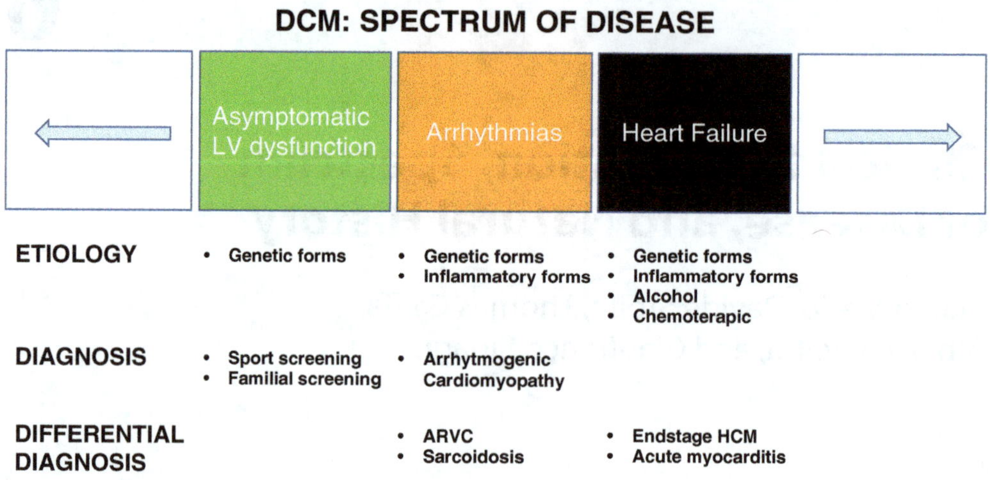

Fig. 6.1 Dilated cardiomyopathy: spectrum of disease

6.1 Spectrum of Disease

Before diagnosing dilated cardiomyopathy (DCM), it is necessary to exclude conditions with phenotypic overlap. A comprehensive integrated approach to patients with a newly diagnosed DCM is essential in order to achieve an accurate early prognostic stratification.

In many DCM individuals, there is a preclinical phase without cardiac expression that subsequently progresses toward mild cardiac abnormalities, such as isolated left ventricular (LV) dilatation, subtle systolic dysfunction, or arrhythmogenic features (ventricular or supraventricular arrhythmia or conduction defects) that can be observed in myocarditis [1, 2] or in the early phase of genetic diseases [3]. The overt phase of systolic dysfunction is usually associated with LV dilatation, but this may be absent in some cases causing diagnostic confusion (described in Lamin A/C gene mutation carriers [4, 5] and also in some patients without a known genetic cause [6–8] (Fig. 6.1).

Thus, in this context every effort has to be made to obtain an accurate diagnosis (cardiac magnetic resonance (CMR), endomyocardial biopsy (EMB), biomarkers, etc.), with the aim to personalize patient management according to specific etiology.

The prognosis of DCM has improved in the course of the past years [9] with the use of evidence-based therapies, both pharmacological and non-pharmacological [10–12], and also due to the constant effort to diagnose this cardiomyopathy in the early stages (Figs. 6.2, 6.3, and 6.4) [13]. Identifying patients with DCM in an asymptomatic phase is equivalent to early diagnosis and guarantees a better long-term survival for the patients [14].

Fig. 6.2 Cause specific KM: survival free from all-cause mortality/heart transplant in IDCM patients according to the decade of enrolment. From Merlo et al., Long-term prognostic impact of therapeutic strategies in patients with idiopathic dilated cardiomyopathy: changing mortality over the last 30 years, Eur J Heart Fail, 2014; 16(3):317–24

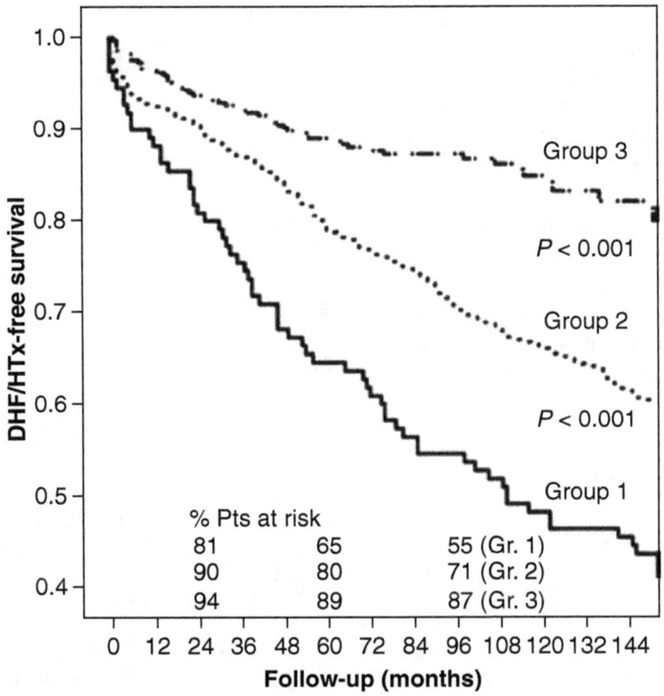

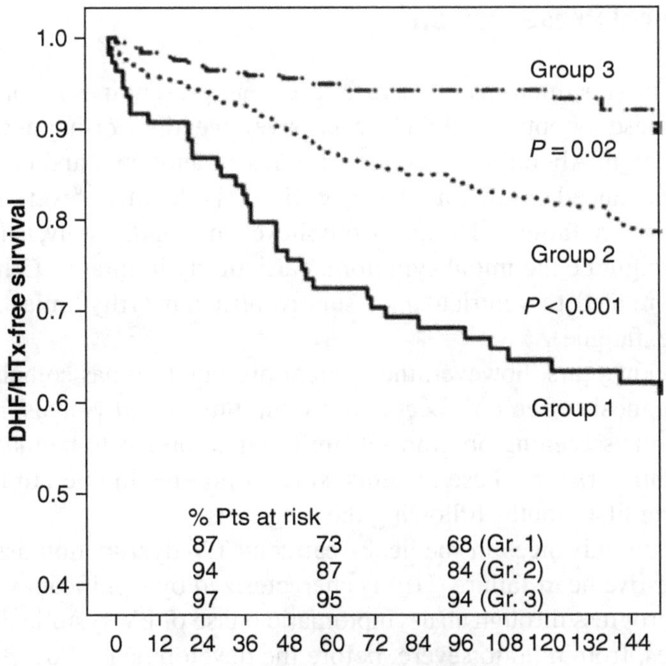

Fig. 6.3 Cause-specific KM curves: survival free from pump failure death/heart transplant in IDCM patients according to the decade of enrolment. From Merlo et al., Long-term prognostic impact of therapeutic strategies in patients with idiopathic dilated cardiomyopathy: changing mortality over the last 30 years, Eur J Heart Fail, 2014; 16(3):317–24

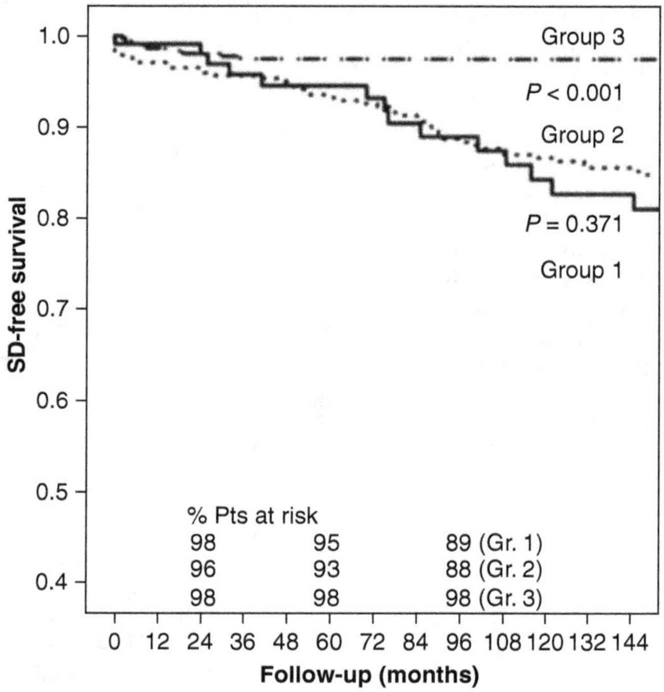

Fig. 6.4 Cause-specific KM curves: survival free from sudden death in IDCM patients according to the decade of enrolment. From Merlo et al., Long-term prognostic impact of therapeutic strategies in patients with idiopathic dilated cardiomyopathy: changing mortality over the last 30 years, Eur J Heart Fail, 2014; 16(3):317–24

6.2 Clinical Presentation

In old series, initial symptoms of heart failure were present in 80% of patients with DCM [15]. These symptoms include excessive sweating, orthopnea, and fatigue after mild exertion. Abdominal discomfort, nausea, anorexia, and cachexia can be prominent in advanced cases. Circulatory collapse is the most severe manifestation of congestive heart failure. Thromboembolic events and, rarely, sudden cardiac death (SCD) might be the initial symptom, particularly in infants. Other symptoms include those related to ventricular or supraventricular arrhythmias (i.e., palpitations, syncope, fatigue).

In more recent years, however, the clinical presentation has somehow changed. In fact, the diagnosis often now occurs in asymptomatic individuals, mostly due to family and sports screening programs. Careful attention has to be made in evaluating the arrhythmic risk of these patients, since a non-negligible number of events can occur in the first months following the diagnosis.

Despite recent advances in medical treatment, LV dysfunction associated with signs of congestive heart failure (HF) is characterized by significant mortality [16]. Patients may progress through an asymptomatic phase of LV systolic dysfunction of various degrees, from mild to severe, before the development of overt HF [17–19]. LV dysfunction has frequently a progressive nature, and that is the reason for increasing interest regarding its preclinical state.

Most patients affected by DCM who present clinically with HF show symptoms and signs due to excess fluid accumulation (dyspnea, orthopnea, edema, pain from hepatic congestion, and abdominal discomfort due to ascites), sometimes associated with those due to a reduction in cardiac output (fatigue, weakness) [20].

In most patients with HF who require hospitalization, the reason for admission is volume overload. In clinical practice, four signs are commonly used to predict elevated filling pressures: jugular venous distention/abdominojugular reflux, presence of an S3 and/or S4, rales, and pedal edema. According to current international guidelines on HF [21, 22], the patient with HF can be clinically assessed along two basic axes—volume status ("dry" or "wet") and perfusion status ("warm" or "cold")—as a useful guide to therapy.

This approach has prognostic usefulness, particularly in assessing patients at discharge after admission for heart failure. For example, such patients discharged with a "wet" or "cold" profile experience worse outcomes (HR, 1.5; 95% CI, 1.1–12.1; $P = 0.017$) compared with those discharged "warm and dry" (HR 0.9; 95% CI, 0.7–2.1; $P = 0.5$) [23].

In chronic presentations (months), symptoms as peripheral edema, abdominal distension, and anorexia may be more pronounced than dyspnea.

On the other hand, a decompensated chronic HF can lead to low-output symptoms.

Four major findings suggest severity of the cardiac dysfunction and low output: resting sinus tachycardia, narrow pulse pressure, diaphoresis, and peripheral vasoconstriction.

An irregularly irregular pulse is suggestive of atrial fibrillation which frequently accompanies HF. Pulsus alternans is a sign of severe left ventricular (LV) systolic failure. This phenomenon is characterized by evenly spaced alternating strong and weak peripheral pulses.

A laterally displaced apical impulse that is past the midclavicular line is usually indicative of LV enlargement.

An S3 gallop is associated with left atrial pressures exceeding 20 mmHg and increased LV end-diastolic pressures (>15 mmHg).

An apical systolic murmur is associated with mitral regurgitation, often present in these patients.

Patients with chronic HF often develop secondary pulmonary hypertension, which can contribute to dyspnea as pulmonary pressures rise with exertion. These patients may also complain of substernal chest pressure, typical of angina. In this setting, elevated right ventricular end-diastolic pressure leads to secondary right ventricular subendocardial ischemia. Physical signs of pulmonary hypertension can include increased intensity of P2, a murmur of pulmonary insufficiency, a parasternal lift, and a palpable pulmonic tap (felt in the left second intercostal space) [20].

In patients with arrhythmic presentation, the onset of the disease may be the presence of palpitations, syncopal or near-syncopal episodes, or in some of them SCD. Thus, arrhythmic risk stratification is a major concern, as discussed in the following chapters.

6.3 Natural History

In the past, the prognosis of DCM was considered ominous [24], and the disease was frequently progressive to death due to HF or heart transplantation.

By time the patients are diagnosed, they often have severe contractile dysfunction and remodeling of the ventricles, reflecting a long period of asymptomatic silent disease progression.

However, implementation of optimal pharmacological and non-pharmacological treatments has dramatically improved the prognosis of DCM [25] with an estimated survival free from death or heart transplantation up to 85% at 10 years [13, 26, 27] (Table 6.1).

Table 6.1 Occurrence of major events in patients with DCM according to the decade of enrolment

	First decade (1978–1987) (110 patients)	Second decade (1988–1997) (376 patients)	Third decade (1998–2007) (367 patients)	*P*-value		
				First vs. second decade	first vs. third decade	second vs. third decade
Mean follow-up (months)	151 ± 29	153 ± 82	93 ± 41	0.389	**0.03**	**<0.001**
All-cause mortality/ heart transplant, *n* (%)	77 (70)	178 (47)	53 (14)	**<0.001**	**<0.001**	**<0.001**
Incidence (events/100 patients/year)	5.6	3.9	1.9			
Heart transplant, *n* (%)	6 (6)	51 (14)	17 (5)	**0.02**	0.724	**<0.001**
Incidence (events/100 patients/year)	0.4	1.1	0.6			
Cardiovascular death, *n* (%)	57 (52)	91 (24)	18 (5)	**<0.001**	**<0.001**	**<0.001**
Incidence (events/100 patients/year)	4.1	2.0	0.6			
Pump-failure death, *n* (%)	38 (35)	32 (9)	6 (2)	**<0.001**	**<0.001**	**<0.001**
Incidence (events/100 patients/year)	2.8	0.7	0.2			
Unexpected sudden death, *n* (%)	16 (15)	51 (14)	9 (3)	0.793	**<0.001**	**<0.001**
Incidence (events/100 patients/year)	1.2	1.1	0.3			
Unknown cause death, *n* (%)	13 (12)	31 (9)	16 (4)	0.338	**0.004**	**0.014**
Incidence (events/100 patients/year)	1.0	0.7	0.6			
Appropriate intervention of ICD (% of Implanted patients)	0	32	38	NC*	NC*	0.499
Incidence (events/100 implanted patients/ year)	NC	2.4	4.8			

From Merlo et al., Long-term prognostic impact of therapeutic strategies in patients with idiopathic dilated cardiomyopathy: changing mortality over the last 30 years, Eur J Heart Fail, 2014; 16(3):317–24

P-value <0.05 are in bold type

ICD Implanted cardioverter–defibrillator, *NC* not calculable

*P-value not calculated; only two patients implanted with ICD in the first decade

Moreover, the lower prevalence of comorbidities when compared to most patients with other forms of systolic LV dysfunction suggests that individuals with DCM tend to have fewer non-cardiovascular events [25]. In hypertensive heart disease, for example, there is a lower incidence of arrhythmic events and a greater competitive risk of non-cardiovascular events [28].

The improved outcomes in DCM are paralleled by a higher rate of LV reverse remodeling (LVRR): in recent years several studies revealed that almost 40% of patients experience a significant LVRR when treated with evidence-based pharmacological and device treatments [26].

From a pure mechanistic standpoint, LVRR is the result of either the removal of the noxious stimuli that triggered cardiac dysfunction or of the institution of therapies favorably interfering with the process of LV remodeling. Factors recognized to trigger or amplify LV remodeling include changes in myocardial wall tension and neurohormonal activation. Initially a compensatory process, the release of hypovolemic hormones (such as renin, antidiuretic hormone, and norepinephrine) eventually contributes to the progression of DCM, and pharmacologic therapies that reduce neurohormonal activation have been shown to promote LVRR [29].

The process of LVRR may take up to 2 years following diagnosis. The following aspects, evaluated at baseline and during follow-up, have been demonstrated as influencing the course and the prognosis of the disease and the likelihood of LVRR in the early stages and should be hence systematically assessed:

(a) Right ventricular function at diagnosis is an important prognostic feature in DCM [30]. The recovery of right ventricular function under therapy is frequent and can already be observed at 6 months. It precedes LVRR and is emerging as an early therapeutic target and an independent prognostic predictor [31]. Improvement in right ventricular function is also described in CRT recipients as a secondary expression of hemodynamic improvement very early after resynchronization, with consequently favorable survival rates [32]. In contrast, the development of right ventricular dysfunction during long-term follow-up is an expression of structural progression of the disease and portends a negative outcome [31].
(b) Functional mitral regurgitation conveys important prognostic implications. Moderate to severe mitral regurgitation at diagnosis or persistent despite optimal medical treatment or CRT is associated with poorer outcomes [32, 33]. Patients with DCM and hemodynamically important mitral regurgitation may require invasive therapeutic strategies such as percutaneous repair of the mitral valve, mechanical circulatory support, or even heart transplantation.
(c) Left bundle branch block (LBBB) is a frequent ECG marker at diagnosis and is negatively associated with the likelihood of LVRR [26]. Importantly the development of new LBBB during follow-up is a strong independent prognostic predictor of all-cause mortality [34].

(d) The onset of atrial fibrillation during the follow-up is a sign of structural progression of the disease and negatively impacts on the prognosis of these patients, despite effective treatments [35].
(e) In patients with DCM, the persistence of restrictive filing at 3 months after presentation is associated with a high mortality and transplantation rate. On the other hand, patients with reversible restrictive filling have a high probability of improvement and excellent survival. Thus, reassessment of these patients after 3 months of therapy gives additional prognostic information with respect to the initial evaluation [36].

The implications of these observations are that a multi-parametric approach to diagnosis and long-term follow-up, not limited to the LV systolic function and size alone, appear essential in order to improve the quality of clinical management of DCM patients [37].

In spite of this therapeutic success, emerging evidence suggests that some patients remain vulnerable to SCD and refractory HF requiring heart transplant or mechanical circulatory support [26].

Thus, the outcome of patients with DCM often remains unpredictable, and major adverse events may occur in the first months following the diagnosis [7, 38].

Furthermore, even when there is improvement in LV dysfunction, the potential for later decline in systolic function remains, despite uninterrupted treatment [37].

Sometimes LVRR is pronounced enough to result in a normalization of both LVEF and LV diameters, in a process that has been referred to as "apparent healing" or "myocardial remission" [39]. Nevertheless, in a retrospective observational study, only about 10% of DCM patients showed persistent apparent healing at long term (10 years), but the vast majority of them experienced a recurrence of LV dysfunction in a very long term, thus suggesting that the observed healing was only apparent and that true myocardial recovery is at most a rare event in DCM patients [40, 41].

This last issue emphasizes the pivotal role not only of an accurate and complete initial diagnostic evaluation but also of continuous and tailored, modulated therapy and individualized, long-term accurate surveillance in order to recognize and treat the first signs of late disease progression (Fig. 6.5).

Modern management of HF has increased the survival rates of DCM and has resulted in long periods of clinical stability [25, 42]. Consequently, affected patients followed for beyond 10–15 years are often encountered in clinical practice.

It has to be noted, in addition, that the patients should be continuously and critically reassessed, particularly in the presence of cardiovascular risk factors. Indeed, abrupt worsening of LV function or an increased ventricular arrhythmic burden can be caused not only by the DCM progression but also by the development of new co-pathologies. Therefore, the possible presence of coronary artery disease, hypertensive heart disease, structured valve disease, or an acute myocarditis should be systematically ruled out during the follow-up [37].

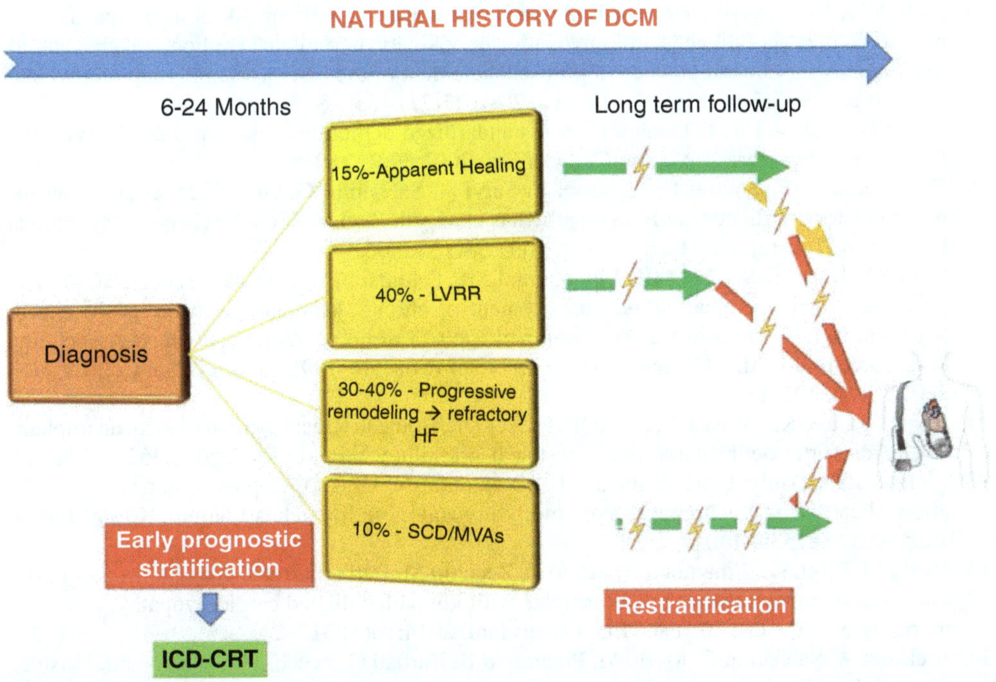

Fig. 6.5 Natural history of dilated cardiomyopathy. Early prognostic stratification and continuous restratification during long-term follow-up are fundamental in order to better identify those at higher risk of sudden cardiac death (arrow)

References

1. Caforio ALP, Pankuweit S, Arbustini E, Basso C, Gimeno-Blanes J, Felix SB, et al. Current state of knowledge on aetiology, diagnosis, management, and therapy of myocarditis: a position statement of the European Society of Cardiology Working Group on Myocardial and Pericardial Diseases. Eur Heart J. 2013;34(33):2636–48, 2648a–d.
2. Schultheiss H-P, Kuhl U, Cooper LT. The management of myocarditis. Eur Heart J. 2011;32(21):2616–25.
3. van Berlo JH, de Voogt WG, van der Kooi AJ, van Tintelen JP, Bonne G, Ben YR, et al. Meta-analysis of clinical characteristics of 299 carriers of LMNA gene mutations: do lamin A/C mutations portend a high risk of sudden death? J Mol Med (Berl). 2005;83(1):79–83.
4. van Tintelen JP, Tio RA, Kerstjens-Frederikse WS, van Berlo JH, Boven LG, Suurmeijer AJH, et al. Severe myocardial fibrosis caused by a deletion of the 5′ end of the lamin A/C gene. J Am Coll Cardiol. 2007;49(25):2430–9.
5. Sanna T, Dello Russo A, Toniolo D, Vytopil M, Pelargonio G, De Martino G, et al. Cardiac features of Emery-Dreifuss muscular dystrophy caused by lamin A/C gene mutations. Eur Heart J. 2003;24(24):2227–36.
6. Keren A, Gottlieb S, Tzivoni D, Stern S, Yarom R, Billingham ME, et al. Mildly dilated congestive cardiomyopathy. Use of prospective diagnostic criteria and description of the clinical course without heart transplantation. Circulation. 1990;81(2):506–17.

7. Pinto YM, Elliott PM, Arbustini E, Adler Y, Anastasakis A, Bohm M, et al. Proposal for a revised definition of dilated cardiomyopathy, hypokinetic non-dilated cardiomyopathy, and its implications for clinical practice: a position statement of the ESC working group on myocardial and pericardial diseases. Eur Heart J. 2016;37(23):1850–8.
8. Felker GM, Shaw LK, O'Connor CM. A standardized definition of ischemic cardiomyopathy for use in clinical research. J Am Coll Cardiol. 2002;39(2):210–8.
9. Di Lenarda A, Pinamonti B, Mestroni L, Salvi A, Sabbadini G, Gregori D, et al. [How the natural history of dilated cardiomyopathy has changed. Review of the Registry of Myocardial Diseases of Trieste]. Ital Heart J Suppl. 2004;5(4):253–66.
10. Hunt SA, Baker DW, Chin MH, Cinquegrani MP, Feldman AM, Francis GS, et al. ACC/AHA guidelines for the evaluation and management of chronic heart failure in the adult: executive summary. A report of the American College of Cardiology/American Heart Association Task Force on Practice Guidelines (Committee to revise the 1995 Guide). J Am Coll Cardiol. 2001;38(7):2101–13.
11. Bardy GH, Lee KL, Mark DB, Poole JE, Packer DL, Boineau R, et al. Amiodarone or an implantable cardioverter-defibrillator for congestive heart failure. N Engl J Med. 2005;352(3):225–37.
12. Cleland JGF, Daubert J-C, Erdmann E, Freemantle N, Gras D, Kappenberger L, et al. The effect of cardiac resynchronization on morbidity and mortality in heart failure. N Engl J Med. 2005;352(15):1539–49.
13. Merlo M, Pivetta A, Pinamonti B, Stolfo D, Zecchin M, Barbati G, et al. Long-term prognostic impact of therapeutic strategies in patients with idiopathic dilated cardiomyopathy: changing mortality over the last 30 years. Eur J Heart Fail. 2014;16(3):317–24.
14. Aleksova A, Sabbadini G, Merlo M, Pinamonti B, Barbati G, Zecchin M, et al. Natural history of dilated cardiomyopathy: from asymptomatic left ventricular dysfunction to heart failure–a subgroup analysis from the Trieste Cardiomyopathy Registry. J Cardiovasc Med (Hagerstown). 2009;10(9):699–705.
15. Dec GW, Fuster V. Idiopathic dilated cardiomyopathy. N Engl J Med. 1994;331(23):1564–75.
16. Levy D, Kenchaiah S, Larson MG, Benjamin EJ, Kupka MJ, Ho KKL, et al. Long-term trends in the incidence of and survival with heart failure. N Engl J Med. 2002;347(18):1397–402.
17. Pfeffer MA, Braunwald E. Ventricular remodeling after myocardial infarction. Experimental observations and clinical implications. Circulation. 1990;81(4):1161–72.
18. Mann DL. Mechanisms and models in heart failure: a combinatorial approach. Circulation. 1999;100(9):999–1008.
19. McMurray JV, McDonagh TA, Davie AP, Cleland JG, Francis CM, Morrison C. Should we screen for asymptomatic left ventricular dysfunction to prevent heart failure? Eur Heart J. 1998;19(6):842–6.
20. Colucci WS. Evaluation of the patient with suspected heart failure. https://www.uptodate.com/contents/evaluation-of-the-patient-with-suspected-heart-failure.
21. Ponikowski P, Voors AA, Anker SD, Bueno H, Cleland JGF, Coats AJS, et al. 2016 ESC Guidelines for the diagnosis and treatment of acute and chronic heart failure: The Task Force for the diagnosis and treatment of acute and chronic heart failure of the European Society of Cardiology (ESC) Developed with the special contribution of the Heart Failure Association (HFA) of the ESC. Eur Heart J. 2016;37(27):2129–200.
22. Yancy CW, Jessup M, Bozkurt B, Butler J, Casey DEJ, Colvin MM, et al. 2017 ACC/AHA/HFSA Focused Update of the 2013 ACCF/AHA Guideline for the Management of Heart Failure: A Report of the American College of Cardiology/American Heart Association Task Force on Clinical Practice Guidelines and the Heart Failure Society of America. Circulation. 2017;136(6):e137–61.
23. Chaudhry A, Singer AJ, Chohan J, Russo V, Lee C. Interrater reliability of hemodynamic profiling of patients with heart failure in the ED. Am J Emerg Med. 2008;26(2):196–201.
24. Gavazzi A, Lanzarini L, Cornalba C, Desperati M, Raisaro A, Angoli L, et al. Dilated (congestive) cardiomyopathy. Follow-up study of 137 patients. G Ital Cardiol. 1984;14(7):492–8.

25. Merlo M, Pyxaras SA, Pinamonti B, Barbati G, Di Lenarda A, Sinagra G. Prevalence and prognostic significance of left ventricular reverse remodeling in dilated cardiomyopathy receiving tailored medical treatment. J Am Coll Cardiol. 2011;57(13):1468–76.
26. Zecchin M, Merlo M, Pivetta A, Barbati G, Lutman C, Gregori D, et al. How can optimization of medical treatment avoid unnecessary implantable cardioverter-defibrillator implantations in patients with idiopathic dilated cardiomyopathy presenting with "SCD-HeFT criteria?". Am J Cardiol. 2012;109(5):729–35.
27. Hazebroek MR, Moors S, Dennert R, van den Wijngaard A, Krapels I, Hoos M, et al. Prognostic relevance of gene-environment interactions in patients with dilated cardiomyopathy: applying the MOGE(S) classification. J Am Coll Cardiol. 2015;66(12):1313–23.
28. Bobbo M, Pinamonti B, Merlo M, Stolfo D, Iorio A, Ramani F, et al. Comparison of patient characteristics and course of hypertensive hypokinetic cardiomyopathy versus idiopathic dilated cardiomyopathy. Am J Cardiol. 2017;119(3):483–9.
29. Merlo M, Caiffa T, Gobbo M, Adamo L, Sinagra G. Reverse remodeling in dilated cardiomyopathy: insights and future perspectives. Int J Cardiol Heart Vasc. 2018;18:52–7.
30. Gulati A, Ismail TF, Jabbour A, Alpendurada F, Guha K, Ismail NA, et al. The prevalence and prognostic significance of right ventricular systolic dysfunction in nonischemic dilated cardiomyopathy. Circulation. 2013;128(15):1623–33.
31. Merlo M, Gobbo M, Stolfo D, Losurdo P, Ramani F, Barbati G, et al. The prognostic impact of the evolution of RV function in idiopathic DCM. JACC Cardiovasc Imaging. 2016;9(9):1034–42.
32. Stolfo D, Merlo M, Pinamonti B, Poli S, Gigli M, Barbati G, et al. Early improvement of functional mitral regurgitation in patients with idiopathic dilated cardiomyopathy. Am J Cardiol. 2015;115(8):1137–43.
33. Stolfo D, Tonet E, Barbati G, Gigli M, Pinamonti B, Zecchin M, et al. Acute hemodynamic response to cardiac resynchronization in dilated cardiomyopathy: effect on late mitral regurgitation. Pacing Clin Electrophysiol. 2015;38(11):1287–96.
34. Aleksova A, Carriere C, Zecchin M, Barbati G, Vitrella G, Di Lenarda A, et al. New-onset left bundle branch block independently predicts long-term mortality in patients with idiopathic dilated cardiomyopathy: data from the Trieste Heart Muscle Disease Registry. Eurospace. 2014;16(10):1450–9.
35. Aleksova A, Merlo M, Zecchin M, Sabbadini G, Barbati G, Vitrella G, et al. Impact of atrial fibrillation on outcome of patients with idiopathic dilated cardiomyopathy: data from the Heart Muscle Disease Registry of Trieste. Clin Med Res. 2010;8(3–4):142–9.
36. Pinamonti B, Zecchin M, Di Lenarda A, Gregori D, Sinagra G, Camerini F. Persistence of restrictive left ventricular filling pattern in dilated cardiomyopathy: an ominous prognostic sign. J Am Coll Cardiol. 1997;29(3):604–12.
37. Merlo M, Cannata A, Gobbo M, Stolfo D, Elliott PM, Sinagra G. Evolving concepts in dilated cardiomyopathy. Eur J Heart Fail. 2018;20(2):228–39.
38. Losurdo P, Stolfo D, Merlo M, Barbati G, Gobbo M, Gigli M, et al. Early arrhythmic events in idiopathic dilated cardiomyopathy. JACC Clin Electrophysiol. 2016;2(5):535–43.
39. Mann DL, Barger PM, Burkhoff D. Myocardial recovery and the failing heart: myth, magic, or molecular target? J Am Coll Cardiol. 2012;60(24):2465–72.
40. Merlo M, Stolfo D, Anzini M, Negri F, Pinamonti B, Barbati G, et al. Persistent recovery of normal left ventricular function and dimension in idiopathic dilated cardiomyopathy during long term follow up: does real healing exist? J Am Heart Assoc. 2015;4(1):e001504.
41. Adamo L, Perry A, Novak E, Makan M, Lindman BR, Mann DL. Abnormal global longitudinal strain predicts future deterioration of left ventricular function in heart failure patients with a recovered left ventricular ejection fraction. Circ Heart Fail 2017;10(6). pii: e003788.
42. Japp AG, Gulati A, Cook SA, Cowie MR, Prasad SK. The diagnosis and evaluation of dilated cardiomyopathy. J Am Coll Cardiol. 2016;67(25):2996–3010.

7

Role of Cardiac Imaging: Echocardiography

Bruno Pinamonti, Elena Abate, Antonio De Luca, Gherardo Finocchiaro, and Renata Korcova

Abbreviations and Acronyms

2D	Two-dimensional
3D	Three-dimensional
AC	Arrhythmogenic cardiomyopathy
CFR	Coronary flow reserve
CMR	Cardiac magnetic resonance
CRT	Cardiac resynchronization therapy
CT	Computed tomography
DCM	Dilated cardiomyopathy
DSE	Dobutamine stress echocardiography
EDV	End-diastolic volume
EF	Ejection fraction
EROA	Effective regurgitant orifice area
ESV	End-systolic volume
FAC	Fractional area change

B. Pinamonti (✉) · A. De Luca · R. Korcova
Cardiovascular Department, Azienda Sanitaria Universitaria Integrata, University of Trieste (ASUITS), Trieste, Italy

E. Abate
Cardiovascular Department, Azienda Sanitaria Universitaria Integrata, University of Trieste (ASUITS), Trieste, Italy

Klinik für Innere Medizin 3, Universitätsklinikum Halle (Saale), Halle (Saale), Germany
e-mail: Elena.Abate@uk-halle.de

G. Finocchiaro
Cardiology Clinical and Academic Group, St George's, University of London, London, UK
e-mail: gfinocch@sgul.ac.uk

GLS	Global longitudinal strain
ICD	Implantable cardioverter defibrillator
LA	Left atrial
LBBB	Left bundle branch block
LGE	Late gadolinium enhancement
LV	Left ventricular
LVRR	Left ventricular reverse remodeling
MR	Mitral regurgitation
MV	Mitral valve
NYHA	New York Heart Association
PISA	Proximal isovelocity surface area
PW	Pulsed wave
RV	Right ventricular
RVol	Regurgitant volume
SDI	Systolic dyssynchrony index
STE	Speckle-tracking echocardiography
TAPSE	Tricuspid annular peak systolic excursion
TDI	Tissue Doppler imaging
TR	Tricuspid regurgitation
WMSI	Wall motion score index

7.1 Echocardiographic Features of Dilated Cardiomyopathy

Echocardiography has crucial importance in the diagnosis of dilated cardiomyopathy (DCM). Indeed, it is still considered as the main tool for both diagnosis and follow-up of patients with DCM. Main echocardiographic features of dilated cardiomyopathy (DCM) are summarized in Table 7.1 [1–3]. DCM is defined in the presence of left ventricular (LV) ejection fraction (EF) <45% and LV end-diastolic diameter >2.7 cm/m^2 or >117% predicted value corrected for age and body surface area [1, 3, 4].

The hallmark of the disease is a global LV dilation (Fig. 7.1). With the progression of the disease, the LV shows a change in its geometry becoming more spherical, with increased short axis/long axis ratio (sphericity index) [5] (Fig. 7.2). In a minority of cases of DCM, the LV end-diastolic diameter is still within 15% of normal values. This entity is classified as "mildly dilated cardiomyopathy" [6].

LV dilation can usually be accompanied by LV eccentric hypertrophy, with normal or only mildly increased LV wall thickness and increased LV mass (due to LV dilation). This feature is important for differential diagnosis between idiopathic DCM and other causes of dysfunction, such as end-stage hypertrophic cardiomyopathy and infiltrative or hypertensive heart disease.

Diffuse hypokinesis is typically seen in DCM, although regional wall motion abnormalities with akinesis or dyskinesis may be noticed, mostly at LV septum or apex, while better contractility is more common in the posterior and lateral walls.

Table 7.1 Echocardiographic features of DCM

Echocardiographic parameters	Cutoff/features	Comments
LV dilatation	LV end-diastolic diameter >2.7 cm/m^2 or >117% predicted value corrected for age and body surface area Increased sphericity index is common	Not necessary for diagnosis (e.g., mildly dilated cardiomyopathy)
LV systolic dysfunction	EF < 45%	Impaired global contractility
LV wall motion abnormalities	Diffuse hypokinesis	Possible regional wall motion abnormalities mostly in LV septum and apex
LV wall thickness	Normal or only mildly increased	Common presence of LV eccentric hypertrophy
LV diastolic dysfunction	"Restrictive pattern" (E < 150 ms and E/A ratio > 2) is related to increased LV stiffness	Useful hallmark of advanced diastolic dysfunction and elevated LV filling pressure. Can vary during follow-up
LV dyssynchrony	Qualitative + quantitative polyparametric evaluation	Frequent if severe LV dysfunction and LBBB; not a selection criteria for CRT
RV dilation and dysfunction	TAPSE < 14 mm, RV FAC < 35%	Secondary of biventricular involvement and/or pulmonary hypertension
LA dilation	End-systolic LA volume index >34 ml/m^2	Associated with diastolic dysfunction, MR, atrial fibrillation
Functional MR	EROA > 0.20 cm^2 identifies a significant functional MR	Contributes to increase of LV filling pressure and decrease of forward stroke volume; increases LV adverse remodeling
Functional TR		Common in presence of RV dilation and dysfunction and pulmonary hypertension
Dobutamine or exercise stress echocardiographic test	Assessment of presence or absence of LV inotropic response; sustained improvement vs. biphasic response	

CRT cardiac resynchronization therapy, *DCM* dilated cardiomyopathy, *EF* ejection fraction, *EROA* effective regurgitant orifice area, *FAC* fractional area change, *LA* left atrial, *LV* left ventricular, *MR* mitral regurgitation, *RV* right ventricular, *TAPSE* tricuspid annular peak systolic excursion, *TR* tricuspid regurgitation

The presence of a coronary artery distribution of wall motion abnormalities raises the suspicion of coronary artery disease. "Idiopathic LV aneurysms" are rarely seen in DCM and should be distinguished from cases of myocarditis, sarcoidosis, or left-dominant arrhythmogenic cardiomyopathy (AC) [7].

As in other cardiac diseases, the main parameter adopted to evaluate LV systolic dysfunction with standard echocardiography is LV EF assessed with two-dimensional (2D) biplane modified Simpson's rule (Fig. 7.3), with the use of contrast agents in the case of poor baseline image quality. Moreover, dP/dT and cardiac

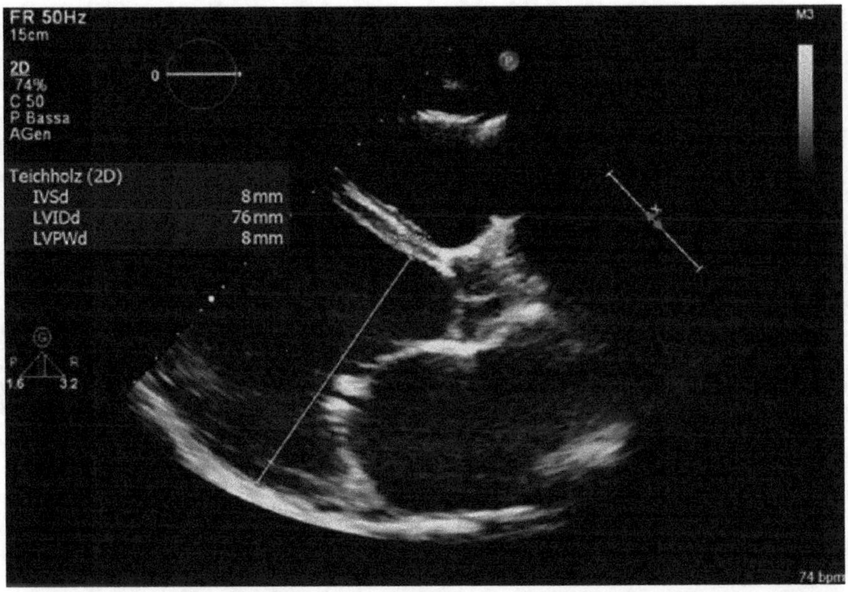

Fig. 7.1 Transthoracic echocardiography of dilated cardiomyopathy, parasternal long axis view with evidence of significant left ventricular (LV) dilatation. Of note, mitral valve annular dilatation, with leaflet tethering and reduced coaptation, is also present

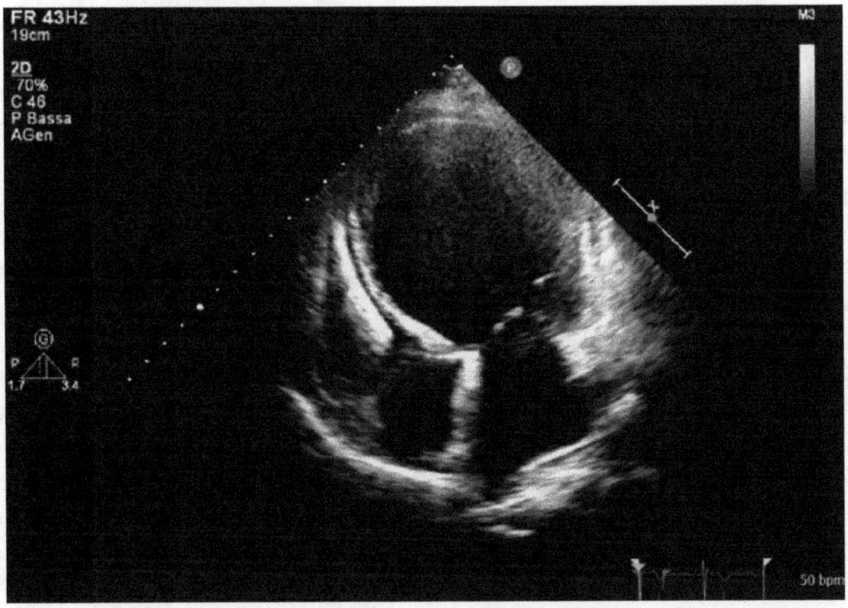

Fig. 7.2 Two-dimensional transthoracic echocardiography of dilated cardiomyopathy, apical four-chamber view. Significant left ventricular remodeling with increased sphericity and presence of implantable defibrillator lead in the right side of the heart are also seen

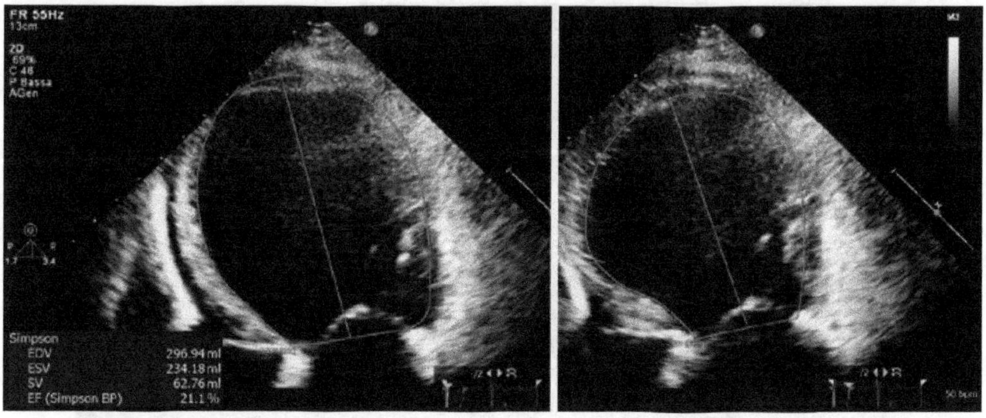

Fig. 7.3 Two-dimensional transthoracic echocardiography of dilated cardiomyopathy, apical four-chamber view. Quantification of left ventricular (LV) volumes and ejection fraction (EF) calculated using the biplane Simpson's method. Quantitative data: LV end-diastolic volume 297 mL, LV end-systolic volume 234 mL, LVEF 21%

output are further load-dependent parameters of LV performance, frequently used in association with LV EF. Tissue Doppler imaging (TDI) mitral annulus velocity can be also reduced showing LV longitudinal dysfunction. Severe LV dilation and dysfunction can trigger development of spontaneous echocontrast and LV thrombi formation, increasing the risk of systemic thromboembolism [8].

Diastolic dysfunction is frequent in DCM, reflecting structural LV wall pathology (particularly fibrosis), and chamber remodeling. Both abnormal relaxation and increased LV stiffness are present in the disease, with resulting increased LV filling pressure. LV diastolic dysfunction can be evaluated with several echocardiographic parameters. In particular, a "restrictive LV filling pattern" (Fig. 7.4) characterized by a short deceleration time of E (<150 ms) and an increased E/A ratio (>2) at transmitral inflow pulsed Doppler tracing is related to increased LV stiffness and filling pressures and usually reflects a more advanced stage of the disease. Frequently the restrictive filling pattern is associated with severe LV dilation, systolic dysfunction, left atrial (LA) dilation, right ventricular (RV) involvement, and functional MR [9]. On another side, an increased E/E' ratio (i.e., early diastolic mitral filling E/early diastolic mitral annular velocity E' at TDI) strongly correlates with diastolic dysfunction and increased LV filling pressure.

Additional indices useful to evaluate diastolic dysfunction are the response of the mitral flow pattern to Valsalva maneuver, the pattern of pulmonary venous Doppler curve, and LA dilation (Fig. 7.5). The latter is frequent in DCM and depends on multiple factors (severity and duration of the disease, LV filling pressure, presence and severity of MR, presence of atrial fibrillation). Changes in diastolic pattern can be seen during the course of the disease, i.e., worsening or improvement after optimal treatment [10].

LV mechanical dyssynchrony is another important aspect that can be evaluated with echocardiography in DCM patients with heart failure, LV systolic dysfunction, and left bundle branch block (LBBB). Echocardiography provides a multiparametric

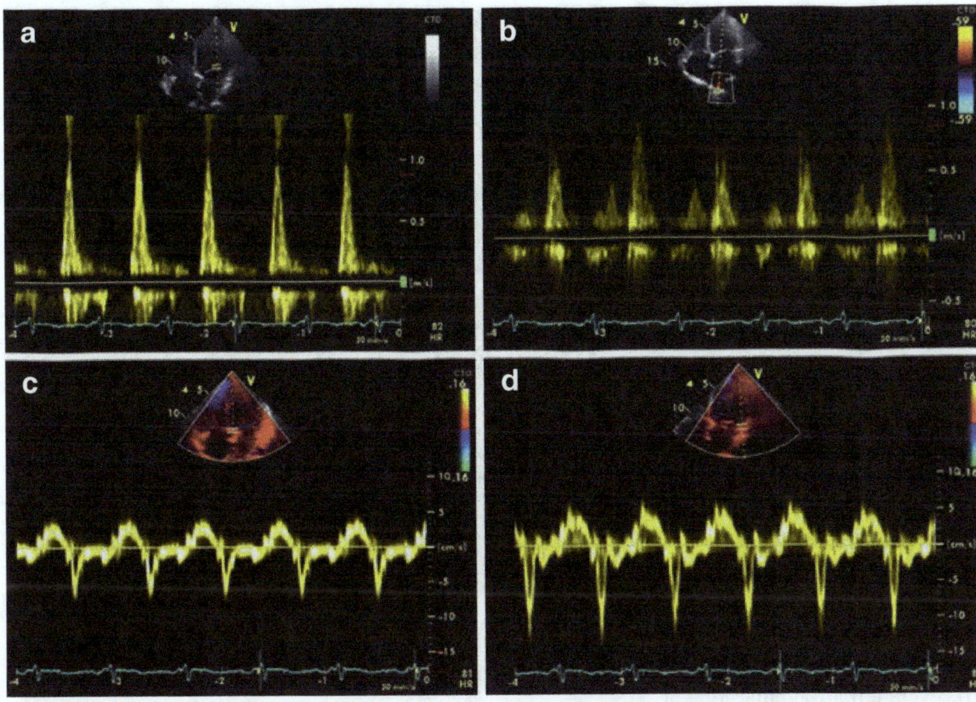

Fig. 7.4 Case of dilated cardiomyopathy with severe diastolic dysfunction. Panel (**a**) pulsed-wave Doppler at mitral valve inflow. Predominant *E* wave with rapid deceleration time and increased *E*/*A* ratio, consistent with restrictive filling pattern. Quantitative data: *E* wave 1.1 m/s, *E* wave deceleration time 100 ms, *A* wave 0.2 m/s, *E*/*A* ratio 5.5. Panel (**b**) pulsed-wave Doppler of the pulmonary vein flow, with predominance of diastolic flow, compatible with increased LV filling pressure. Quantitative data: *S* wave 0.4 m/s, *D* wave 0.9 ms, *S*/*D* ratio 0.4, systolic fraction of the pulmonary vein velocity-time integral 0.3. Panel (**c**) and (**d**) medial and lateral tissue Doppler velocities for the estimation of the left ventricular filling pressure. Quantitative data: medial *S′* wave 0.04 m/s, medial *E′* wave 0.07 m/s, medial *A′* wave 0.03 m/s, lateral *S′* 0.05 m/s, lateral *E′* 0.12 m/s, lateral *A′* 0.03 m/s, *E*/*E′* (medial) ratio 16

qualitative and quantitative approach for assessment of LV mechanical dyssynchrony [11]. The "apical rocking" motion of the LV yields a first qualitative diagnostic hint, which should be confirmed by other indices, as "septal flash," septal to posterior wall motion delay at M-mode, and TDI-derived indices (intervals from QRS to peak systolic velocities of wall motion of different LV segments, assessing the delay between opposite LV walls). Also the presence of significant interventricular dyssynchrony, demonstrated by the time delay between the LV and RV ejections at pulsed-wave (PW) Doppler, was proven to be associated with higher probability of favorable response to CRT in DCM patients [12]. However, echo-Doppler indexes of dyssynchrony are scarcely reliable [13, 14], and therefore, current guidelines do not recommend echocardiography as selection criteria for CRT [15].

Functional MR in DCM is secondary to several concurrent factors. LV enlargement and mitral annulus dilation cause papillary muscle displacement and systolic retraction of mitral valve (MV) leaflets toward the LV apex resulting in leaflet malcoaptation [16] (Fig. 7.6). On the other side, MR itself increases the LV and LA

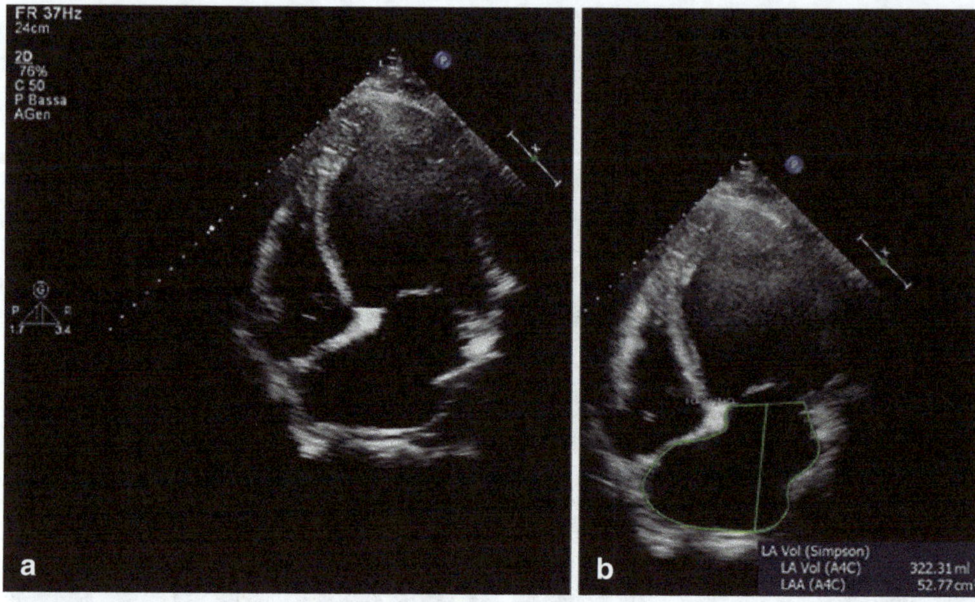

Fig. 7.5 Two-dimensional transthoracic echocardiography of an advanced case of dilated cardiomyopathy, apical four-chamber view. Panel (**a**) extreme remodeling of the heart chambers. Panel (**b**) severe left atrial enlargement

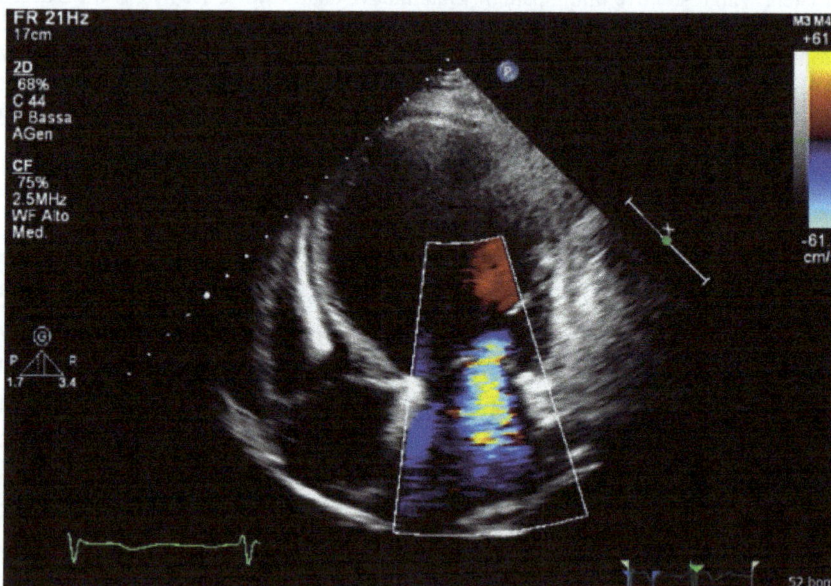

Fig. 7.6 Two-dimensional transthoracic echocardiography of dilated cardiomyopathy, apical four-chamber view, color Doppler study. Presence of significant functional mitral regurgitation due to dilatation of the mitral valve annulus and tethering of mitral valve leaflets

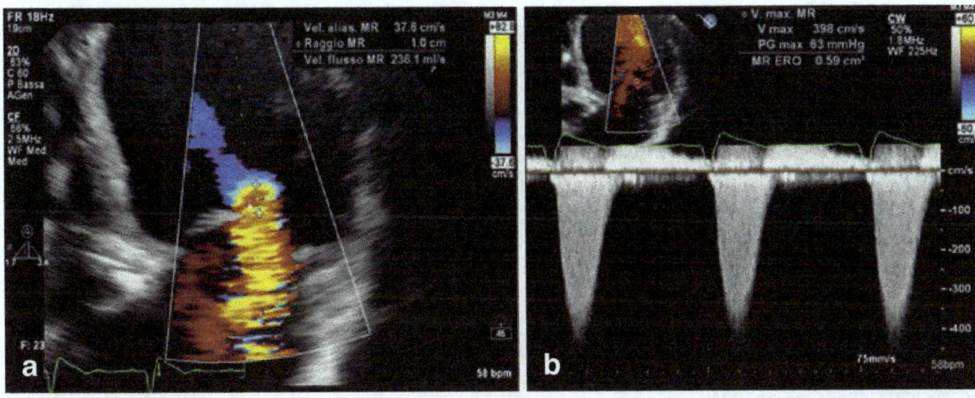

Fig. 7.7 Two-dimensional transthoracic echocardiography of dilated cardiomyopathy with severe mitral regurgitation (MR). Quantification of the effective regurgitant orifice area (EROA) with the proximal isovelocity surface area (PISA) method. Panel (**a**) apical four-chamber view focused on mitral regurgitation jet origin for the measurement of the PISA radius. Panel (**b**) continuous wave Doppler of the regurgitant jet with low velocity and a triangular profile, suggestive of severe MR. Quantitative data: PISA radius 1 cm, EROA 59 mm^2

volume overload causing further LV dilation and remodeling, which consecutively escalates the degree of MR. Hemodynamically significant MR contributes to increase LA pressure and decreases LV forward stroke volume, worsening the patients' status. According to the current guidelines, a cutoff of effective regurgitant orifice area (EROA) >0.20 cm^2 identifies a significant functional MR [17] (Fig. 7.7).

Echocardiography is pivotal to assess MV morphology, quantify mitral annulus dilation, and rule out the presence of structural leaflet disease. Furthermore, it is important to evaluate MR severity with a multiparametric approach [17]. To increase sensitivity and specificity in detecting the severity of MR, transesophageal echocardiography provides the best accuracy. Indeed, transesophageal echocardiograms are capable of providing a more accurate estimation of morphological (MV annulus dilation, quantification of systolic leaflet retraction, coaptation depth, and tenting area) and functional (EROA calculated with proximal isovelocity surface area [PISA], regurgitant volume [RVol]) parameters.

RV dilation and systolic dysfunction are frequent in DCM and can represent biventricular involvement of the disease (30% of DCM cases) and/or are secondary to RV pressure overload due to left-side disease [18, 19]. RV dysfunction correlates with worse functional status and more advanced heart failure [20]. The presence of RV dilation is usually assessed with 2D echocardiography from standard echo views (Fig. 7.8). RV systolic function is estimated with various parameters, as fractional area change (FAC), tricuspid annular peak systolic excursion (TAPSE), TDI, systolic tricuspid annular velocity, and RV myocardial performance index [21] (Fig. 7.9).

In the presence of RV dilation and dysfunction, functional tricuspid regurgitation (TR) and pulmonary hypertension are quite common in DCM. Pulmonary hypertension is more frequently associated with the severity of functional MR and LV

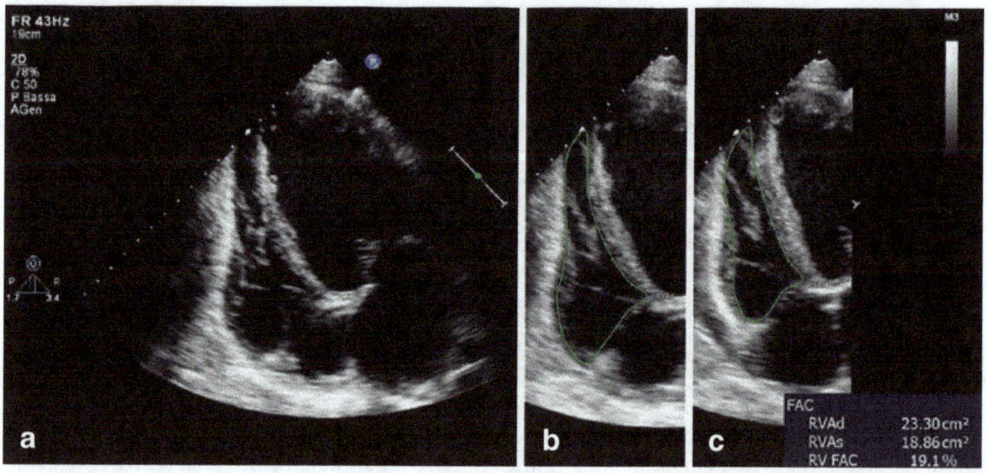

Fig. 7.8 Two-dimensional transthoracic echocardiography of dilated cardiomyopathy, apical four-chamber view focused on the right ventricle (Panel **a**) for RV systolic function evaluation with fractional area change (FAC) method. Panel (**b**) RV end-diastolic area contour. Panel (**c**) end-systolic area contour. Quantitative data: RV end-diastolic area 23.3 cm^2, RV end-systolic area 18.86 cm^2, RV FAC 19.1%, consistent with severe RV systolic dysfunction

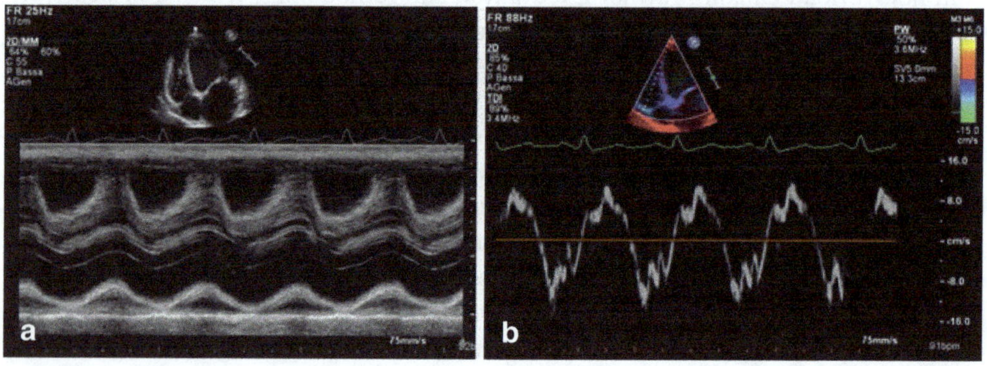

Fig. 7.9 Transthoracic echocardiography of dilated cardiomyopathy with associated right ventricular (RV) dysfunction. Assessment of right ventricular longitudinal function with M-mode tricuspid annular peak systolic excursion – TAPSE – (Panel **a**) and tissue Doppler *S*′ wave velocity (Panel **b**). Quantitative data: TAPSE 17 mm, *S*′ 10 cm/s, consistent with mild RV systolic dysfunction

diastolic dysfunction than with the degree of LV systolic dysfunction [19]. In particular, patients with "restrictive" or pseudonormal mitral inflow patterns have a higher pulmonary artery systolic pressure, and the improvement to an impaired relaxation pattern appears to be followed by a significant reduction of pulmonary artery pressure [22].

Stress echocardiography can be useful in DCM to assess the myocardial contractile reserve and the presence of inducible ischemia and to evaluate the coronary flow reserve (CFR) [23]. However, to date there is no standardized protocol for stress echocardiography in patients with LV dysfunction, and the preferred stress technique (dobutamine, dipyridamole, or exercise) is chosen depending on the indication of the test, the exercise ability of each patient, image quality, and expertise of the center.

Exercise is the most physiological stress test, which should be used if the patient is able to exercise. However, the most used test in DCM patients is dobutamine stress echocardiography (DSE) [24]. Low-dose dobutamine is the method of choice for assessment of myocardial contractile reserve. Also dipyridamole is a feasible test that can be used to assess the contractile response; it is less arrhythmogenic and better tolerated [23]. A LV EF increase >20% or a wall motion score index (WMSI) >0.44 from baseline recognizes patients with preserved contractile reserve. A biphasic response in at least two segments and/or extensive ischemic response during high-dose dobutamine or exercise stress can help to identify ischemic cardiomyopathy, whereas idiopathic DCM is characterized by sustained improvement of LV function. Absence of inotropic response identifies patients with severe cardiomyopathy [23].

Dipyridamole stress test allows a combined assessment of contractile reserve and CFR on left anterior descending artery (defined by the ratio of hyperemic to rest peak diastolic flow velocity, normal value >2.5). CFR is often reduced in DCM, and it is associated with the functional class and the oxygen consumption.

DSE can also be useful to unmask a significant LV intraventricular dyssynchrony [25] and helps to identify potential responders to CRT (together with the presence of contractile reserve). Furthermore, it can be used to discriminate between true aortic valve stenosis and pseudo-stenosis combined with DCM [23]. However, to date, indications for stress echocardiography in the setting of functional MR in idiopathic DCM are controversial [26].

Importantly, many of the aforementioned echocardiographic parameters, evaluated at baseline and at follow-up, are crucial for the prognostic stratification of DCM patients (see paragraph on prognostic role of echocardiography in DCM) and are useful to evaluate the progression of the disease and the response to therapy.

7.2 Role of New Echocardiographic Techniques

Technological advances in the field of cardiac ultrasound have led to new noninvasive techniques, such as 3D echocardiography, TDI, and speckle-tracking echocardiography (STE). These techniques have demonstrated a significant incremental value over basic echocardiography [2, 27–29].

Accurate LV volume and EF quantification is crucial in the echocardiographic evaluation of patients with DCM. However, it is well known that M-mode and 2D evaluation of LV volumes and EF have limitations [30]. LV volume measurement by 2D echocardiography is highly dependent on user's experience (in manually tracing of endocardium and in visualization of perpendicular imaging planes), and this approach relies on geometrical assumption about the shape of the LV. The greatest advantage of 3D echocardiography in the evaluation of the LV includes independence from geometric assumption, semiautomatic delineation of the endocardium border, and the absence of errors deriving from "foreshortening" of the LV apex [31, 32].

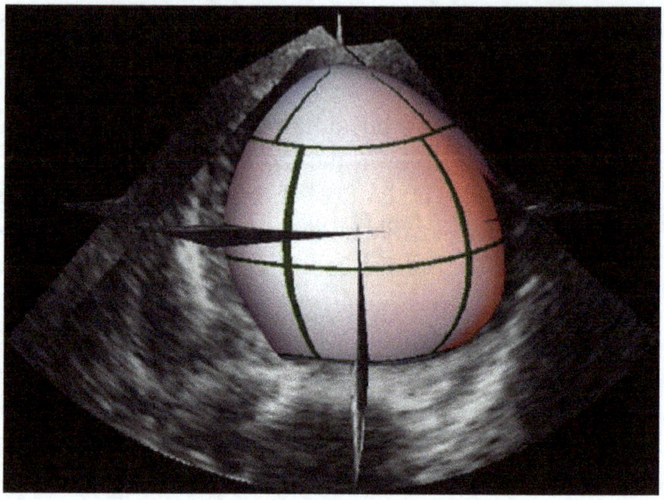

Fig. 7.10 Three-dimensional reconstruction of left ventricular (LV) volumes. Severe LV dilatation and remodeling. Quantitative data: LV end-diastolic volume 307 mL, LV end-systolic volume 234 mL, LV ejection fraction 24%, 3D global longitudinal strain (GLS) −8.4%

With 3D echocardiography, only one acquisition is needed to obtain volumes and EF and provides the possibility for quantitative assessment of LV regional wall motion by measuring the volume change of each segment in the cardiac cycle (Fig. 7.10). Three-dimensional measurements and reporting of LV volumes are recommended when feasible, depending on image quality and center expertise. Three-dimensional echocardiography demonstrated high feasibility in DCM patients [33] and has been extensively validated against cardiac magnetic resonance (CMR). It has been demonstrated to be more time-saving, reproducible, and accurate than conventional 2D echocardiography for LV volumes, mass, and EF measurements, with lower inter- and intra-observer variability [34–37]. Three-dimensional echocardiography slightly underestimates both LV EDV and ESV in comparison with those measured with CMR. A recent meta-analysis of 23 studies comparing 3D echocardiography with CMR volumes and EF demonstrated biases of -19 ± 34 mL, -10 ± 30 mL, and $-1 \pm 12\%$ for LV EDV and ESV and EF, respectively [38]. The lower spatial resolution of 3D echocardiography compared to CMR is responsible for this underestimation. With 3D echocardiography, it is often difficult to identify the endocardial-trabecular border and the blood-trabecular interface. In a review of sources of error, it was shown that the agreement between 3D echocardiography and CMR improved when the trabeculae were excluded from the LV cavity [39].

Technological advances in the field of cardiac ultrasound have led to further new noninvasive techniques, such as TDI and STE, for assessing cardiac mechanics and segmental and global LV function. The peak systolic myocardial velocity S', a simple TDI index of systolic longitudinal function, is a marker of impaired subendocardial fiber contraction and correlates with myocardial fibrosis [40]. STE has emerged as a novel technology to detect myocardial abnormalities. Strain analysis allows discrimination between active and passive movement of myocardial segments and permits separate assessment of distinct components of myocardial deformation (longitudinal and circumferential shortening, radial thickening, rotation, and twisting). Patients with DCM have an increased LV mass and volume and typically decreased contractility of the LV walls [41]. These changes lead to impaired strain in all direction (longitudinal, radial, and circumferential) [42–45].

Strain echocardiography is important for the arrhythmic risk stratification of patients with DCM since global longitudinal strain (GLS) is a promising marker of arrhythmias. Mechanical dispersion predicted arrhythmic events in patients with DCM independently of LV EF [46]. Speckle-tracking longitudinal deformation has also a potential role in assessing fibrosis as detected by contrast CMR late gadolinium enhancement (LGE), but the relationship between myocardial fibrosis and segmental strain is still not well established, especially in setting of DCM. In a small prospective study, abnormal 3D speckle-tracking GLS could detect LGE-determinant myocardial fibrosis with a sensitivity of 85%, a specificity of 85%, a positive predictive value of 69%, and a negative predictive value of 93%, considering an optimal GLS cutoff value of −15.25% [47].

LV twist and torsion have been investigated with different measurement methods during the past two decades, using tagged CMR as the gold standard [48]. Many studies using different echocardiographic techniques, like TDI, STE, velocity vector imaging, and 3D STE, showed that LV torsion (twisting and untwisting) represents an important mechanism for both ejection and filling. LV twist/torsion indexes are significantly impaired in patients with DCM correlating with worse functional capacity and LV function [42, 49, 50]. Reduced LV torsion in patients with DCM was found to be a predictor of response to CRT and increased after 8 months of therapy [51].

The accuracy of LV mass determined by 3D echocardiography is similar to that of CMR in most patients, showing only a slight overestimation [37, 52, 53].

Advanced indices of LV intraventricular mechanical dyssynchrony are based on TDI, speckle-tracking imaging, and 3D echocardiography [11]. As stated in the previous paragraph, the role of echocardiography in assessing LV mechanic dyssynchrony in DCM patients remains controversial to date. The Predictors of Response to Cardiac Resynchronization Therapy (PROSPECT) trial examined the predictive value of 12 echocardiographic parameters of dyssynchrony, including both conventional- and TDI-based methods, showing only a modest sensitivity and specificity of these markers [54]. Three-dimensional echocardiography has been used as a technique for dyssynchrony quantification. The systolic dyssynchrony index (SDI) is calculated as the standard deviation of regional ejection time (time to reach minimal volume). Three-dimensional echocardiography allows evaluating all LV segments simultaneously, displaying a "bull's eye" map, which demonstrates the time required to each segment to reach minimal volume. Three-dimensional echocardiography-derived LV SDI was described as highly predictive of response to CRT at 48 h [55], 6 months [56, 57], and 1 year of follow-up [58]. Benefits from CRT have been defined as a ≥15% reduction in LV ESV at follow-up [56–58], which can also readily be measured by 3D echocardiography.

Several groups have addressed analysis of LV strain of opposite walls by STE as the ideal technique for the assessment of LV intraventricular dyssynchrony [14, 59, 60]. Radial strain values were demonstrated to be reliable indexes of LV mechanical dyssynchrony useful to identify potential responders to CRT [59]. The Speckle Tracking and Resynchronization (STAR) study demonstrated that radial and transverse LV strain values were significantly related to LV EF response and long-term outcome after CRT [60]. On the other hand, absence of radial or transverse dyssynchrony (≥130 ms time difference in peak strain values between opposing segments) at baseline was an adverse prognostic factor after CRT [60]. In one study pacing at the site of the latest mechanical activation, as determined by speckle-tracking radial strain analysis, resulted in superior echocardiographic response after 6 months of CRT and better prognosis during long-term follow-up. Moreover, the demonstration of scar tissue by speckle-tracking GLS was found to be an independent predictor of lack of response to CRT and was related to the total scar burden assessed with CMR [61]. Furthermore, 3D speckle-tracking strain indices have been studied to quantify dyssynchrony before and after CRT [62].

For the echocardiographic assessment of LV diastolic dysfunction in patients with DCM, the ratio of early diastolic transmitral flow velocity to early diastolic annular velocity (*E*/*E*′) is frequently used to predict an increase in LV filling pressure. This approach, however, has several limitations, and its accuracy is questionable, particularly in patients with advanced DCM and severe heart failure. A study with invasive hemodynamic assessment as gold standard showed that *E*/*E*′ ratio had a weak correlation with LV filling pressure in DCM, particularly those with severe LV dilatation and after CRT [63]. Other new indices for LV diastolic dysfunction evaluation obtained by speckle-tracking techniques analysis are promising. Circumferential strain and strain rate during late diastolic LV filling, *E*/circumferential strain rate at early diastolic LV filling, and *E*/circumferential strain at the time of peak *E* wave had greater area under the curve than the *E*/*E*′ ratio for the prediction of pulmonary capillary wedge pressure >12 mmHg [64].

Importantly, 2D LA strain assessment with speckle-tracking technique demonstrated a better correlation than other Doppler indices, such as *E*/*E*′ ratio, with LV filling pressure as measured by right catheterization, in patients with advanced systolic heart failure [65]. In particular, the peak atrial longitudinal strain that corresponds to LA expansion during the reservoir phase is reduced in the presence of an increased LA pressure, and this parameter could be useful in the multiparametric assessment of LV filling pressure. In addition, LA strain represents a promising noninvasive technique to assess left atrial pump function in patients with DCM. Two-dimensional STE-based LA function is impaired in patients with nonischemic DCM [66]. In a study with 134 patients with either idiopathic or ischemic DCM, LA systolic deformation was more depressed in idiopathic compared with ischemic DCM and was closely associated with functional capacity during effort. LA lateral wall systolic strain and LA volume were powerful independent predictors of peak oxygen consumption during cardiopulmonary exercise testing [67].

Quantification of MR is challenging and should be performed by using 2D or 3D vena contracta and PISA method [17, 68]. It is well known that the 2D vena contracta and PISA method have several limitations. These methods assume the EROA is nearly circular, and the exact shape and size might not be accurately assessed due to the limited scan plane orientation of 2D echocardiography. Real-time 3D echocardiography is now available to overcome this limitation, which is particularly relevant in patients with functional MR, in whom EROA geometry is usually complex and asymmetric [69–71]. The direct measurement of the regurgitation orifice area with 3D echocardiography avoids the underestimation of its size, independently from the eccentricity of the MR jet or from cardiac rhythm [72, 73]. Quantification of RVol of functional MR with 3D echocardiography showed excellent correlation with RVol measured by CMR ($r = 0.94$), without a significant difference between these techniques (mean difference = −0.08 mL/beat). Conversely, 2D echocardiography approach from the four-chamber view significantly underestimated RVol ($r = 0.006$) as compared with CMR (mean difference = 2.9 mL/beat) [73]. Currently, dedicated MV analysis softwares allow a fast, complete, and reproducible evaluation of MV anatomy and function (MV annulus dimensions, MV annulus displacement, MV leaflet surface, tenting volume, aortomitral angle, and papillary muscle geometry) [74–76]. Furthermore, 3D transesophageal echocardiography plays an important role in the selection of patients for MitraClip, in the echocardiographic guidance of the procedure and in the pre- and post-procedural MR quantification [77].

Multiparametric advanced echocardiographic assessment of RV includes the measurement of volumes and EF by 3D technology and semiautomatic software quantification and analysis of RV longitudinal strain by 2D and 3D speckle-tracking technology (Fig. 7.11). Reduced RV strain and 3D RV EF are associated with decreased exercise capacity in DCM [78, 79].

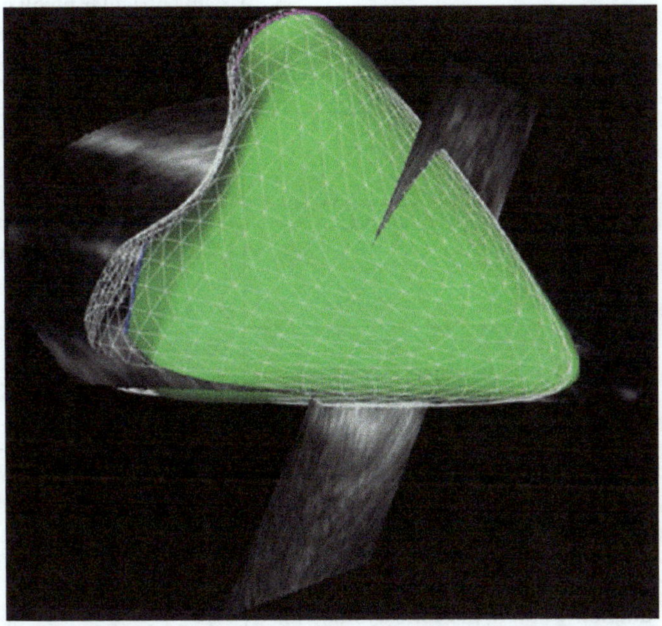

Fig. 7.11 Three-dimensional reconstruction of right ventricular (RV) volumes. Severe RV dysfunction. Quantitative data: RV end-diastolic volume 109 mL, RV end-systolic volume 92 mL, RV ejection fraction 15%, 3D longitudinal strain of the free-wall −11.5%

7.3 Clinical Echocardiography in DCM: Advantages and Limitations in Clinical Practice

Echocardiography is the first-level imaging tool, which plays a valuable role in many steps of the clinical management of patients with DCM. These include primarily the diagnosis of DCM and its differentiation from other diseases causing LV dysfunction in heart failure patients (Table 7.2) [1, 2, 27, 28]. The echocardiographic demonstration of LV dilation and systolic dysfunction is diagnostic for DCM but only after exclusion of other specific causes of heart disease. The differential

Table 7.2 Echocardiographic clues in differential diagnosis of DCM

Echocardiographic features	Possible differential diagnosis vs. DCM
Associated significant LV hypertrophy	1. Advanced hypertrophic cardiomyopathy 2. Advanced infiltrative/storage cardiomyopathy 3. Advanced hypertensive heart disease
Segmental wall motion abnormalities with coronary artery distribution	Ischemic cardiomyopathy
Biphasic response in at least two LV segments and/or extensive ischemic response during high-dose dobutamine or exercise stress	Ischemic cardiomyopathy
Wall motion abnormalities with non-coronary distribution/idiopathic LV aneurysms	1. Left-dominant or biventricular AC 2. Myocarditis 3. Cardiac sarcoidosis
Prevalent RV dilation and dysfunction	1. Arrhythmogenic RV cardiomyopathy with biventricular involvement 2. Congenital heart disease 3. Pulmonary hypertension
Presence of RV/LV aneurysms	AC
Low-gradient aortic valve stenosis + LV dysfunction	True severe aortic valve stenosis vs. pseudo-severe aortic stenosis + DCM > differentiation by response to DSE
Significant MR + LV dysfunction	Functional MR+DCM vs. organic MR + secondary LV dysfunction > through transthoracic + transesophageal echocardiography assessment of MV
LV dysfunction without severe dilation, LV hypertrophy, non-coronary wall motion abnormalities, LV thrombi	Myocarditis
Reversibility of pathological echocardiographic parameters once the causal factors are removed	Other cardiomyopathies: inflammatory, alcoholic, tachycardia-induced, stress-induced, chemotherapy-induced, peripartum
Mild/moderate LV systolic dysfunction without significant dilation + severe diastolic dysfunction	Mildly dilated cardiomyopathy vs. restrictive cardiomyopathy

AC arrhythmogenic cardiomyopathy, *DCM* dilated cardiomyopathy, *DSE* dobutamine stress echocardiography, *LV* left ventricular, *MV* mitral valve, *MR* mitral regurgitation, *RV* right ventricular diagnosis of various possible causes of heart failure is particularly challenging for the clinician. Therefore echocardiography provides relevant help recognizing "red flags" and directing further second-level imaging techniques, in order to obtain the final diagnosis [80, 81].

"Red flags" echocardiographic clues can raise the suspicion of a diagnosis but are however not totally specific for a definitive etiology. For example, documentation of LV dysfunction, not necessarily associated with LV hypertrophy, in patients with history of systemic hypertension may clarify the cause of LV dysfunction as end-stage dilated and hypokinetic phase of hypertensive heart disease that may mimic a DCM [82]. Also multivessel coronary heart disease can be indistinguishable by echocardiography from DCM, and sometimes only coronary angiography clarifies the diagnosis. In some cases, a diagnostic hint originates from the evidence of segmental wall motion abnormalities with coronary distribution, as well as the proof of an ischemic "biphasic" response at DSE. Other noninvasive imaging techniques, as CMR which evaluates the LGE pattern, single-photon emission computed tomography (CT) which assesses perfusion abnormalities, and CT which depicts the coronary anatomy, are useful to differentiate ischemic from nonischemic DCM.

Regarding the differential diagnosis in the case of DCM associated with valve disease, low-dose dobutamine stress test is particularly valuable in the differentiation between a true severe aortic valve stenosis with consequent LV dysfunction and a pseudo-aortic valve stenosis in the presence of DCM. Also a severe MR can lead to advanced LV dysfunction: in this case transthoracic and transesophageal echocardiographic assessment of MV apparatus is valuable in excluding organic MV disease.

Several other cardiomyopathies can mimic the morphological features of DCM. Echocardiography can give diagnostic hints but remains often limited in defining DCM etiology, thus suggesting the use of second-level imaging investigations, primarily CMR which can recognize distinct LGE distribution in different cardiomyopathies. Myocarditis is echocardiographically characterized by LV dysfunction frequently without severe dilation, sometimes LV hypertrophy due to interstitial edema, wall motion abnormalities with non-coronary distribution, and possible presence of LV thrombi [83]. CMR in these cases facilitates the diagnosis detecting myocardial edema, but the diagnostic gold standard remains endomyocardial biopsy. AC with biventricular or "left-dominant" involvement can be suspected by echocardiography in presence of biventricular dysfunction and in presence of RV/LV aneurysms [84]. Again, the diagnostic imaging tool of choice in suspected AC is CMR [85]. Also advanced hypertrophic cardiomyopathy in hypokinetic-dilated end-stage has echocardiographic features similar to DCM with LV spherical remodeling and apparent regression of LV hypertrophy [86]. The presence of previous echocardiographic exams with documentation of severe LV hypertrophy typical of hypertrophic cardiomyopathy may help the diagnosis in these extreme cases. Of note, evidence of significant LV hypertrophy may also suggest advanced stages of infiltrative/storage cardiomyopathy [87]. Hemochromatosis causes a restrictive cardiomyopathy which progresses to an end-stage DCM with echocardiographic features undistinguishable from idiopathic DCM. Therefore, CMR is the imaging modality of choice to detect the iron overload in the myocardium. Also the differential diagnosis between LV non-compaction and DCM with conspicuous trabeculations secondary to LV remodeling is often possible only with CMR. Finally, other cardiomyopathies (inflammatory, alcoholic, tachycardia-induced [88], stress-induced, chemotherapy-induced, peripartum) usually show a reversibility of pathological echocardiographic parameters once the causal factors have resolved; therefore echocardiography is extremely valuable in follow-up of these patients.

Echocardiography is also important in the early diagnosis of DCM in patients with positive familiar history and/or in presence of a positive genetic mutation [4, 89, 90]. The diagnosis of DCM is obtained in presence of two or more affected family members or in presence of a first-degree relative of a DCM patient with unexplained sudden death at <35 years [1]. Familiar screening including history, physical examination, ECG, and echocardiography is indicated in probands and first-degree relatives. LV dilation and reduced fractional shortening are common in asymptomatic relatives of patients with DCM and are associated with a significant risk for disease progression [90]. Advanced echocardiographic techniques as myocardial deformation imaging might permit the detection of latent DCM (with reduced strain) earlier than LV enlargement and depression of EF [91]. In controversial cases other imaging techniques as CMR, as well as follow-up reassessment, are indicated.

In addition, several echocardiographic parameters, assessed at baseline and at follow-up, are relevant for prognostic stratification of DCM patients (see paragraph about prognostic role of echocardiography in DCM) and help the clinician in assessing the progression of the disease and the response to treatment. They also guide in taking decisions not only about pharmacological therapy but also indication for invasive treatments as implantable device therapy (implantable cardioverter defibrillators (ICD), CRT, and correction of valvulopathy [92–95]). Documentation of LV EF < 30%, severe LV dilatation, and LV thrombosis suggests the indication for anticoagulation therapy in order to lower the risk of thromboembolism. Echocardiographic LV EF measurement is an important parameter for determining the appropriateness of ICD and CRT implantation. LV EF ≤ 35% in association with advanced New York Heart Association (NYHA) class despite optimal medical therapy for at least 3 months is considered in the indication for ICD and, if prolonged QRS is present, is an echo criterion for the selection of patients for CRT. Accurate MV echocardiographic evaluation is becoming increasingly more relevant due to the emerging role of percutaneous procedures to treat functional MR. In particular, the percutaneous mitral valve edge-to-edge repair with MitraClip implantation in heart failure patients with severe functional MR and high risk for surgery is a new therapeutic possibility. Echocardiography is fundamental not only in the selection of patients [96] but also in guiding the procedure and in the follow-up. Echocardiography can also provide assistance in the implantation of ventricular assist devices and the evaluation for heart transplantation in end-stage heart failure patients.

In conclusion, echocardiography is the first-line imaging exam in patients with DCM, and it has a pivotal role in assessing its morphological and functional features and in piloting treatment options. However, sometimes echocardiographic data are not sufficient, and they should guide further and more specific cardiac diagnostic investigations. General advantages of echocardiography over other imaging techniques in clinical everyday practice are its extensive availability, accessibility, and low cost. Furthermore, it is noninvasive, safe, and free from radiations and can be performed in patients with heart devices who cannot undergo magnetic fields. Limitations of echocardiography include inadequate image quality and unfeasibility for tissue characterization. Moreover, as other imaging techniques, the operators require a learning curve and adequate expertise and familiarity with the disease.

7.4 Prognostic Role of Echocardiographic Data in DCM

The natural history of DCM has dramatically improved in the last 20 years as a result of the introduction in clinical practice of beta-blockers, ACE inhibitors, and mineralocorticoid receptor antagonists which showed not only a reduction in mortality and morbidity but also significant improvements in terms of LV reverse remodeling (LVRR) [27, 28, 97, 98]. Therefore, studies on the prognostic role of echocardiography should be contextualized in their historical phase of conception, keeping in mind that during the last three decades, the gradual optimization of medical therapy has paralleled a significant improvement in survival [99].

The main echocardiographic parameters useful to assess the prognosis in patients with DCM are summarized in Table 7.3.

LV dilatation and systolic dysfunction are the hallmarks of the disease and markers of adverse outcome [2, 18, 27, 28, 100]. Remodeling in DCM includes other features as dyssynchronous ventricular contraction, functional MR, dilatation of other chambers, and myocardial fibrosis. Conversely, LVRR, characterized by a decrease in LV dimensions and the normalization of shape associated with a significant improvement of systolic function, is a therapeutic goal (nowadays achieved in almost 40% of patients in optimal medical and device treatment) and adds prognostic value for the stratification of long-term risk [92]. Therefore, although baseline LV EF is an independent predictor or outcome both in adults and children with idiopathic DCM [101], a serial thorough assessment of LV size and systolic function, especially after medical treatment optimization, is pivotal in the management of these patients. At approximately 24 months after diagnosis and establishment of optimal medical therapy, LVRR is considered completed; nonetheless, possible disease progression indicates the need for continuous follow-up, lifelong therapy, and evaluation of potential negative prognostic factors (including atrial fibrillation, LV restrictive filling, RV dysfunction, LBBB, functional MR) [27].

Severe LV diastolic dysfunction, characterized by restrictive filling pattern, has been demonstrated a powerful adverse prognostic sign specifically in patients with DCM, as in other patients with heart failure [9]. Furthermore, persistence of LV restrictive filling pattern is associated with high mortality and transplantation rate, while patients with reversible restrictive filling have a high probability of improvement and excellent survival [10]. Early diastolic mitral filling *E*/early diastolic mitral

Table 7.3 Main echocardiographic parameters clinically useful to assess prognosis in patients with DCM

	Echo parameters	Comments	References
At first assessment	LV dilatation	Larger indexed LV ESV is predictor of early arrhythmic events	[27, 120]
	LV EF	Independent predictor of outcome	[101]
	LV diastolic dysfunction	Independent prognostic indicator of poor outcome or heart transplantation	[9]
	Functional MR	Independently associated with a poor prognosis	[92, 106]
	RV dysfunction	Correlates with worse functional status, more advanced LV failure, and has prognostic importance. Biventricular dilation is associated with a worse prognosis as compared to isolated LV dilation	[20]
	LA enlargement	Correlates with ↓exercise tolerance and ↑pro-BNP	[105]
	Pulmonary artery pressure	Peak TR velocity >2.5 m/s is associated with increased mortality, increased hospitalization, and higher incidence of heart failure	[115]
	LV GLS	Independent predictor of arrhythmogenic events in DCM	[46]
	Contractile reserve at DSE	Predicts outcome	[24]
At follow-up	LVRR	Characterized by a decrease in LV dimensions and normalization of LV shape associated with a significant improvement of systolic function. It is one of the main determinants of prognosis	[27, 92]
	Persistent vs. reversible LV restrictive filling pattern	Associated with subsequent mortality and transplantation rate	[10]
	Improvement of functional MR	Early improvement is a favorable independent prognostic factor	[107, 108]
	Regression vs. persistence or new development of RV systolic dysfunction	Independent risk factor of subsequent outcome	[112, 113]

DCM dilated cardiomyopathy, *DSE* dobutamine stress echocardiography, *EF* ejection fraction, *ESV* end-systolic volume, *FAC* fractional area change, *GLS* global longitudinal strain, *LA* left atrial, *LV* left ventricular, *LVRR* left ventricular reverse remodeling, *MR* mitral regurgitation, *RV* right ventricular, *TR* tricuspid regurgitation annular velocity E' at TDI (E/E' ratio) is associated with exercise capacity in DCM [102]. E/E' ratio was also demonstrated to be a powerful predictor of clinical outcome in DCM patients [103]. Furthermore, baseline lateral E/E' ratio was an independent predictor for cardiac events in patients with heart failure treated with CRT [104].

LA enlargement is often observed in DCM as a consequence of LV diastolic dysfunction, functional MR, and atrial fibrillation. LA volume has incremental prognostic value in patients with DCM and correlates with exercise tolerance and pro-BNP [105].

Functional MR is independently associated with a poor prognosis in patients with LV dysfunction [16, 92, 106]. Improvement of functional MR in response to pharmacological therapy and CRT has been previously demonstrated [107]. Stolfo et al. [108] showed that in patients with DCM receiving optimal medical treatment, early improvement of functional MR is frequent (more than half of the cases) and is a favorable independent prognostic factor. Furthermore, early improvement of functional MR is frequently documented after CRT implantation in DCM and is associated with improved transplant-free survival [109]. With the emergence of percutaneous transcatheter MV procedures for the treatment of MR (MitraClip repair), the prognostic importance of correction of functional MR in DCM is likely to increase [110].

Concomitant RV dysfunction, in particular TAPSE < 14 mm, represents an adverse prognostic marker in DCM [111].

The serial assessment of RV function by echocardiography is useful, particularly after optimization of medical therapy or after CRT. A regression of RV dysfunction is associated with a favorable transplant-free survival, whereas the persistence or the new development of RV systolic dysfunction is an independent risk factor of adverse outcome [112–114].

Functional TR is often associated with RV dilatation, RV dysfunction, or pulmonary hypertension. Pulmonary artery pressure measured from TR velocity provides additional prognostic information as peak TR velocity of more than 2.5 m/s is associated with increased mortality, increased hospitalization, and higher incidence of heart failure [115].

A significant prolongation of QRS duration in the context of LBBB is the main marker of ventricular dyssynchrony used in trials of CRT [116]. Echocardiographic techniques may also detect mechanical dyssynchrony in some patients without significant QRS prolongation. However, in a large series of patients with systolic heart failure, echocardiographic evidence of LV dyssynchrony and a QRS duration of less than 130 ms, CRT did not reduce the rate of death or hospitalization for heart failure and may increase mortality [117]. Therefore, assessment of dyssynchrony should not be part of the routine echocardiographic evaluation for patients with DCM and should be used in selected cases only.

Recent data demonstrated that the reversion after CRT treatment of simple qualitative echocardiographic signs of LV intraventricular dyssynchrony (septal flash and apical rocking) is a favorable prognostic sign and is associated with frequent improvement of LV function [118].

Few data are presently available about prognostic value of evaluation of LV strain by STE in DCM. LV subendocardial longitudinal function is often early deranged in DCM, and LV GLS is markedly decreased in DCM when compared with healthy controls [119]. As showed by Haugaa et al., LV GLS may be a valuable tool in the selection of candidates for CRT and independent predictor of arrhythmogenic events in DCM [46].

As previously stated, approximately one third of patients with DCM exhibit an improvement of LV function on optimal medical therapy. Merlo et al. [92] showed on a large cohort of patients with idiopathic DCM that LVRR (defined as a normalization or improvement of LV systolic function and a significant decrease in LV size) is related with more favorable outcomes in the long term. In this study, baseline independent predictors of LVRR were higher systolic blood pressure and the absence of LBBB. Notably, no baseline echocardiographic parameters were predictive of subsequent LVRR.

The implantation of an ICD in selected patients with DCM may prevent sudden cardiac death. Current international guidelines recommend ICD implantation in patients and previous cardiac arrest (secondary prevention) or in patients with severely reduced EF (≤35%) and NYHA II/III despite optimal medical therapy (primary prevention) with a life expectancy >1 year [15]. It is recommended that patients should receive at least 3 months of optimal medical therapy before considering ICD implantation in primary prevention, as LVRR with recovery of systolic function may lead to unnecessary implantation. Patients that experience sudden death or major ventricular arrhythmias within the 6 months window after diagnosis are approximately 2%; larger indexed LV ESV and QRS duration are predictors of early arrhythmic events [120].

Assessment of contractile reserve by DSE may be a useful tool to predict outcome in patients with DCM [121]. There is no general consensus on the definition of positive response to dobutamine in this specific context, but generally an increase in LVEF from rest to peak stress by ≥5 points or a percentage change from baseline of ≥20% indicates the presence of contractile reserve [122]. Pinamonti et al. [24] investigated 51 patients with DCM with DSE and found that the addition of DSE-derived information added a moderate but significant improvement of sensitivity to a model based only on rest echocardiography, with a general low predictive power. In addition, a reduced CFR during dipyridamole vasodilator test together with absence of contractile reserve provides additional negative prognostic value in DCM patients. CFR on left anterior descending artery less than 2 yields the worse prognosis [123].

In conclusion, echocardiography remains an extremely useful tool for the prognostic stratification of patients with DCM. The approach to echocardiographic interpretation should be holistic and not focused only on the LV systolic function or the regional wall motion abnormalities but also on the possible coexistence of diastolic impairment, valvular defects as functional MR, and other chamber dilatation. A serial echocardiographic assessment is mandatory in patients with DCM in order to capture possible improvements due to medical treatment and adverse progression of the disease, to clarify the possible presence of specific etiologies often characterized by reversibility of the systolic function (as myocarditis or alcoholic cardiomyopathy), and finally to select patients that may benefit from device therapy.

References

1. Mestroni L, Maisch B, McKenna WJ, Schwartz K, Charron P, Rocco C, et al. Guidelines for the study of familial dilated cardiomyopathies. Collaborative Research Group of the European Human and Capital Mobility Project on Familial Dilated Cardiomyopathy. Eur Heart J. 1999;20:93–102.
2. Abate E, Pinamonti B, Porto A. Basic echocardiography in dilated cardiomyopathy. In: Pinamonti B, Sinagra G, editors. Clinical echocardiography and other imaging techniques in cardiomyopathies. New York: Springer; 2014.
3. Pinto YM, Elliott PM, Arbustini E, Adler Y, Anastasakis A, Böhm M, et al. Proposal for a revised definition of dilated cardiomyopathy, hypokinetic non-dilated cardiomyopathy, and its implications for clinical practice: a position statement of the ESC working group on myocardial and pericardial diseases. Eur Heart J. 2016;37:1850–8. https://doi.org/10.1093/eurheartj/ehv727.
4. McNally EM, Mestroni L. Dilated cardiomyopathy: genetic determinants and mechanisms. Circ Res. 2017;121:731–48. https://doi.org/10.1161/CIRCRESAHA.116.309396.
5. Douglas PS, Morrow R, Ioli A, Reichek N. Left ventricular shape, afterload and survival in idiopathic dilated cardiomyopathy. J Am Coll Cardiol. 1989;13:311–5.
6. Gigli M, Stolfo D, Merlo M, Barbati G, Ramani F, Brun F, et al. Insights into mildly dilated cardiomyopathy: temporal evolution and long-term prognosis. Eur J Heart Fail. 2017;19:531–9. https://doi.org/10.1002/ejhf.608.
7. Mestroni L, Morgera T, Miani D, Pinamonti B, Sinagra G, Tanganelli P, et al. Idiopathic left ventricular aneurysm: a clinical and pathological study of a new entity in the spectrum of cardiomyopathies. Postgrad Med J. 1994;70(Suppl 1):S13–20.
8. Günthard J, Stocker F, Bolz D, Jäggi E, Ghisla R, Oberhänsli I, et al. Dilated cardiomyopathy and thrombo-embolism. Eur J Pediatr. 1997;156:3–6.
9. Pinamonti B, Di Lenarda A, Sinagra G, Camerini F. Restrictive left ventricular filling pattern in dilated cardiomyopathy assessed by Doppler echocardiography: clinical, echocardiographic and hemodynamic correlations and prognostic implications. Heart Muscle Disease Study Group. J Am Coll Cardiol. 1993;22:808–15.
10. Pinamonti B, Zecchin M, Di Lenarda A, Gregori D, Sinagra G, Camerini F. Persistence of restrictive left ventricular filling pattern in dilated cardiomyopathy: an ominous prognostic sign. J Am Coll Cardiol. 1997;29:604–12.
11. Gorcsan J III, Abraham T, Agler DA, Bax JJ, Derumeaux G, Grimm RA, et al. Echocardiography for cardiac resynchronization therapy: recommendations for performance and reporting – a report from the American Society of Echocardiography Dyssynchrony Writing Group endorsed by the Heart Rhythm Society. J Am Soc Echocardiogr. 2008;21:191–213. https://doi.org/10.1016/j.echo.2008.01.003.
12. Richardson M, Freemantle N, Calvert MJ, Cleland JG, Tavazzi L, CARE-HF Study Steering Committee and Investigators. Predictors and treatment response with cardiac resynchronization therapy in patients with heart failure characterized by dyssynchrony: a pre-defined analysis from the CARE-HF trial. Eur Heart J. 2007;28:1827–34.
13. De Boeck BW, Meine M, Leenders GE, Teske AJ, van Wessel H, Kirkels JH, et al. Practical and conceptual limitations of tissue Doppler imaging to predict reverse remodelling in cardiac resynchronisation therapy. Eur J Heart Fail. 2008;10:281–90. https://doi.org/10.1016/j.ejheart.2008.02.003.
14. Gorcsan J III. Role of echocardiography to determine candidacy for cardiac resynchronization therapy. Curr Opin Cardiol. 2008;23:16–22. https://doi.org/10.1097/HCO.0b013e3282f2e260.
15. Ponikowski P, Voors AA, Anker SD, Bueno H, Cleland JGF, Coats AJS, et al. 2016 ESC Guidelines for the diagnosis and treatment of acute and chronic heart failure. Eur Heart J. 2016;37:2129–200. https://doi.org/10.1093/eurheartj/ehw128.
16. Junker A, Thayssen P, Nielsen B, Andersen PE. The hemodynamic and prognostic significance of echo-Doppler-proven mitral regurgitation in patients with dilated cardiomyopathy. Cardiology. 1993;83:14–20.

17. Lancellotti P, Tribouilloy C, Hagendorff A, Popescu BA, Edvardsen T, Pierard LA, et al. Recommendations for the echocardiographic assessment of native valvular regurgitation: an executive summary from the European Association of Cardiovascular Imaging. Eur Heart J Cardiovasc Imaging. 2013;14:611–44. https://doi.org/10.1093/ehjci/jet105.
18. Thomas DE, Wheeler R, Yousef ZR, Masani ND. The role of echocardiography in guiding management in dilated cardiomyopathy. Eur J Echocardiogr. 2009;10:iii15–21. https://doi.org/10.1093/ejechocard/jep158.
19. Enriquez-Sarano M, Rossi A, Seward JB, Bailey KR, Tajik AJ. Determinants of pulmonary hypertension in left ventricular dysfunction. J Am Coll Cardiol. 1997;29:153–9.
20. Puwanant S, Priester TC, Mookadam F, Bruce CJ, Redfield MM, Chandrasekaran K. Right ventricular function in patients with preserved and reduced ejection fraction heart failure. Eur J Echocardiogr. 2009;10:733–7. https://doi.org/10.1093/ejechocard/jep052.
21. Pavlicek M, Wahl A, Rutz T, de Marchi SF, Hille R, Wustmann K, et al. Right ventricular systolic function assessment: rank of echocardiographic methods vs. cardiac magnetic resonance imaging. Eur J Echocardiogr. 2011;12:871–80. https://doi.org/10.1093/ejechocard/jer138.
22. Dini FL, Nuti R, Barsotti L, Baldini U, Dell'Anna R, Micheli G. Doppler-derived mitral and pulmonary venous flow variables are predictors of pulmonary hypertension in dilated cardiomyopathy. Echocardiography. 2002;19:457–65.
23. Lancellotti P, Pellikka PA, Budts W, Chaudhry FA, Donal E, Dulgheru R, et al. The clinical use of stress echocardiography in non-ischaemic heart disease: recommendations from the European Association of Cardiovascular Imaging and the American Society of Echocardiography. J Am Soc Echocardiogr. 2017;30:101–38.
24. Pinamonti B, Perkan A, Di Lenarda A, Gregori D, Sinagra G. Dobutamine echocardiography in idiopathic dilated cardiomyopathy: clinical and prognostic implications. Eur J Heart Fail. 2002;4:49–61.
25. Parsai C, Bijnens B, Sutherland GR, Baltabaeva A, Claus P, Marciniak M, et al. Toward understanding response to cardiac resynchronization therapy: left ventricular dyssynchrony is only one of multiple mechanisms. Eur Heart J. 2009;30:940–9. https://doi.org/10.1093/eurheartj/ehn481.
26. Ennezat PV, Maréchaux S, Huerre C, Deklunder G, Asseman P, Jude B, et al. Exercise does not enhance the prognostic value of Doppler echocardiography in patients with left ventricular systolic dysfunction and functional mitral regurgitation at rest. Am Heart J. 2008;155:752–7. https://doi.org/10.1016/j.ahj.2007.11.022.
27. Merlo M, Cannatà A, Gobbo M, Stolfo D, Elliott PM, Sinagra G. Evolving concepts in dilated cardiomyopathy. Eur J Heart Fail. 2018;20:228–39. https://doi.org/10.1002/ejhf.1103.
28. Japp AG, Gulati A, Cook SA, Cowie MR, Prasad SK. The diagnosis and evaluation of dilated cardiomyopathy. J Am Coll Cardiol. 2016;67:2996–3010. https://doi.org/10.1016/j.jacc.2016.03.590.
29. Jan MF, Tajik AJ. Modern imaging techniques in cardiomyopathies. Circ Res. 2017;121:874–91. https://doi.org/10.1161/CIRCRESAHA.117.309600.
30. Otterstad JE, Froeland G, Sutton SJ, Holme I. Accuracy and reproducibility of biplane two-dimensional echocardiograph measurements of left ventricular dimensions and function. Eur Heart J. 1997;18:507–13.
31. Lang RM, Badano LP, Tsang W, Adams DH, Agricola E, Buck T, et al. EAE/ASE recommendation for image acquisition and display using three dimensional echocardiography. Eur Heart J Cardiovasc Imaging. 2012;13:1–46. https://doi.org/10.1016/j.echo.2011.11.010.
32. Lang RM, Badano LP, Mor-Avi V, Afilalo J, Armstrong A, Ernande L, et al. Recommendation for cardiac chamber quantification by echocardiograph in adults: an update from American Society of Echocardiography and the European Association of Cardiovascular Imaging. J Am Soc Echocardiogr. 2015;28:1–39. https://doi.org/10.1016/j.echo.2014.10.003.
33. Mu Y, Chen L, Tang Q, Ayoufu G. Real time three-dimensional echocardiographic assessment of left ventricular regional systolic function and dyssynchrony in patients with dilated cardiomyopathy. Echocardiography. 2010;27:415–20. https://doi.org/10.1111/j.1540-8175.2009.01028.x.

34. Gutiérrez-Chico JL, Zamorano JL, Pérez de Isla L, Orejas M, Almería C, Rodrigo JL, et al. Comparison of left ventricular volumes and ejection fraction measured by three-dimensional echocardiography versus by two-dimensional echocardiography and cardiac magnetic resonance in patient with various cardiomyopathies. Am J Cardiol. 2005;95:809–13.
35. Shiota T, McCarthy PM, White RD, Qin JX, Greenberg NL, Flamm SD, et al. Initial clinical experience of real-time three-dimensional echocardiography in patients with ischemic and idiopathic dilated cardiomyopathy. Am J Cardiol. 1999;84:1068–73.
36. Gopal AS, Schnellbaecher MJ, Shen Z, Boxt LM, Katz J, King DL. Freehand three-dimensional echocardiography for determination of left ventricular volume and mass in patients with abnormal ventricles: comparison with magnetic resonance imaging. J Am Soc Echocardiogr. 1997;10:853–61.
37. Mor-Avi V, Sugeng L, Weinert L, MacEneaney P, Caiani EG, Koch R, et al. Fast measurements of left ventricular mass with real-time three-dimensional echocardiography: comparison with magnetic resonance imaging. Circulation. 2004;110:1814–8.
38. Shimada YJ, Shiota T. A meta-analysis and investigation for the source of bias of left ventricular volumes and function by three-dimensional echocardiography in comparison with magnetic resonance imaging. Am J Cardiol. 2011;107:126–38. https://doi.org/10.1016/j.amjcard.2010.08.058.
39. Mor-Avi V, Jenkins C, Kühl HP, Nesser HJ, Marwick T, Franke A, et al. Real-time 3-dimensional echocardiography quantification of left ventricular volumes: multicenter study for validation with magnetic resonance imaging and investigation of source of error. J Am Coll Cardiol Img. 2008;1:413–23. https://doi.org/10.1016/j.jcmg.2008.02.009.
40. Shan K, Bick RJ, Poindexter BJ, Shimoni S, Letsou GV, Reardon MJ, et al. Relation of tissue Doppler derived myocardial velocities to myocardial structure and beta-adrenergic receptor density in humans. J Am Coll Cardiol. 2011;36:891–6.
41. Takamura T, Dohi K, Onishi K, Tanabe M, Sugiura E, Nakajima H, et al. Left ventricular contraction-relaxation coupling in normal, hypertrophic and failing myocardium quantified by speckle-tracking global strain and strain rate imaging. J Am Soc Echocardiogr. 2010;23:747–54. https://doi.org/10.1016/j.echo.2010.04.005.
42. Meluzin J, Spinarova L, Hude P, Krejci J, Poloczkova H, Podrouzkova H, et al. Left ventricular mechanics in idiopathic dilated cardiomyopathy: systolic-diastolic coupling and torsion. J Am Soc Echocardiogr. 2009;22:486–93. https://doi.org/10.1016/j.echo.2009.02.022.
43. Zeng S, Zhou QC, Peng QH, Cao DM, Tian LQ, Ao K, et al. Assessment of regional myocardial function in patients with dilated cardiomyopathy by velocity vector imaging. Echocardiography. 2009;26:163–70. https://doi.org/10.1111/j.1540-8175.2008.00797.x.
44. Jasaityte R, Dandel M, Lehmkuhl H, Hetzer R. Prediction of short-term outcomes in patients with idiopathic dilated cardiomyopathy referred for transplantation using standard echocardiography and strain imaging. Transplant Proc. 2009;41:277–80. https://doi.org/10.1016/j.transproceed.2008.10.083.
45. Friedberg MK, Slorach C. Relation between left ventricular regional radial function and radial wall motion abnormalities using two-dimensional speckle tracking in children with idiopathic dilated cardiomyopathy. Am J Cardiol. 2008;102:335–9. https://doi.org/10.1016/j.amjcard.2008.03.064.
46. Haugaa KH, Goebel B, Dahlslett T, Meyer K, Jung C, Lauten A, et al. Risk assessment of ventricular arrhythmias in patients with nonischemic dilated cardiomyopathy by strain echocardiography. J Am Soc Echocardiogr. 2012;25:667–73. https://doi.org/10.1016/j.echo.2012.02.004.
47. Spartera M, Damascelli A, Mozes F, De Cobelli F, La Canna G. Three-dimensional speckle tracking longitudinal strain is related to myocardial fibrosis determined by late-gadolinium enhancement. Int J Cardiovasc Imaging. 2017;33:1351–60. https://doi.org/10.1007/s10554-017-1115-1.
48. Russel IK, Gotte MJ, Bronzwaer JG, Knaapen P, Paulus WJ, van Rossum AC. Left ventricular torsion: an expanding role in the analysis of myocardial dysfunction. JACC Cardiovasc Imaging. 2009;2:648–55. https://doi.org/10.1016/j.jcmg.2009.03.001.

49. Sveric KM, Ulbrich S, Rady M, Ruf T, Kvakan H, Strasser RH, et al. Three-dimensional left ventricular torsion in patients with dilated cardiomyopathy. Circ J. 2017;81:529–36. https://doi.org/10.1253/circj.CJ-16-0965.
50. Matsumoto K, Tanaka H, Tatsumi K, Miyoshi T, Hiraishi M, Kaneko A, et al. Left ventricular dyssynchrony using three-dimensional speckle-tracking imaging as a determinant of torsional mechanics in patients with idiopathic dilated cardiomyopathy. Am J Cardiol. 2012;109:1197–205. https://doi.org/10.1016/j.amjcard.2011.11.059.
51. Sade LE, Demir Ö, Atar I, Müderrinsoglu H, Özin B. Effect of mechanical dyssynchrony and cardiac resynchronization therapy on the left ventricular rotational mechanics. Am J Cardiol. 2008;101:1163–9. https://doi.org/10.1016/j.amjcard.2007.11.069.
52. Jenkins C, Bricknell K, Hanekom L, Marwick TH. Reproducibility of accuracy of echocardiographic measurements of left ventricular parameters using real-time three-dimensional echocardiography. J Am Coll Cardiol. 2004;44:878–86.
53. Qin JX, Jones M, Travaglini A, Song JM, Li J, White RD, et al. The accuracy of left ventricular mass determined by real-time three-dimensional echocardiography in chronic animal and clinical studies: a comparison with postmortem examination and magnetic resonance imaging. J Am Soc Echocardiogr. 2005;18:1037–43.
54. Chung ES, Leon AR, Tavazzi L, Sun JP, Nihoyannopoulos P, Merlino J, et al. Results of the Predictors of Response to CRT (PROSPECT) trial. Circulation. 2008;117:2608–16. https://doi.org/10.1161/CIRCULATIONAHA.107.743120.
55. Marsan NA, Bleeker GB, Ypenburg C, Ghio S, van de Veire NR, Holman ER, et al. Real-time three-dimensional echocardiography permits quantification of left ventricular mechanical dyssynchrony and predicts acute response to cardiac resynchronization therapy. J Cardiovasc Electrophysiol. 2008;19:392–9. https://doi.org/10.1111/j.1540-8167.2007.01056.x.
56. Marsan NA, Bleeker GB, Ypenburg C, Van Bommel RJ, Ghio S, Van de Veire NR, et al. Real-time three-dimensional echocardiography as a novel approach to assess left ventricular and left atrium reverse remodeling and to predict response to cardiac resynchronization therapy. Heart Rhythm. 2008;5:1257–64. https://doi.org/10.1016/j.hrthm.2008.05.021.
57. Kleijn SA, van Dijk J, de Cock CC, Allaart CP, van Rossum AC, Kamp O. Assessment of intraventricular mechanical dyssynchrony and prediction of response to cardiac resynchronization therapy: comparison between tissue Doppler imaging and real-time three-dimensional echocardiography. J Am Soc Echocardiogr. 2009;22:1047–54. https://doi.org/10.1016/j.echo.2009.06.012.
58. Soliman OI, Geleijnse ML, Theuns DA, van Dalen BM, Vletter WB, Jordaens LJ, et al. Usefulness of left ventricular systolic dyssynchrony by real-time three-dimensional echocardiography to predict long-term response to cardiac resynchronization therapy. Am J Cardiol. 2009;103:1586–91. https://doi.org/10.1016/j.amjcard.2009.01.372.
59. Delgado V, Ypenburg C, van Bommel RJ, Tops LF, Mollema SA, Marsan NA, et al. Assessment of left ventricular dyssynchrony by speckle tracking strain imaging comparison between longitudinal, circumferential, and radial strain in cardiac resynchronization therapy. J Am Coll Cardiol. 2008;51:1944–52. https://doi.org/10.1016/j.jacc.2008.02.040.
60. Tanaka H, Nesser HJ, Buck T, Oyenuga O, Jánosi RA, Winter S, et al. Dyssynchrony by speckle-tracking echocardiography and response to cardiac resynchronization therapy: results of the Speckle Tracking and Resynchronization (STAR) study. Eur Heart J. 2010;31:1690–700. https://doi.org/10.1093/eurheartj/ehq213.
61. D'Andrea A, Caso P, Scarafile R, Riegler L, Salerno G, Castaldo F, et al. Effects of global longitudinal strain and total scar burden on response to cardiac resynchronization therapy in patients with ischaemic dilated cardiomyopathy. Eur J Heart Fail. 2009;11:58–67. https://doi.org/10.1093/eurjhf/hfn010.
62. Tanaka H, Hara H, Saba S, Gorcsan J III. Usefulness of three-dimensional speckle tracking strain to quantify dyssynchrony and the site of latest mechanical activation. Am J Cardiol. 2010;105:235–42. https://doi.org/10.1016/j.amjcard.2009.09.010.
63. Mullens W, Borowski AG, Curtin RJ, Thomas JD, Tang WH. Tissue Doppler imaging in the estimation of intracardiac filling pressure in decompensated patients with

advanced systolic heart failure. Circulation. 2009;119:62–70. https://doi.org/10.1161/CIRCULATIONAHA.108.779223.

64. Meluzin J, Spinarova L, Hude P, Krejci J, Podrouzkova H, Pesl M, et al. Estimation of left ventricular filling pressure by speckle tracking echocardiography in patients with idiopathic dilated cardiomyopathy. Eur J Echocardiogr. 2011;12:11–8. https://doi.org/10.1093/ejechocard/jeq088.
65. Cameli M, Lisi M, Mondillo S, Padeletti M, Ballo P, Tsioulpas C, et al. Left atrial longitudinal strain by speckle tracking echocardiography correlates well with left ventricular filling pressures in patients with heart failure. Cardiovasc Ultrasound. 2010;8:14. https://doi.org/10.1186/1476-7120-8-14.
66. Guler A, Tigen KM, Dundar C, Karaahmet T, Karabay CY, Aung SM, et al. Left atrial deformation and nonischaemic dilated cardiomyopathy. A 2D speckle-tracking imaging study. Herz. 2014;39:251–7. https://doi.org/10.1007/s00059-013-3817-z.
67. D'Andrea A, Caso P, Romano S, Scarafile R, Cuomo S, Salerno G, et al. Association between left atrial myocardial function and exercise capacity in patients with either idiopathic or ischemic dilated cardiomyopathy: a two-dimensional speckle strain study. Int J Cardiol. 2009;132:354–63. https://doi.org/10.1016/j.ijcard.2007.11.102.
68. Thavendiranathan P, Phelan D, Collier P, Thomas JD, Flamm SD, Marwick TH. Quantitative assessment of mitral regurgitation: how best to do it. JACC Cardiovasc Imaging. 2012;5:1161–75. https://doi.org/10.1016/j.jcmg.2012.07.013.
69. Kahlert P, Plicht B, Schenk IM, Janosi RA, Erbel R, Bluck T. Direct assessment of size and shape of non circular vena contracta area in functional versus organic mitral regurgitation using real-time three-dimensional echocardiography. J Am Soc Echocardiogr. 2008;21:912–21. https://doi.org/10.1016/j.echo.2008.02.003.
70. Otsuji Y, Handschumacher MD, Schwammenthal E, Jiang L, Song JK, Guerrero JL, et al. Insight from three-dimensional echocardiography into the mechanism of functional mitral regurgitation: direct in vivo demonstration of altered leaflet tethering geometry. Circulation. 1997;96:1999–2008.
71. Buck T, Plicht B. Real-time three dimensional echocardiographic assessment of severity of mitral regurgitation using proximal isovelocity surface area and vena contracta area method. lesson we learned and clinical implication. Curr Cardiovasc Imaging Rep. 2015;8:38.
72. Iwakura K, Ito H, Kawano S, Okamura A, Kurotobi T, Date M, et al. Comparison of orifice area by transthoracic three-dimensional Doppler echocardiography versus proximal isovelocity surface area (PISA) method for assessment of mitral regurgitation. Am J Cardiol. 2006;97:1630–7.
73. Marsan NA, Westenberg JJ, Ypenburg C, Delgado V, van Bommel RJ, Roes SD, et al. Quantification of functional mitral regurgitation by real-time 3D echocardiography. JACC Cardiovasc Imaging. 2009;2:1245–52. https://doi.org/10.1016/j.jcmg.2009.07.006.
74. Acquila I, Fernandéz-Golfín C, Rincon LM, Gonzales A, Garcia-Martin A, Hinojar R, et al. Fully automated software for mitral annulus evaluation in chronic mitral regurgitation by 3-dimensional transesophageal echocardiography. Medicine (Baltimore). 2015;95:e5387. https://doi.org/10.1097/MD.0000000000005387.
75. Acquila I, González A, Fernandéz-Golfín C, Rincon LM, Casas E, Garcia A, et al. Reproducibility of a novel echocardiographic 3D automated software for the assessment of mitral valve anatomy. Cardiovasc Ultrasound. 2016;14:17. https://doi.org/10.1186/s12947-016-0061-8.
76. Lancellotti P, Zamorano JL, Vannan M. Imaging challenges in secondary mitral regurgitation: unsolved issue and perspectives. Circ Cardiovasc Imaging. 2014;7:735–46. https://doi.org/10.1161/CIRCIMAGING.114.000992.
77. Wunderlich NC, Siegel RJ. Peri-interventional echo assessment for the MitraClip procedure. Eur Heart J Cardiovasc Imaging. 2013;14:935–49. https://doi.org/10.1093/ehjci/jet060.
78. Salerno G, D'Andrea A, Bossone E, Scarafile R, Riegler L, Di Salvo G, et al. Association between right ventricular two-dimensional strain and exercise capacity in patients with either idiopathic or ischemic dilated cardiomyopathy. J Cardiovasc Med (Hagerstown). 2011;12:625–34. https://doi.org/10.2459/JCM.0b013e328349a268.

79. D'Andrea A, Gravino R, Riegler L, Salerno G, Scarafile R, Romano M, et al. Right ventricular ejection fraction and left ventricular dyssynchrony by 3D echo correlate with functional impairment in patients with dilated cardiomyopathy. J Card Fail. 2011;17:309–17. https://doi.org/10.1016/j.cardfail.2010.11.005.
80. Rapezzi C, Arbustini E, Caforio AL, Charron P, Gimeno-Blanes J, Heliö T, et al. Diagnostic work-up in cardiomyopathies: bridging the gap between clinical phenotypes and final diagnosis. A position statement from the ESC Working Group on Myocardial and Pericardial Diseases. Eur Heart J. 2013;34:1448–58. https://doi.org/10.1093/eurheartj/ehs397.
81. Bozkurt B, Colvin M, Cook J, Cooper LT, Deswal A, Fonarow GC, et al. Current diagnostic and treatment strategies for specific dilated cardiomyopathies: a scientific statement from the American Heart Association. Circulation. 2016;134:579–646.
82. Bobbo M, Pinamonti B, Merlo M, Stolfo D, Iorio A, Ramani F, et al. Comparison of patient characteristics and course of hypertensive hypokinetic cardiomyopathy versus idiopathic dilated cardiomyopathy. Am J Cardiol. 2017;119:483–9. https://doi.org/10.1016/j.amjcard.2016.10.014.
83. Pinamonti B, Alberti E, Cigalotto A, Dreas L, Salvi A, Silvestri F, et al. Echocardiographic findings in myocarditis. Am J Cardiol. 1988;62:285–91.
84. Dragos AM, Pinamonti B, Abate E. Basic echocardiography in arrhythmogenic right ventricular cardiomyopathy. In: Pinamonti B, Sinagra G, editors. Clinical echocardiography and other imaging techniques in cardiomyopathies. New York: Springer; 2014.
85. Blake LM, Scheinman MM, Higgins CB. MR features of arrhythmogenic right ventricular dysplasia. AJR Am J Roentgenol. 1994;162:809–12.
86. Finocchiaro G, Pinamonti B, Abate E. Basic echocardiography in hypertrophic cardiomyopathy. In: Pinamonti B, Sinagra G, editors. Clinical echocardiography and other imaging techniques in cardiomyopathies. New York: Springer; 2014.
87. Moretti M, Fabris E, Finocchiaro G, et al. Infiltrative/storage cardiomyopathies: clinical assessment and imaging in diagnosis and patient management. In: Pinamonti B, Sinagra G, editors. Clinical echocardiography and other imaging techniques in cardiomyopathies. New York: Springer; 2014.
88. Martin CA, Lambiase PD. Pathophysiology, diagnosis and treatment of tachycardiomyopathy. Heart. 2017;103:1543–52. https://doi.org/10.1136/heartjnl-2016-310391.
89. Moretti M, Merlo M, Barbati G, Di Lenarda A, Brun F, Pinamonti B, et al. Prognostic impact of familial screening in dilated cardiomyopathy. Eur J Heart Fail. 2010;12:922–7. https://doi.org/10.1093/eurjhf/hfq093.
90. Mahon NG, Murphy RT, MacRae CA, Caforio AL, Elliott PM, McKenna WJ. Echocardiographic evaluation in asymptomatic relatives of patients with dilated cardiomyopathy reveals preclinical disease. Ann Intern Med. 2005;143:108–15.
91. Murtaza G, Virk HUH, Khalid M, Rahman Z, Sitwala P, Schoondyke J, et al. Role of speckle tracking echocardiography in dilated cardiomyopathy: a review. Cureus. 2017;9:e1372. https://doi.org/10.7759/cureus.1372.
92. Merlo M, Pyxaras SA, Pinamonti B, Barbati G, Di Lenarda A, Sinagra G. Prevalence and prognostic significance of left ventricular reverse remodeling in dilated cardiomyopathy receiving tailored medical treatment. J Am Coll Cardiol. 2011;57:1468–76. https://doi.org/10.1016/j.jacc.2010.11.030.
93. Merlo M, Pivetta A, Pinamonti B, Stolfo D, Zecchin M, Barbati G, et al. Long-term prognostic impact of therapeutic strategies in patients with idiopathic dilated cardiomyopathy: changing mortality over the last 30 years. Eur J Heart Fail. 2014;16:317–24. https://doi.org/10.1002/ejhf.16.
94. Zecchin M, Lenarda AD, Bonin M, Mazzone C, Zanchi C, Di Chiara C, et al. Incidence and predictors of sudden cardiac death during long-term follow-up in patients with dilated cardiomyopathy on optimal medical therapy. Ital Heart J. 2001;2:213–21.
95. Zecchin M, Merlo M, Pivetta A, Barbati G, Lutman C, Gregori D, et al. How can optimization of medical treatment avoid unnecessary implantable cardioverter-defibrillator implantations in patients with idiopathic dilated cardiomyopathy presenting with "SCD-HeFT criteria?". Am J Cardiol. 2012;109:729–35. https://doi.org/10.1016/j.amjcard.2011.10.033.

96. Stolfo D, De Luca A, Morea G, Merlo M, Vitrella G, Caiffa T, et al. Predicting device failure after percutaneous repair of functional mitral regurgitation in advanced heart failure: implications for patient selection. Int J Cardiol. 2018;257:182–7. https://doi.org/10.1016/j.ijcard.2018.01.009.
97. Di Lenarda A, Secoli G, Perkan A, Gregori D, Lardieri G, Pinamonti B, et al. Changing mortality in dilated cardiomyopathy. The Heart Muscle Disease Study Group. Br Heart J. 1994;72(6 Suppl):S46–51.
98. Sinagra G, Sabbadini G, Di Lenarda A, Gortan R, Massa L, Carniel E, et al. [Changes in medical treatment of heart failure in the light of large clinical trials]. Ital Heart J Suppl. 2001;2:97–115.
99. Di Lenarda A, Pinamonti B, Mestroni L, Salvi A, Sabbadini G, Gregori D, et al. [The natural history of dilated cardiomyopathy: a review of the Heart Muscle Disease Registry of Trieste]. Ital Heart J Suppl. 2004;5:253–66.
100. Faris R, Coats AJ, Henein MY. Echocardiography-derived variables predict outcome in patients with nonischemic dilated cardiomyopathy with or without a restrictive filling pattern. Am Heart J. 2002;144:343–50.
101. Puggia I, Merlo M, Barbati G, Rowland TJ, Stolfo D, Gigli M et al. Natural history of dilated cardiomyopathy in children. J Am Heart Assoc. 2016;5(7). https://doi.org/10.1161/JAHA.116.003450.
102. Zambon E, Iorio A, Di Nora C, Carriere C, Abate E, Merlo M, et al. Left ventricular function and exercise performance in idiopathic dilated cardiomyopathy: role of tissue Doppler imaging. J Cardiovasc Med (Hagerstown). 2017;18:230–6. https://doi.org/10.2459/JCM.0000000000000411.
103. Galrinho A, Branco L, Soares R, Timóteo A, Abreu J, Leal A, et al. Prognostic implications of tissue Doppler in patients with dilated cardiomyopathy. Rev Port Cardiol. 2006;25:781–93.
104. Soliman OI, Theuns DA, ten Cate FJ, Anwar AM, Nemes A, Vletter WB, et al. Baseline predictors of cardiac events after cardiac resynchronization therapy in patients with heart failure secondary to ischemic or nonischemic etiology. Am J Cardiol. 2007;100:464–9.
105. Galrinho A, Branco LM, Soares RM, Miranda F, Leal A, Ferreira RC. Left atrial volume: an old echocardiographic measure with renewed prognostic significance: a study in patients with dilated cardiomyopathy. Rev Port Cardiol. 2009;28:1049–60.
106. Rossi A, Dini FL, Faggiano P, Agricola E, Cicoira M, Frattini S, et al. Independent prognostic value of functional mitral regurgitation in patients with heart failure. A quantitative analysis of 1256 patients with ischaemic and non-ischaemic dilated cardiomyopathy. Heart. 2011;97:1675–80. https://doi.org/10.1136/hrt.2011.225789.
107. van Bommel RJ, Marsan NA, Delgado V, Borleffs CJ, van Rijnsoever EP, Schalij MJ, et al. Cardiac resynchronization therapy as a therapeutic option in patients with moderate-severe functional mitral regurgitation and high operative risk. Circulation. 2011;124:912–9. https://doi.org/10.1161/CIRCULATIONAHA.110.009803.
108. Stolfo D, Merlo M, Pinamonti B, Poli S, Gigli M, Barbati G, et al. Early improvement of functional mitral regurgitation in patients with idiopathic dilated cardiomyopathy. Am J Cardiol. 2015;115:1137–43. https://doi.org/10.1016/j.amjcard.2015.01.549.
109. Stolfo D, Tonet E, Barbati G, Gigli M, Pinamonti B, Zecchin M, et al. Acute hemodynamic response to cardiac resynchronization in dilated cardiomyopathy: effect on late mitral regurgitation. Pacing Clin Electrophysiol. 2015;38:1287–96. https://doi.org/10.1111/pace.12731.
110. Kamperidis V, van Wijngaarden SE, van Rosendael PJ, Kong WKF, Regeer MV, van der Kley F, et al. Mitral valve repair for secondary mitral regurgitation in non-ischaemic dilated cardiomyopathy is associated with left ventricular reverse remodelling and increase of forward flow. Eur Heart J Cardiovasc Imaging. 2018;19:208–15. https://doi.org/10.1093/ehjci/jex011.
111. Ghio S, Recusani F, Klersy C, Sebastiani R, Laudisa ML, Campana C, et al. Prognostic usefulness of the tricuspid annular plane systolic excursion in patients with congestive heart failure secondary to idiopathic or ischemic dilated cardiomyopathy. Am J Cardiol. 2000;85:837–42.
112. Merlo M, Gobbo M, Stolfo D, Losurdo P, Ramani F, Barbati G, et al. The prognostic impact of the evolution of RV function in idiopathic DCM. JACC Cardiovasc Imaging. 2016;9:1034–42. https://doi.org/10.1016/j.jcmg.2016.01.027.

113. Pueschner A, Chattranukulchai P, Heitner JF, Shah DJ, Hayes B, Rehwald W, et al. The prevalence, correlates, and impact on cardiac mortality of right ventricular dysfunction in nonischemic cardiomyopathy. JACC Cardiovasc Imaging. 2017;10(10 Pt B):1225–36. https://doi.org/10.1016/j.jcmg.2017.06.013.
114. Stolfo D, Tonet E, Merlo M, Barbati G, Gigli M, Pinamonti B, et al. Early right ventricular response to cardiac resynchronization therapy: impact on clinical outcomes. Eur J Heart Fail. 2016;18:205–13. https://doi.org/10.1002/ejhf.450.
115. Hung J, Koelling T, Semigran MJ, Dec GW, Levine RA, Di Salvo TG. Usefulness of echocardiographic determined tricuspid regurgitation in predicting event-free survival in severe heart failure secondary to idiopathic-dilated cardiomyopathy or to ischemic cardiomyopathy. Am J Cardiol. 1998;82:1301–3, A10.
116. Cleland JG, Daubert JC, Erdmann E, Freemantle N, Gras D, Kappenberger L, et al. The effect of cardiac resynchronization on morbidity and mortality in heart failure. N Engl J Med. 2005;352:1539–49.
117. Ruschitzka F, Abraham WT, Singh JP, Bax JJ, Borer JS, Brugada J, et al. Cardiac-resynchronization therapy in heart failure with a narrow QRS complex. N Engl J Med. 2013;369:1395–405. https://doi.org/10.1056/NEJMoa1306687.
118. Stankovic I, Prinz C, Ciarka A, Daraban AM, Kotrc M, Aarones M, et al. Relationship of visually assessed apical rocking and septal flash to response and long-term survival following cardiac resynchronization therapy (PREDICT-CRT). Eur Heart J Cardiovasc Imaging. 2016;17:262–9. https://doi.org/10.1093/ehjci/jev288.
119. Abduch MC, Salgo I, Tsang W, Vieira ML, Cruz V, Lima M, et al. Myocardial deformation by speckle tracking in severe dilated cardiomyopathy. Arq Bras Cardiol. 2012;99:834–43.
120. Losurdo P, Stolfo D, Merlo M, Barbati G, Gobbo M, Gigli M et al. Early arrhythmic events in idiopathic dilated cardiomyopathy. JACC Clin Electrophysiol. 2016;2(5). https://doi.org/10.1016/j.jacep.2016.05.002.
121. Drozd J, Krzeminska-Pakula M, Plewka M, Ciesielczyk M, Kasprzak JD. Prognostic value of low-dose dobutamine echocardiography in patients with dilated cardiomyopathy. Chest. 2002;121:1216–22.
122. Neskovic AN, Otasevic P. Stress-echocardiography in idiopathic dilated cardiomyopathy: instructions for use. Cardiovasc Ultrasound. 2005;3:3. https://doi.org/10.1186/1476-7120-3-3.
123. Rigo F, Gherardi S, Galderisi M, Pratali L, Cortigiani L, Sicari R, et al. The prognostic impact of coronary flow reserve assessed by Doppler echocardiography in non ischemic dilated cardiomyopathy. Eur Heart J. 2006;27:1319–23.

8

Role of Cardiac Imaging: Cardiac Magnetic Resonance and Cardiac Computed Tomography

Giancarlo Vitrella, Giorgio Faganello, Gaetano Morea, Lorenzo Pagnan, Manuel Belgrano, and Maria Assunta Cova

Abbreviations and Acronyms

2D	Two-dimensional
CAD	Coronary artery disease
CCT	Cardiac computed tomography
CMR	Cardiac magnetic resonance
CRT	Cardiac resynchronization therapy
CT	Computed tomography
CTCA	Computed tomography coronary angiography
DCM	Dilated cardiomyopathy
ECV	Extracellular volume
FFR	Fractional flow reserve
GRE	Global relative enhancement
HF	Heart failure
ICD	Implantable cardioverter-defibrillator
LAV	Left atrial volume
LGE	Late gadolinium enhancement
LIE	Late iodine enhancement
LLC	Lake Louise criteria
LV	Left ventricular
LVEF	Left ventricular ejection fraction

G. Vitrella (✉) · G. Faganello · G. Morea
Cardiovascular Department, Azienda Sanitaria Universitaria Integrata di Trieste (ASUITS), Trieste, Italy
e-mail: giorgio.faganello@asuits.sanita.fvg.it

L. Pagnan · M. Belgrano · M. A. Cova
Diagnostic and Interventional Radiology Department, Azienda Sanitaria Universitaria Integrata di Trieste (ASUITS), Trieste, Italy
e-mail: manuel.belgrano@asuits.sanita.fvg.it; cova@gnbts.univ.trieste.it

LVRR	Left ventricular reverse remodeling
MOLLI	Modified look-locker inversion recovery
RV	Right ventricular
RVEF	Right ventricular ejection fraction
SAPPHIRE	Saturation pulse prepared heart rate-independent inversion recovery
SASHA	Saturation recovery single-shot acquisition
SCD	Sudden cardiac death
Sh-MOLLI	Shortened modified look-locker inversion recovery
SSFP	Steady-state free precession
STIR	Short tau inversion recovery

8.1 Cardiac Magnetic Resonance

Cardiac magnetic resonance (CMR) has become an extensively validated noninvasive diagnostic imaging tool. Through its ability to assess cardiac morphology and function, and to characterize myocardial tissue in a reliable and reproducible fashion, it plays a pivotal role in the management of patients with dilated cardiomyopathy (DCM). In particular, it increases diagnostic accuracy and it aids in determining the etiology of left ventricular (LV) dysfunction and in prognostic stratification.

8.2 Diagnostic Accuracy

Steady-state free precession (SSFP) sequences are cornerstone sequences in CMR. Owing to their elevated spatial, temporal, and contrast resolution and lesser approximation in delineating endocardial borders than two-dimensional (2D) echocardiography, they minimize operator dependence and variability of intra- and interobserver reproducibility. SSFP cine imaging is currently regarded as the gold standard imaging technique for the evaluation of LV volume and systolic function [1, 2], as it is not affected by the geometric assumptions used in 2D echocardiography for the LV (such as the area-length method) [3] (Fig. 8.1). In addition, the precise identification of endocardial borders allows more accurate and reliable evaluation of the extent of non-compacted myocardium than does 2D echocardiography, thus allowing a more precise diagnosis of myocardial non-compaction [4] (Fig. 8.2). CMR also allows for accurate and reproducible, noninvasive measurement of the left atrial [5, 6] and right ventricular volume and function [7, 8].

LV thrombus is a potential complication of severe LV dysfunction. Late gadolinium enhancement (LGE) CMR imaging is the most accurate imaging modality to detect left ventricular thrombus [9], in particular when acquiring LGE sequences with a long inversion time (compared to that needed to null normal myocardium) in order to selectively null the avascular thrombus [10] (Fig. 8.3).

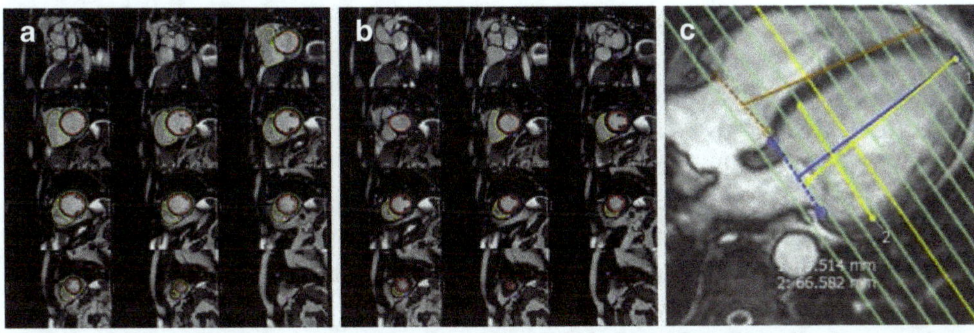

Fig. 8.1 Calculation of LV- and RVEF in MR with SSFP cine sequences. Diastolic (**a**) and systolic (**b**) endocardial contours are outlined in multislice short-axis cine runs covering the entirety of the ventricles (**c**); slices are 8–10mm apart. Diastolic and systolic volumes are thus obtained

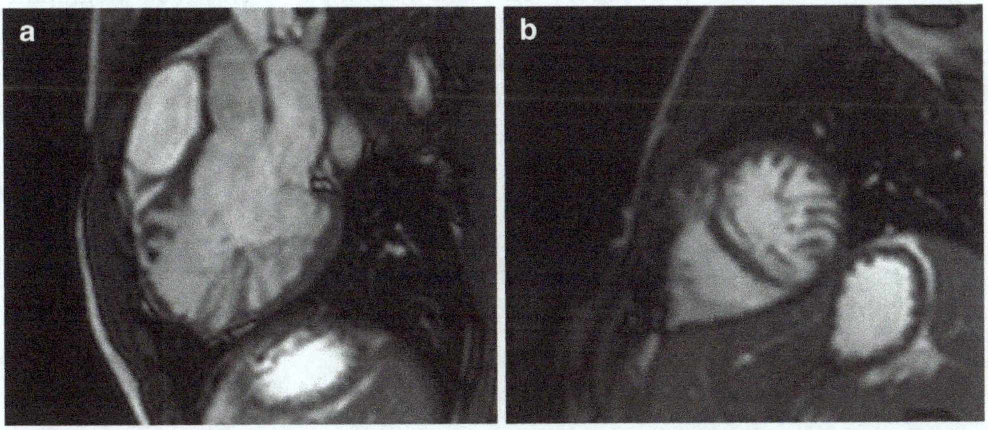

Fig. 8.2 SSFP imaging of left ventricular non-compaction in three-chamber (**a**) and short-axis (**b**) views

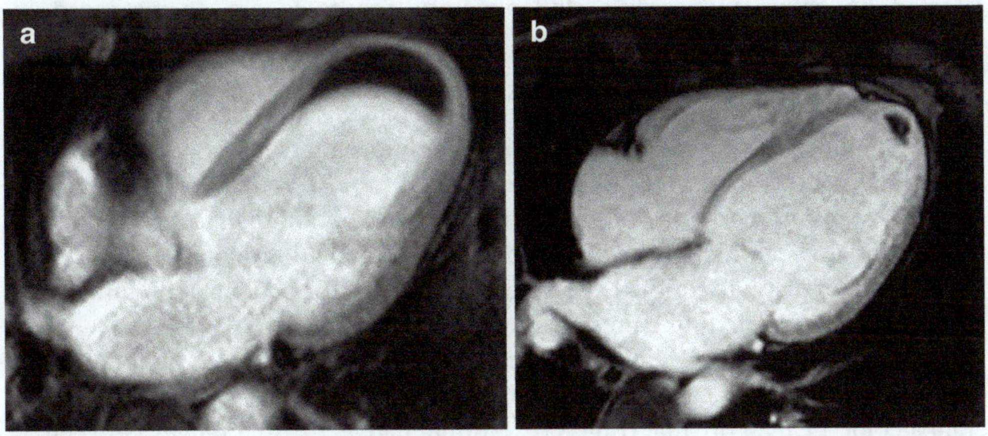

Fig. 8.3 Inversion recovery images with long inversion time in four chamber of the left ventricular thrombus in patients with left ventricular dysfunction secondary to myocardial infarction (**a**), and myocarditis presenting as heart failure (**b**)

8.3 Differential Diagnosis

DCM is a condition characterized by LV dilatation and dysfunction and may represent the end stage of multiple cardiac disease processes of different etiology. The origin may be ischemic, inflammatory, infectious, hypertensive, or idiopathic. Accurate diagnostic characterization of DCM is of foremost importance in order to guide tailored treatment for patients affected by this condition. CMR is an important noninvasive imaging tool that helps to characterize the etiology of DCM. This is achieved by evaluating the presence and distribution of macroscopic myocardial fibrosis with LGE sequences (Fig. 8.3 differential diagnosis). In particular, LGE is usually found in patients with LV dysfunction secondary to coronary artery disease. The pattern of distribution follows coronary perfusion territories, and the scar may be subendocardial or transmural. In patients presenting with de novo acute heart failure (HF) and no clinical or electrocardiographic suggestion of ischemic etiology, LGE-CMR is sensitive and specific for the presence of underlying significant coronary artery disease (CAD) [11, 12]. Conversely, LGE is absent in most patients with left ventricular dysfunction of nonischemic origin. If present in DCM, LGE is typically found in a mid-wall distribution without an apparent correlation to coronary perfusion territories [13, 14] (Fig. 8.4). Mid-wall LGE was found in 10–28% of patients with DCM [13, 15]. Coexistent subendocardial LGE may indicate ischemic contribution to HF etiology despite the absence of angina and significant stenoses on coronary angiography, as infarction may follow coronary spasm or embolism, followed by spontaneous coronary recanalization [13, 16, 17].

8.4 Myocarditis Presenting as Left Ventricular Dysfunction

Patients presenting with HF and LV dysfunction with or without dilatation may be affected by active myocarditis. Inflammatory processes are characterized by increased water content due to edema. CMR may show edema at T2-weighted sequences such as short tau inversion recovery (STIR), diffuse hyperemia at global relative enhancement (GRE) sequences or T1-weighted sequences early after gadolinium administration, or LGE with a myocarditic pattern (patchy subepicardial and/or mid-wall) (Fig. 8.5). Finding at least two of the aforementioned three criteria, the Lake Louise criteria (LLC) was found to have good diagnostic accuracy in identifying myocarditis presenting with chest pain and troponin release [18]. However, the sensitivity of the LLC criteria is greatest for patients with infarct-like rather than HF or arrhythmic presentations [19, 20].

Recently, T2-mapping sequences were designed to obtain a T2 signal intensity decay curve of the myocardium, in order to estimate myocardial T2 value and generate a color T2 map off-line (Fig. 8.6). Normal native T2 time ranges between 39 and 59 ms. T2 relaxation time is increased in conditions characterized by myocardial edema [21]. In a recent study, patients with recent-onset HF and clinically suspected myocarditis revealed higher median global myocardial T2 values in those

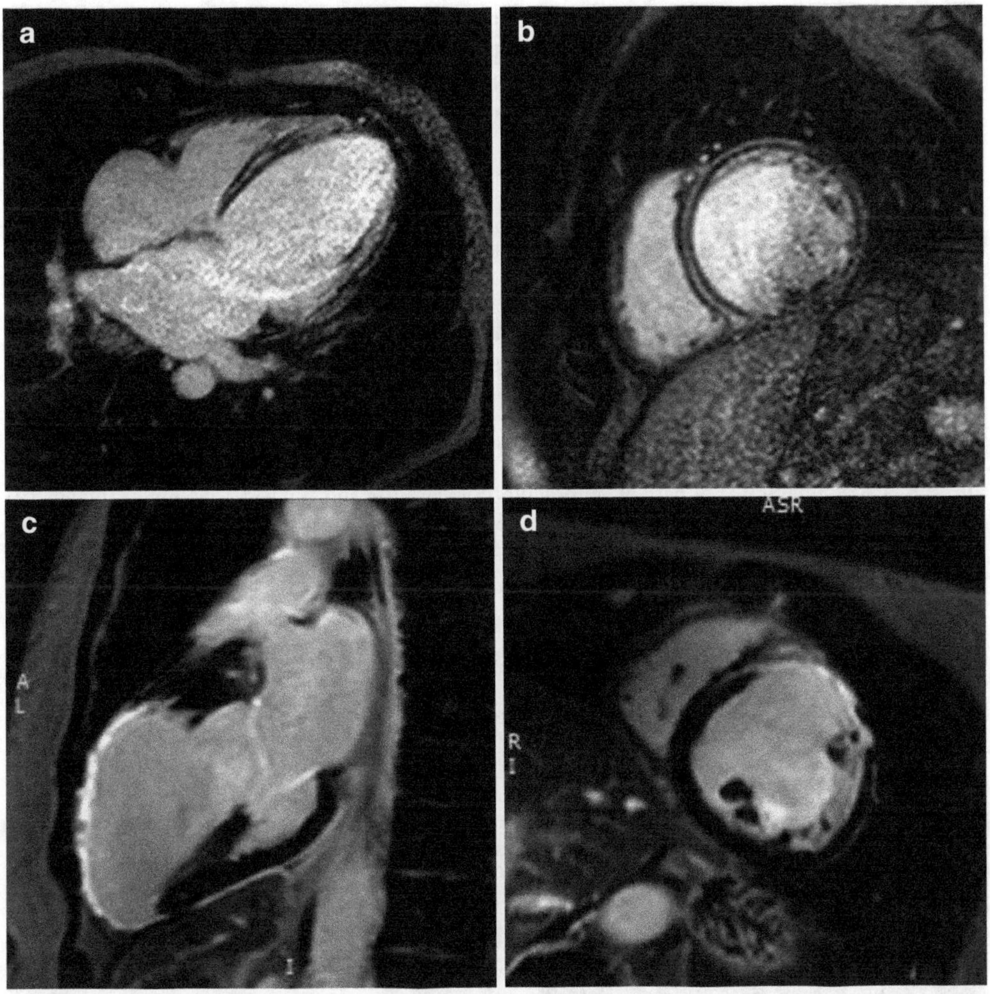

Fig. 8.4 Late gadolinium enhancement imaging in a case of DCM in four-chamber (**a**) and short-axis (**b**) views showing patchy distribution of LGE (septal intramural and subepicardial free wall). LGE imaging in a case of LV dysfunction secondary to prior anterior myocardial infarction in two-chamber (**c**) and short-axis (**d**) views, showing transmural LGE in the left anterior descending territory

with biopsy-proven active myocarditis at T2 mapping, while there were no significant differences in native or post-contrast global myocardial T1 [22]. Caution must be applied when interpreting these results as T2 values may differ according to sequences and field strength [23, 24]. Furthermore, increased T2 values may be found in DCM patients without inflammation. Finally, differences between normal and pathological subjects can be very subtle and reported in the range of 10–20 ms, sometimes even overlapping normal T2 values, making it therefore difficult to define precise cutoff values [23, 25]. Nevertheless, despite these limitations T2 mapping can overcome the T2 or STIR sequence artifacts and is the only mapping sequence that allows for discrimination between inflammatory and noninflammatory cardiomyopathies [26].

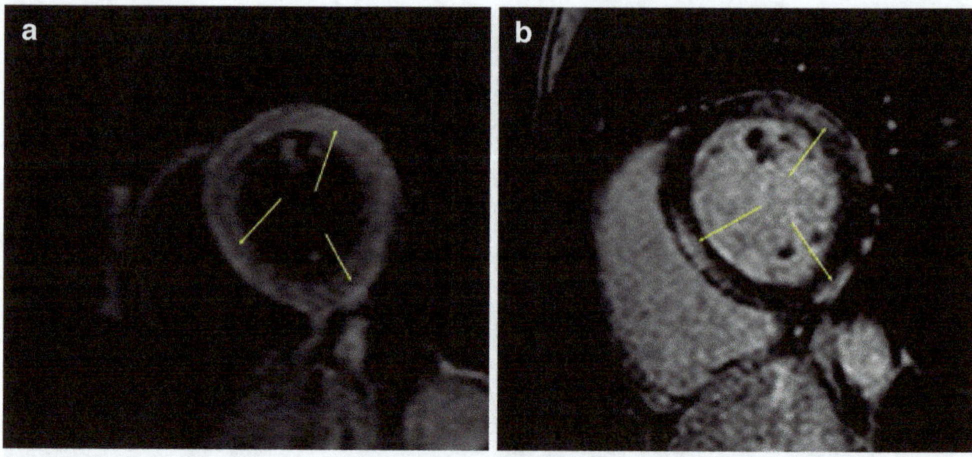

Fig. 8.5 CMR imaging in a patient with acute myocarditis: short-axis T2-weighted images (**a**) show edema, and short-axis LGE images (**b**) show patchy subepicardial LGE in the septum, inferior and anterolateral walls

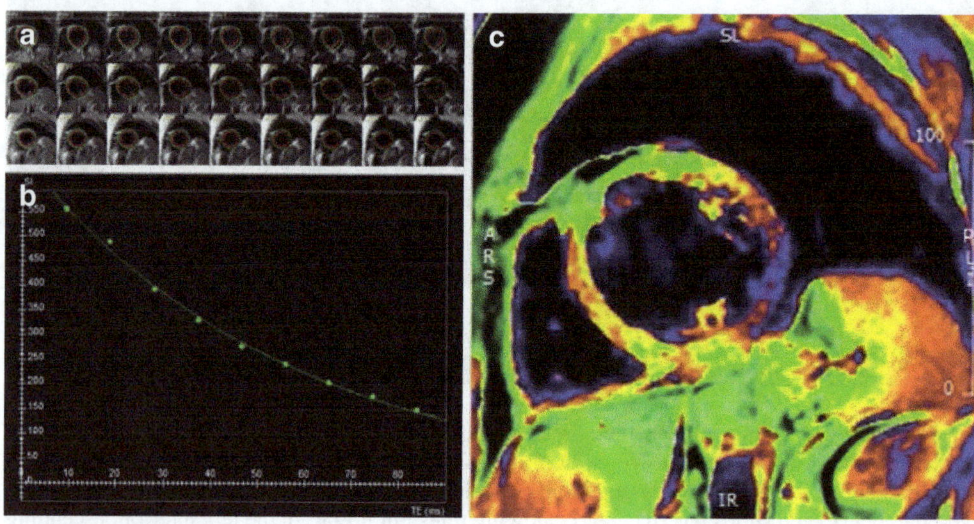

Fig. 8.6 T2 mapping with multi-echo spin-echo sequence: endocardial and epicardial contours are traced in all slices for each echo time (**a**). A T2 decay curve fit is obtained, and the T2 value is calculated for the region of interest (**b**). Results can also be depicted in color-coded maps (**c**)

As native T1 values increase with increasing myocardial water content, native T1 mapping may serve as a complementary technique to T2-weighted imaging for assessing myocardial edema in myocarditis presenting as infarct-like syndrome [22, 27] or where gadolinium is contraindicated. However, since native T1 values increase both with water content and with diffuse fibrosis, it is not able to discriminate between inflammatory and noninflammatory cardiomyopathies in patients presenting with heart failure [28].

8.5 Other Secondary Forms of DCM

CMR may help in diagnosing Chagas cardiomyopathy, caused by *Trypanosoma cruzi* infection, which results in LV dysfunction, HF, and ventricular arrhythmias. Its typical pattern is characterized by DCM with aneurysm formation with preferential sites at the apex and infero-lateral walls, which can be easily detected with SSFP cine imaging. The pattern of LGE is variable and may involve any or all layers of the myocardial wall [29, 30]. CMR was also found to identify the early stages of the disease [29].

Cardiac involvement of sarcoidosis may manifest itself as LV dilatation and dysfunction. Patients with sarcoidosis develop large areas of LGE with variable distribution, which can precede the occurrence of LV dilatation, frequently involving the mid-wall of the basal septum, basal and lateral segments of the LV, and papillary muscles, unrelated to vascular territories [31].

8.6 Prognostic Stratification

Risk stratification is of foremost importance in DCM, particularly regarding the risk of sudden arrhythmic cardiac death (SCD). LV ejection fraction (LVEF) is the strongest predictor of progression to HF [32], while LV volume and mass are independently correlated with mortality and morbidity. Therefore, accurate quantification of all these parameters is essential to adequately evaluate patients and to monitor progression of disease and response to different therapeutic agents [33]. LVEF is the main criterion to select patients for primary prevention of SCD with implantable cardioverter-defibrillator (ICD) [34–36]. However, LVEF has low sensitivity and low specificity for the prediction of SCD [34, 37]. The use of low LVEF alone as an indicator for ICD placement is associated with both a low event rate of SCD in the control and treatment groups and a significant number of inappropriate ICD shocks [38]. Risk stratification for SCD among patients with nonischemic cardiomyopathy remains inadequate, causing ongoing clinical challenges in the appropriate identification of candidates for primary prevention ICDs [39].

In DCM, the remodeling process is characterized by changes in the extracellular matrix and interstitial fibrosis. The fibrous tissue constitutes a substrate for ventricular arrhythmias by inducing slow and heterogeneous conduction, favoring reentrant circuits, and producing vulnerability to life-threatening ventricular tachyarrhythmias [40]. Areas of LGE detected by CMR correlate well with histologically detected regional myocardial fibrosis in animal models and human explanted hearts [41, 42].

Several studies demonstrated that LGE is associated with an increased risk of adverse remodeling, hospitalization for HF, ventricular arrhythmia induction, and SCD in patients with DCM [43–52]. A recent meta-analysis showed that LGE was present in a considerable proportion of patients with DCM (44%), and it had a strong and significant association with the risk for ventricular arrhythmias and SCD. This association was consistently observed in patients at different stages of their cardiomyopathy and was independent of LVEF [53]. In DCM patients undergoing ICD placement for primary prevention of SCD, the presence of myocardial fibrosis is also predictive of appropriate device therapy [46, 54] regardless of LVEF. Mid-wall LGE may also identify a subgroup at high risk of SCD despite mild or moderate LV systolic impairment, not meeting conventional criteria for ICD implantation [55, 56]. Moreover, LGE extent is also associated with adverse outcomes [44]. However, LGE extent is variably described in studies, and there is no current consensus on the best method of LGE quantification [50]. A relationship between patterns of myocardial scar and arrhythmogenesis was also suggested: a scar with a transmurality of 26–75% is predictive of inducible ventricular tachycardia [43]. The detailed characterization of the heterogeneous boundary zone surrounding the LGE-CMR base scar has been linked to all-cause mortality and the most frequent ventricular arrhythmias although its role in DCM patients is still controversial [57]. Despite the abovementioned strong evidences, however, current guidelines from European Society of Cardiology [35] and more recently from American College of Cardiology/American Heart Association/Heart Rhythm Society [36] do not mention arrhythmic risk stratification with LGE-CMR.

The presence and extent of LGE in patients with DCM also predicts a lack of improvement in LV function despite optimal medical treatment compared to a significant improvement in patients without LGE [48, 58–61]. Furthermore, LGE detected at CMR correlates with LV diastolic function evaluated by Doppler echocardiography. Patients with DCM and positive LGE have indices of higher diastolic filling pressure [62–64]. The presence and extent of LGE also correlates with echocardiographic measures of LV systolic dyssynchrony, an indicator of poor clinical outcome [65].

Scar burden was also found to be predictive of poor response to cardiac resynchronization therapy (CRT) [66]. Specifically, pacing over scar was associated with a higher risk of cardiac mortality or HF hospitalizations compared with pacing viable myocardium [67, 68]. Moreover, pacing a transmural scar was associated with a worse outcome than pacing a subendocardial scar [69]. Scar in the vicinity of right ventricular (RV) lead during CRT may also be associated with suboptimal left ventricular reverse remodeling (LVRR) [70]. However, the strategy avoiding myocardial scar in lead implantation has not been evaluated by multicenter, randomized, controlled trials.

8.7 Macroscopic vs. Diffuse Fibrosis

Myocardial scar is the main substrate for ventricular arrhythmias, but not all patients with DCM have identifiable scars, especially in cases of diffuse fibrosis. In most patients with DCM, myocardial fibrosis does not progress focally but instead gradually and randomly, leading to irreversible replacement fibrosis [42, 71]. LGE sequences are designed to improve signal contrast differences between zones of normal myocardium and zones with focal fibrosis or necrosis [72, 73]. The technique is however very limited in the quantification of widespread tissue fibrosis [72, 74, 75]. This impairment has been nowadays overcome with the introduction of another family of sequences (MOLLI, Sh-MOLLI, SASHA, and SAPPHIRE) that are able to quantitatively identify real myocardial T1 recovery time, native and post-contrast, and to quantify extracellular volume (ECV). It is also possible to assess all the collected data in color maps (Fig. 8.7) [76–78]. T1-mapping techniques correlate with myocardial histology [79–82] and may allow the early differentiation of diseased myocardium from healthy myocardium, in the absence of LGE [80, 83]. Native T1 and ECV are increased, and post-contrast T1 is decreased in nonischemic DCM patients [81, 83, 84]. All T1-mapping measures have been linked to prognosis in nonischemic DCM patients [85–88]. However, native T1 was found to be the sole independent predictor of all-cause and HF composite endpoints in a recent large prospective multicenter observational study [86]. Native T1 has also shown a strong relationship with markers of structural and functional LV remodeling, diastolic impairment, and the severity of functional mitral regurgitation [89–91].

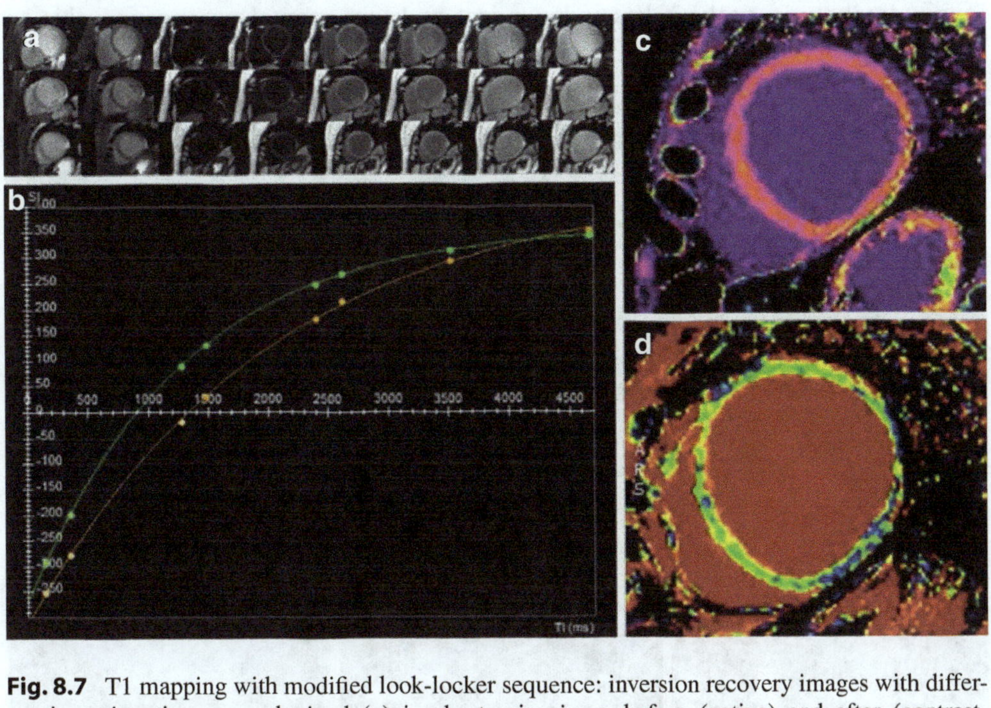

Fig. 8.7 T1 mapping with modified look-locker sequence: inversion recovery images with different inversion times are obtained **(a)** in short-axis views, before (native) and after (contrast-enhanced) gadolinium administration. The signal intensity is measured in each image, and a T1 relaxation curve **(b)** is obtained for the myocardium (green) and blood (orange). Results can be depicted as color-coded maps of native myocardial T1 **(c)** and ECV **(d)**

8.8 Strain Analysis

In DCM, the occurrence of nonhomogeneous fibrous substitution of cardiomyocytes may alter mechanical activity in these areas [92], thus leading to a heterogeneous compromise of regional contractile function [93]. Myocardial deformation analysis can supply useful information for the evaluation of global and regional myocardial function [94, 95]. CMR tagging is considered a reference standard for the assessment of myocardial regional function [96]. By adding grids or lines to the imaging plane through selective saturation pulses, and following them throughout the cardiac cycle, myocardial deformation can be quantitatively analyzed. However, the need for additional acquisition sequences and time-consuming protocols have limited its clinical application. Recently, new CMR feature tracking technology, which agrees well with CMR tagging, has allowed for the assessment of global and regional myocardial strain by tracking patterns of features or irregularities comprised between the endocardial and epicardial borders during cardiac cycle using SSFP long-axis and short-axis cine images (Fig. 8.8). This technology, similar to speckle tracking, can be applied to routine cine-CMR acquisitions, thus avoiding the need for dedicated pulse sequences [97]. Global longitudinal, circumferential, and radial strain are significantly impaired in patients with DCM [98]. More importantly, there is growing evidence that CMR-derived strain analysis is a predictor of adverse events in patients with nonischemic DCM [99–101]. In particular, global longitudinal strain analysis has independent and incremental prognostic value to

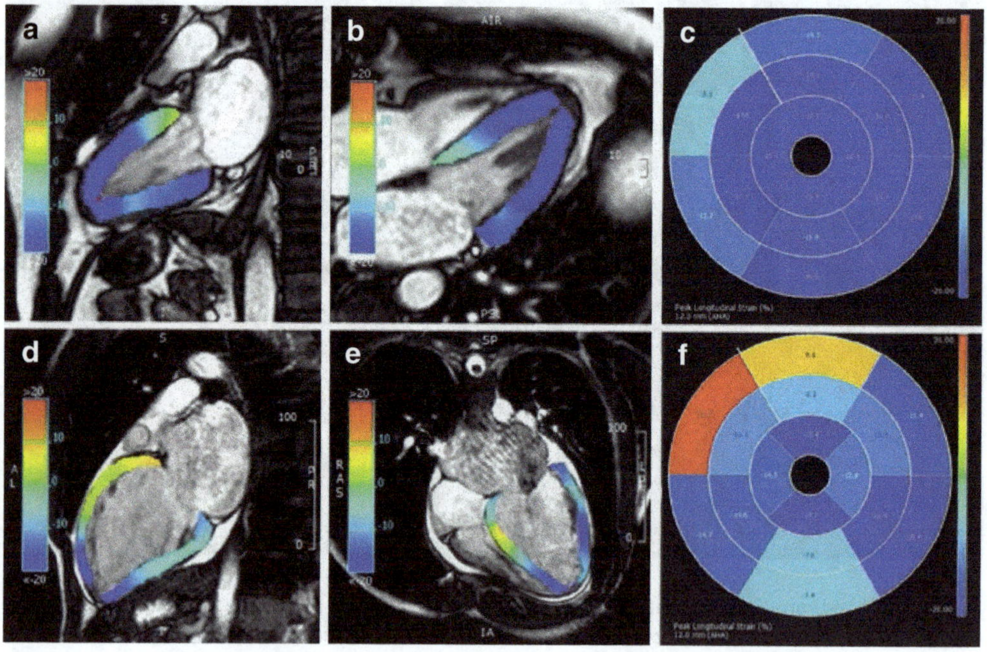

Fig. 8.8 Strain analysis in a normal subject (**a–c**) and in a patient with DCM (**d–f**) at 1.5T. Color-coded maps of peak longitudinal strain in two-chamber (**a**, **d**) and four-chamber (**b**, **e**) views. Bull's-eye graphic depicting peak longitudinal strain values in all AHA segments (**c**, **f**)

other risk factors including LVEF, LGE, and ECV [99–103]. Peak circumferential strain in association with the absence of LGE and LV mass were found to be predictive of LVRR [104].

Cardiac dyssynchrony assessed by CMR strain analysis, associated with LGE imaging, was also suggested to better predict improvement in functional class after CRT implantation [105], compared to currently recommended parameters for patient selection [106].

8.9 Other Prognostic Indicators

Biventricular involvement in DCM identifies a subset of patients with poor outcome [107, 108]. CMR is considered the gold standard for noninvasive assessment of RV function [7, 8]. RV ejection fraction (RVEF) ≤45% was shown to be independently associated with adverse outcome in nonischemic DCM patients [109]. Furthermore, RV longitudinal strain is also an independent predictor of outcome and offers additional prognostic information over RVEF [110].

Left atrial enlargement is associated with adverse outcome in patients with DCM [111, 112]. Left atrial volume (LAV) provides the most accurate estimate of left atrial size compared to linear dimension in M-mode and area in 2D echocardiography [113]. Echocardiographic measures systematically underestimate LAV compared to CMR [6], even though both methods are reproducible and have limited intra- or interobserver variability. A LAV index >72 mL/m^2, measured with the biplane area-length method, was found to be an independent predictor of adverse events in DCM [114]. Conversely, LAV index<38 mL/m^2 is predictive of LVRR [115].

Finally, RV dysfunction [109], but not greater degrees of trabeculation [116], is an independent predictor of survival and HF outcomes in patients with DCM.

8.10 Computed Tomography

Cardiac computed tomography (CCT) is a noninvasive cardiac imaging technique that is increasingly gaining importance in DCM patients. It is mainly used to test for the presence of CAD but may also play a role in the evaluation of cardiac volumes and function, characterization of the type of cardiomyopathy, and treatment planning.

Calcium score may be useful in excluding CAD as the etiology for HF. In patients with HF, an Agatston score of 0 has been shown to have 100% specificity in excluding left main or ≥2-vessel coronary artery disease [117, 118]. Computed tomography coronary angiography (CTCA) (Fig. 8.9) is a highly accurate diagnostic modality for excluding CAD in patients with DCM of undetermined cause [119–122], especially in the low- to intermediate-risk population due to its high specificity (95–98%) and negative predictive value (95–100%) [123–125].

Prospective ECG triggering is the preferred CTCA mode to minimize radiation dose, although this is possible only if the heart rate is slow and regular. Retrospective

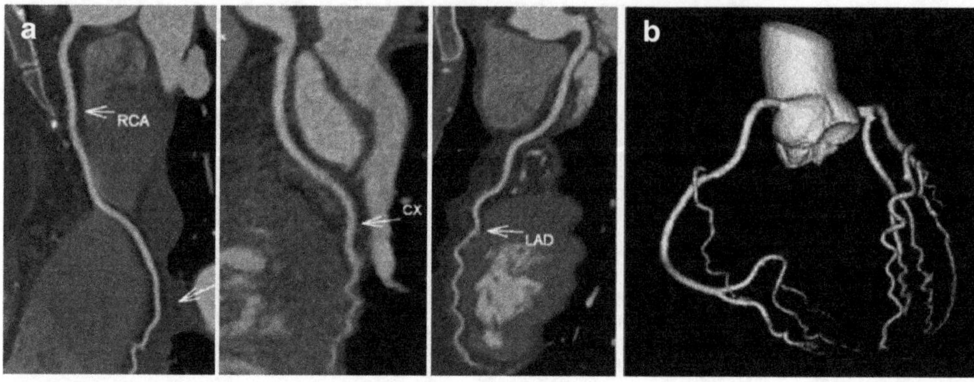

Fig. 8.9 Curved multiplanar reconstructions (cMPR) of the right coronary (RCA), left circumflex (CX), and left anterior descending (LAD) arteries obtained from a coronary CTA in a patient with normal coronary arteries (**a**). Three-dimensional volume reconstruction (3DVR) is shown in panel (**b**)

ECG gating must be used if the heart rate is high or irregular. This mode is also used for the evaluation of cardiac function and volumes, wall motion, and valvular abnormalities, with good correlation with CMR and contrast-enhanced echocardiography [2, 126–129]. Latest technologies such as CT perfusion and CT-FFR may give additional important information on the hemodynamic significance of coronary artery disease [130–135].

There is increasing evidence supporting the usefulness of CCT for the detection of myocardial fibrosis in patients with hypertrophic cardiomyopathy [136] and after myocardial infarction [137, 138] through late iodine enhancement (LIE), although CMR remains more sensitive. However, data in DCM patients are still limited. Initial data suggest that LIE-CCT correlates well with LGE-CMR and electroanatomic mapping [139, 140]. LIE may also be used for ECV assessment [141]. It has good correlation with T1-mapping methods and is associated with increased LV volume and reduced EF and circumferential strain [142]. Dual-energy CT reduces imaging artifacts and increases contrast to noise ratio and thus may improve LIE images compared to conventional CT [143, 144].

A number of challenges still remain, relating to the required contrast dose, image quality, and radiation exposure. CTCA has been given a high appropriateness rating for the evaluation of ischemic etiology in patients presenting with HF [145, 146]. However, for all other indications, CCT should still be reserved for patients with contraindications or suboptimal results of other imaging tests.

References

1. Bellenger NG, Burgess MI, Ray SG, Lahiri A, Coats AJ, Cleland JG, et al. Comparison of left ventricular ejection fraction and volumes in heart failure by echocardiography, radionuclide ventriculography and cardiovascular magnetic resonance; are they interchangeable? Eur Heart J. 2000;21(16):1387–96.
2. Greupner J, Zimmermann E, Grohmann A, Dubel HP, Althoff TF, Borges AC, et al. Head-to-head comparison of left ventricular function assessment with 64-row computed tomography,

biplane left cineventriculography, and both 2- and 3-dimensional transthoracic echocardiography: comparison with magnetic resonance imaging as the reference standard. J Am Coll Cardiol. 2012;59(21):1897–907.

3. Moon JC, Lorenz CH, Francis JM, Smith GC, Pennell DJ. Breath-hold FLASH and FISP cardiovascular MR imaging: left ventricular volume differences and reproducibility. Radiology. 2002;223(3):789–97.
4. Thuny F, Jacquier A, Jop B, Giorgi R, Gaubert JY, Bartoli JM, et al. Assessment of left ventricular non-compaction in adults: side-by-side comparison of cardiac magnetic resonance imaging with echocardiography. Arch Cardiovasc Dis. 2010;103(3):150–9.
5. Anderson JL, Horne BD, Pennell DJ. Atrial dimensions in health and left ventricular disease using cardiovascular magnetic resonance. J Cardiovasc Magn Reson. 2005;7(4):671–5.
6. Whitlock M, Garg A, Gelow J, Jacobson T, Broberg C. Comparison of left and right atrial volume by echocardiography versus cardiac magnetic resonance imaging using the area-length method. Am J Cardiol. 2010;106(9):1345–50.
7. Grothues F, Moon JC, Bellenger NG, Smith GS, Klein HU, Pennell DJ. Interstudy reproducibility of right ventricular volumes, function, and mass with cardiovascular magnetic resonance. Am Heart J. 2004;147(2):218–23.
8. Mooij CF, de Wit CJ, Graham DA, Powell AJ, Geva T. Reproducibility of MRI measurements of right ventricular size and function in patients with normal and dilated ventricles. J Magn Reson Imaging. 2008;28(1):67–73.
9. Roifman I, Connelly KA, Wright GA, Wijeysundera HC. Echocardiography vs. cardiac magnetic resonance imaging for the diagnosis of left ventricular thrombus: a systematic review. Can J Cardiol. 2015;31(6):785–91.
10. Goyal P, Weinsaft JW. Cardiovascular magnetic resonance imaging for assessment of cardiac thrombus. Methodist Debakey Cardiovasc J. 2013;9(3):132–6.
11. Casolo G, Minneci S, Manta R, Sulla A, Del Meglio J, Rega L, et al. Identification of the ischemic etiology of heart failure by cardiovascular magnetic resonance imaging: diagnostic accuracy of late gadolinium enhancement. Am Heart J. 2006;151(1):101–8.
12. Valle-Munoz A, Estornell-Erill J, Soriano-Navarro CJ, Nadal-Barange M, Martinez-Alzamora N, Pomar-Domingo F, et al. Late gadolinium enhancement-cardiovascular magnetic resonance identifies coronary artery disease as the aetiology of left ventricular dysfunction in acute new-onset congestive heart failure. Eur J Echocardiogr. 2009;10(8):968–74.
13. McCrohon JA, Moon JC, Prasad SK, McKenna WJ, Lorenz CH, Coats AJ, et al. Differentiation of heart failure related to dilated cardiomyopathy and coronary artery disease using gadolinium-enhanced cardiovascular magnetic resonance. Circulation. 2003;108(1):54–9.
14. Mahrholdt H, Wagner A, Deluigi CC, Kispert E, Hager S, Meinhardt G, et al. Presentation, patterns of myocardial damage, and clinical course of viral myocarditis. Circulation. 2006;114(15):1581–90.
15. Soriano CJ, Ridocci F, Estornell J, Jimenez J, Martinez V, De Velasco JA. Noninvasive diagnosis of coronary artery disease in patients with heart failure and systolic dysfunction of uncertain etiology, using late gadolinium-enhanced cardiovascular magnetic resonance. J Am Coll Cardiol. 2005;45(5):743–8.
16. Bello D, Shah DJ, Farah GM, Di Luzio S, Parker M, Johnson MR, et al. Gadolinium cardiovascular magnetic resonance predicts reversible myocardial dysfunction and remodeling in patients with heart failure undergoing beta-blocker therapy. Circulation. 2003;108(16):1945–53.
17. Karamitsos TD, Francis JM, Myerson S, Selvanayagam JB, Neubauer S. The role of cardiovascular magnetic resonance imaging in heart failure. J Am Coll Cardiol. 2009;54(15):1407–24.
18. Friedrich MG, Sechtem U, Schulz-Menger J, Holmvang G, Alakija P, Cooper LT, et al. Cardiovascular magnetic resonance in myocarditis: a JACC White Paper. J Am Coll Cardiol. 2009;53(17):1475–87.
19. Gutberlet M, Spors B, Thoma T, Bertram H, Denecke T, Felix R, et al. Suspected chronic myocarditis at cardiac MR: diagnostic accuracy and association with immunohistologically detected inflammation and viral persistence. Radiology. 2008;246(2):401–9.

20. Francone M, Chimenti C, Galea N, Scopelliti F, Verardo R, Galea R, et al. CMR sensitivity varies with clinical presentation and extent of cell necrosis in biopsy-proven acute myocarditis. J Am Coll Cardiol Img. 2014;7(3):254–63.
21. Kim PK, Hong YJ, Im DJ, Suh YJ, Park CH, Kim JY, et al. Myocardial T1 and T2 mapping: techniques and clinical applications. Korean J Radiol. 2017;18(1):113–31.
22. Lurz P, Luecke C, Eitel I, Fohrenbach F, Frank C, Grothoff M, et al. Comprehensive cardiac magnetic resonance imaging in patients with suspected myocarditis: the myoracer-trial. J Am Coll Cardiol. 2016;67(15):1800–11.
23. Wassmuth R, Prothmann M, Utz W, Dieringer M, von Knobelsdorff-Brenkenhoff F, Greiser A, et al. Variability and homogeneity of cardiovascular magnetic resonance myocardial T2-mapping in volunteers compared to patients with edema. J Cardiovasc Magn Reson. 2013;15:27.
24. Baessler B, Schaarschmidt F, Stehning C, Schnackenburg B, Maintz D, Bunck AC. Cardiac T2-mapping using a fast gradient echo spin echo sequence - first in vitro and in vivo experience. J Cardiovasc Magn Reson. 2015;17:67.
25. Thavendiranathan P, Walls M, Giri S, Verhaert D, Rajagopalan S, Moore S, et al. Improved detection of myocardial involvement in acute inflammatory cardiomyopathies using T2 mapping. Circ Cardiovasc Imaging. 2012;5(1):102–10.
26. Verhaert D, Thavendiranathan P, Giri S, Mihai G, Rajagopalan S, Simonetti OP, et al. Direct T2 quantification of myocardial edema in acute ischemic injury. JACC Cardiovasc Imaging. 2011;4(3):269–78.
27. Ferreira VM, Piechnik SK, Dall'Armellina E, Karamitsos TD, Francis JM, Choudhury RP, et al. Non-contrast T1-mapping detects acute myocardial edema with high diagnostic accuracy: a comparison to T2-weighted cardiovascular magnetic resonance. J Cardiovasc Magn Reson. 2012;14:42.
28. Bohnen S, Radunski UK, Lund GK, Kandolf R, Stehning C, Schnackenburg B, et al. Performance of t1 and t2 mapping cardiovascular magnetic resonance to detect active myocarditis in patients with recent-onset heart failure. Circ Cardiovasc Imaging. 2015;8(6). pii: e003073.
29. Rochitte CE, Oliveira PF, Andrade JM, Ianni BM, Parga JR, Avila LF, et al. Myocardial delayed enhancement by magnetic resonance imaging in patients with Chagas' disease: a marker of disease severity. J Am Coll Cardiol. 2005;46(8):1553–8.
30. Regueiro A, Garcia-Alvarez A, Sitges M, Ortiz-Perez JT, De Caralt MT, Pinazo MJ, et al. Myocardial involvement in Chagas disease: insights from cardiac magnetic resonance. Int J Cardiol. 2013;165(1):107–12.
31. Schatka I, Bengel FM. Advanced imaging of cardiac sarcoidosis. J Nucl Med. 2014;55(1):99–106.
32. Grzybowski J, Bilinska ZT, Ruzyllo W, Kupsc W, Michalak E, Szczesniewska D, et al. Determinants of prognosis in nonischemic dilated cardiomyopathy. J Card Fail. 1996;2(2):77–85.
33. Lehrke S, Lossnitzer D, Schob M, Steen H, Merten C, Kemmling H, et al. Use of cardiovascular magnetic resonance for risk stratification in chronic heart failure: prognostic value of late gadolinium enhancement in patients with non-ischaemic dilated cardiomyopathy. Heart. 2011;97(9):727–32.
34. Buxton AE, Lee KL, Hafley GE, Pires LA, Fisher JD, Gold MR, et al. Limitations of ejection fraction for prediction of sudden death risk in patients with coronary artery disease: lessons from the MUSTT study. J Am Coll Cardiol. 2007;50(12):1150–7.
35. Priori SG, Blomstrom-Lundqvist C, Mazzanti A, Blom N, Borggrefe M, Camm J, et al. 2015 ESC Guidelines for the management of patients with ventricular arrhythmias and the prevention of sudden cardiac death: The Task Force for the Management of Patients with Ventricular Arrhythmias and the Prevention of Sudden Cardiac Death of the European Society of Cardiology (ESC). Endorsed by: Association for European Paediatric and Congenital Cardiology (AEPC). Eur Heart J. 2015;36(41):2793–867.

36. Al-Khatib SM, Stevenson WG, Ackerman MJ, Bryant WJ, Callans DJ, Curtis AB, et al. AHA/ACC/HRS Guideline for management of patients with ventricular arrhythmias and the prevention of sudden cardiac death: executive summary: a report of the American College of Cardiology/American Heart Association Task Force on Clinical Practice Guidelines and the Heart Rhythm Society. Circulation. 2017, 2017; https://doi.org/10.1161/CIR.0000000000000548.
37. Kober L, Thune JJ, Nielsen JC, Haarbo J, Videbaek L, Korup E, et al. Defibrillator implantation in patients with nonischemic systolic heart failure. N Engl J Med. 2016;375(13):1221–30.
38. Kadish A, Dyer A, Daubert JP, Quigg R, Estes NA, Anderson KP, et al. Prophylactic defibrillator implantation in patients with nonischemic dilated cardiomyopathy. N Engl J Med. 2004;350(21):2151–8.
39. Arbustini E, Disertori M, Narula J. Primary prevention of sudden arrhythmic death in dilated cardiomyopathy: current guidelines and risk stratification. JACC Heart Fail. 2017;5(1):39–43.
40. Pogwizd SM, McKenzie JP, Cain ME. Mechanisms underlying spontaneous and induced ventricular arrhythmias in patients with idiopathic dilated cardiomyopathy. Circulation. 1998;98(22):2404–14.
41. Kim RJ, Fieno DS, Parrish TB, Harris K, Chen EL, Simonetti O, et al. Relationship of MRI delayed contrast enhancement to irreversible injury, infarct age, and contractile function. Circulation. 1999;100(19):1992–2002.
42. Iles LM, Ellims AH, Llewellyn H, Hare JL, Kaye DM, McLean CA, et al. Histological validation of cardiac magnetic resonance analysis of regional and diffuse interstitial myocardial fibrosis. Eur Heart J Cardiovasc Imaging. 2015;16(1):14–22.
43. Nazarian S, Bluemke DA, Lardo AC, Zviman MM, Watkins SP, Dickfeld TL, et al. Magnetic resonance assessment of the substrate for inducible ventricular tachycardia in nonischemic cardiomyopathy. Circulation. 2005;112(18):2821–5.
44. Assomull RG, Prasad SK, Lyne J, Smith G, Burman ED, Khan M, et al. Cardiovascular magnetic resonance, fibrosis, and prognosis in dilated cardiomyopathy. J Am Coll Cardiol. 2006;48(10):1977–85.
45. Wu KC, Weiss RG, Thiemann DR, Kitagawa K, Schmidt A, Dalal D, et al. Late gadolinium enhancement by cardiovascular magnetic resonance heralds an adverse prognosis in nonischemic cardiomyopathy. J Am Coll Cardiol. 2008;51(25):2414–21.
46. Klem I, Weinsaft JW, Bahnson TD, Hegland D, Kim HW, Hayes B, et al. Assessment of myocardial scarring improves risk stratification in patients evaluated for cardiac defibrillator implantation. J Am Coll Cardiol. 2012;60(5):408–20.
47. Gulati A, Jabbour A, Ismail TF, Guha K, Khwaja J, Raza S, et al. Association of fibrosis with mortality and sudden cardiac death in patients with nonischemic dilated cardiomyopathy. JAMA. 2013;309(9):896–908.
48. Kubanek M, Sramko M, Maluskova J, Kautznerova D, Weichet J, Lupinek P, et al. Novel predictors of left ventricular reverse remodeling in individuals with recent-onset dilated cardiomyopathy. J Am Coll Cardiol. 2013;61(1):54–63.
49. Neilan TG, Coelho-Filho OR, Danik SB, Shah RV, Dodson JA, Verdini DJ, et al. CMR quantification of myocardial scar provides additive prognostic information in nonischemic cardiomyopathy. JACC Cardiovasc Imaging. 2013;6(9):944–54.
50. Kuruvilla S, Adenaw N, Katwal AB, Lipinski MJ, Kramer CM, Salerno M. Late gadolinium enhancement on cardiac magnetic resonance predicts adverse cardiovascular outcomes in nonischemic cardiomyopathy: a systematic review and meta-analysis. Circ Cardiovasc Imaging. 2014;7(2):250–8.
51. Perazzolo Marra M, De Lazzari M, Zorzi A, Migliore F, Zilio F, Calore C, et al. Impact of the presence and amount of myocardial fibrosis by cardiac magnetic resonance on arrhythmic outcome and sudden cardiac death in nonischemic dilated cardiomyopathy. Heart Rhythm. 2014;11(5):856–63.
52. Disertori M, Rigoni M, Pace N, Casolo G, Mase M, Gonzini L, et al. Myocardial fibrosis assessment by LGE is a powerful predictor of ventricular tachyarrhythmias in isch-

emic and nonischemic LV dysfunction: a meta-analysis. JACC Cardiovasc Imaging. 2016;9(9):1046–55.

53. Di Marco A, Anguera I, Schmitt M, Klem I, Neilan TG, White JA, et al. Late gadolinium enhancement and the risk for ventricular arrhythmias or sudden death in dilated cardiomyopathy: systematic review and meta-analysis. JACC Heart Fail. 2017;5(1):28–38.
54. Iles L, Pfluger H, Lefkovits L, Butler MJ, Kistler PM, Kaye DM, et al. Myocardial fibrosis predicts appropriate device therapy in patients with implantable cardioverter-defibrillators for primary prevention of sudden cardiac death. J Am Coll Cardiol. 2011;57(7):821–8.
55. Venero JV, Doyle M, Shah M, Rathi VK, Yamrozik JA, Williams RB, et al. Mid wall fibrosis on CMR with late gadolinium enhancement may predict prognosis for LVAD and transplantation risk in patients with newly diagnosed dilated cardiomyopathy-preliminary observations from a high-volume transplant centre. ESC Heart Fail. 2015;2(4):150–9.
56. Halliday BP, Gulati A, Ali A, Guha K, Newsome S, Arzanauskaite M, et al. Association between midwall late gadolinium enhancement and sudden cardiac death in patients with dilated cardiomyopathy and mild and moderate left ventricular systolic dysfunction. Circulation. 2017;135(22):2106–15.
57. Jablonowski R, Chaudhry U, van der Pals J, Engblom H, Arheden H, Heiberg E, et al. Cardiovascular magnetic resonance to predict appropriate implantable cardioverter defibrillator therapy in ischemic and nonischemic cardiomyopathy patients using late gadolinium enhancement border zone: comparison of four analysis methods. Circ Cardiovasc Imaging. 2017;10(9). pii: e006105.
58. Park S, Choi BW, Rim SJ, Shim CY, Ko YG, Kang SM, et al. Delayed hyperenhancement magnetic resonance imaging is useful in predicting functional recovery of nonischemic left ventricular systolic dysfunction. J Card Fail. 2006;12(2):93–9.
59. Leong DP, Chakrabarty A, Shipp N, Molaee P, Madsen PL, Joerg L, et al. Effects of myocardial fibrosis and ventricular dyssynchrony on response to therapy in new-presentation idiopathic dilated cardiomyopathy: insights from cardiovascular magnetic resonance and echocardiography. Eur Heart J. 2012;33(5):640–8.
60. Ikeda Y, Inomata T, Fujita T, Iida Y, Nabeta T, Ishii S, et al. Cardiac fibrosis detected by magnetic resonance imaging on predicting time course diversity of left ventricular reverse remodeling in patients with idiopathic dilated cardiomyopathy. Heart Vessels. 2016;31(11):1817–25.
61. Yingchoncharoen T, Jellis C, Popovic ZB, Wang L, Gai N, Levy WC, et al. Focal fibrosis and diffuse fibrosis are predictors of reversed left ventricular remodeling in patients with non-ischemic cardiomyopathy. Int J Cardiol. 2016;221:498–504.
62. Choi EY, Choi BW, Kim SA, Rhee SJ, Shim CY, Kim YJ, et al. Patterns of late gadolinium enhancement are associated with ventricular stiffness in patients with advanced non-ischaemic dilated cardiomyopathy. Eur J Heart Fail. 2009;11(6):573–80.
63. Nanjo S, Yoshikawa K, Harada M, Inoue Y, Namiki A, Nakano H, et al. Correlation between left ventricular diastolic function and ejection fraction in dilated cardiomyopathy using magnetic resonance imaging with late gadolinium enhancement. Circ J. 2009;73(10):1939–44.
64. Malaty AN, Shah DJ, Abdelkarim AR, Nagueh SF. Relation of replacement fibrosis to left ventricular diastolic function in patients with dilated cardiomyopathy. J Am Soc Echocardiogr. 2011;24(3):333–8.
65. Tigen K, Karaahmet T, Kirma C, Dundar C, Pala S, Isiklar I, et al. Diffuse late gadolinium enhancement by cardiovascular magnetic resonance predicts significant intraventricular systolic dyssynchrony in patients with non-ischemic dilated cardiomyopathy. J Am Soc Echocardiogr. 2010;23(4):416–22.
66. White JA, Yee R, Yuan X, Krahn A, Skanes A, Parker M, et al. Delayed enhancement magnetic resonance imaging predicts response to cardiac resynchronization therapy in patients with intraventricular dyssynchrony. J Am Coll Cardiol. 2006;48(10):1953–60.
67. Chalil S, Foley PW, Muyhaldeen SA, Patel KC, Yousef ZR, Smith RE, et al. Late gadolinium enhancement-cardiovascular magnetic resonance as a predictor of response to cardiac resynchronization therapy in patients with ischaemic cardiomyopathy. Europace. 2007;9(11):1031–7.

68. Leyva F, Foley PW, Chalil S, Ratib K, Smith RE, Prinzen F, et al. Cardiac resynchronization therapy guided by late gadolinium-enhancement cardiovascular magnetic resonance. J Cardiovasc Magn Reson. 2011;13:29.
69. Chalil S, Stegemann B, Muhyaldeen SA, Khadjooi K, Foley PW, Smith RE, et al. Effect of posterolateral left ventricular scar on mortality and morbidity following cardiac resynchronization therapy. Pacing Clin Electrophysiol. 2007;30(10):1201–9.
70. Wong JA, Yee R, Stirrat J, Scholl D, Krahn AD, Gula LJ, et al. Influence of pacing site characteristics on response to cardiac resynchronization therapy. Circ Cardiovasc Imaging. 2013;6(4):542–50.
71. Brooks A, Schinde V, Bateman AC, Gallagher PJ. Interstitial fibrosis in the dilated non-ischaemic myocardium. Heart. 2003;89(10):1255–6.
72. Jellis C, Martin J, Narula J, Marwick TH. Assessment of nonischemic myocardial fibrosis. J Am Coll Cardiol. 2010;56(2):89–97.
73. Mewton N, Liu CY, Croisille P, Bluemke D, Lima JA. Assessment of myocardial fibrosis with cardiovascular magnetic resonance. J Am Coll Cardiol. 2011;57(8):891–903.
74. Schalla S, Bekkers SC, Dennert R, van Suylen RJ, Waltenberger J, Leiner T, et al. Replacement and reactive myocardial fibrosis in idiopathic dilated cardiomyopathy: comparison of magnetic resonance imaging with right ventricular biopsy. Eur J Heart Fail. 2010;12(3):227–31.
75. Francone M. Role of cardiac magnetic resonance in the evaluation of dilated cardiomyopathy: diagnostic contribution and prognostic significance. ISRN Radiol. 2014;2014:365404.
76. Hamlin SA, Henry TS, Little BP, Lerakis S, Stillman AE. Mapping the future of cardiac MR imaging: case-based review of T1 and T2 mapping techniques. Radiographics. 2014;34(6):1594–611.
77. Haaf P, Garg P, Messroghli DR, Broadbent DA, Greenwood JP, Plein S. Cardiac T1 mapping and extracellular volume (ECV) in clinical practice: a comprehensive review. J Cardiovasc Magn Reson. 2016;18(1):89.
78. Salerno M, Sharif B, Arheden H, Kumar A, Axel L, Li D, et al. Recent advances in cardiovascular magnetic resonance: techniques and applications. Circ Cardiovasc Imaging. 2017;10(6). pii: e003951.
79. Sibley CT, Noureldin RA, Gai N, Nacif MS, Liu S, Turkbey EB, et al. T1 mapping in cardiomyopathy at cardiac MR: comparison with endomyocardial biopsy. Radiology. 2012;265(3):724–32.
80. aus dem Siepen F, Buss SJ, Messroghli D, Andre F, Lossnitzer D, Seitz S, et al. T1 mapping in dilated cardiomyopathy with cardiac magnetic resonance: quantification of diffuse myocardial fibrosis and comparison with endomyocardial biopsy. Eur Heart J Cardiovasc Imaging. 2015;16(2):210–6.
81. Inui K, Tachi M, Saito T, Kubota Y, Murai K, Kato K, et al. Superiority of the extracellular volume fraction over the myocardial T1 value for the assessment of myocardial fibrosis in patients with non-ischemic cardiomyopathy. Magn Reson Imaging. 2016;34(8):1141–5.
82. Nakamori S, Dohi K, Ishida M, Goto Y, Imanaka-Yoshida K, Omori T, et al. Native T1 mapping and extracellular volume mapping for the assessment of diffuse myocardial fibrosis in dilated cardiomyopathy. J Am Coll Cardiol Img. 2018;11(1):48–59.
83. Puntmann VO, Voigt T, Chen Z, Mayr M, Karim R, Rhode K, et al. Native T1 mapping in differentiation of normal myocardium from diffuse disease in hypertrophic and dilated cardiomyopathy. J Am Coll Cardiol Img. 2013;6(4):475–84.
84. Iles L, Pfluger H, Phrommintikul A, Cherayath J, Aksit P, Gupta SN, et al. Evaluation of diffuse myocardial fibrosis in heart failure with cardiac magnetic resonance contrast-enhanced T1 mapping. J Am Coll Cardiol. 2008;52(19):1574–80.
85. Kammerlander AA, Marzluf BA, Zotter-Tufaro C, Aschauer S, Duca F, Bachmann A, et al. T1 mapping by CMR imaging: from histological validation to clinical implication. JACC Cardiovasc Imaging. 2016;9(1):14–23.
86. Puntmann VO, Carr-White G, Jabbour A, Yu CY, Gebker R, Kelle S, et al. T1-mapping and outcome in nonischemic cardiomyopathy: all-cause mortality and heart failure. JACC Cardiovasc Imaging. 2016;9(1):40–50.

87. Radenkovic D, Weingartner S, Ricketts L, Moon JC, Captur G. T1 mapping in cardiac MRI. Heart Fail Rev. 2017;22(4):415–30.
88. Youn JC, Hong YJ, Lee HJ, Han K, Shim CY, Hong GR, et al. Contrast-enhanced T1 mapping-based extracellular volume fraction independently predicts clinical outcome in patients with non-ischemic dilated cardiomyopathy: a prospective cohort study. Eur Radiol. 2017;27(9):3924–33.
89. Dass S, Suttie JJ, Piechnik SK, Ferreira VM, Holloway CJ, Banerjee R, et al. Myocardial tissue characterization using magnetic resonance noncontrast t1 mapping in hypertrophic and dilated cardiomyopathy. Circ Cardiovasc Imaging. 2012;5(6):726–33.
90. Puntmann VO, Arroyo Ucar E, Hinojar Baydes R, Ngah NB, Kuo YS, Dabir D, et al. Aortic stiffness and interstitial myocardial fibrosis by native T1 are independently associated with left ventricular remodeling in patients with dilated cardiomyopathy. Hypertension. 2014;64(4):762–8.
91. Kato S, Nakamori S, Roujol S, Delling FN, Akhtari S, Jang J, et al. Relationship between native papillary muscle T1 time and severity of functional mitral regurgitation in patients with non-ischemic dilated cardiomyopathy. J Cardiovasc Magn Reson. 2016;18(1):79.
92. Taylor RJ, Umar F, Lin EL, Ahmed A, Moody WE, Mazur W, et al. Mechanical effects of left ventricular midwall fibrosis in non-ischemic cardiomyopathy. J Cardiovasc Magn Reson. 2016;18:1.
93. Henn MC, Lawrance CP, Kar J, Cupps BP, Kulshrestha K, Koerner D, et al. Dilated cardiomyopathy: normalized multiparametric myocardial strain predicts contractile recovery. Ann Thorac Surg. 2015;100(4):1284–91.
94. Claus P, Omar AMS, Pedrizzetti G, Sengupta PP, Nagel E. Tissue tracking technology for assessing cardiac mechanics: principles, normal values, and clinical applications. J Am Coll Cardiol Img. 2015;8(12):1444–60.
95. Schuster A, Hor KN, Kowallick JT, Beerbaum P, Kutty S. Cardiovascular magnetic resonance myocardial feature tracking: concepts and clinical applications. Circ Cardiovasc Imaging. 2016;9(4):e004077.
96. Jeung MY, Germain P, Croisille P, El ghannudi S, Roy C, Gangi A. Myocardial tagging with MR imaging: overview of normal and pathologic findings. Radiographics. 2012;32(5):1381–98.
97. Pedrizzetti G, Claus P, Kilner PJ, Nagel E. Principles of cardiovascular magnetic resonance feature tracking and echocardiographic speckle tracking for informed clinical use. J Cardiovasc Magn Reson. 2016;18(1):51.
98. Yu Y, Yu S, Tang X, Ren H, Li S, Zou Q, et al. Evaluation of left ventricular strain in patients with dilated cardiomyopathy. J Int Med Res. 2017;45(6):2092–100.
99. Buss SJ, Breuninger K, Lehrke S, Voss A, Galuschky C, Lossnitzer D, et al. Assessment of myocardial deformation with cardiac magnetic resonance strain imaging improves risk stratification in patients with dilated cardiomyopathy. Eur Heart J Cardiovasc Imaging. 2015;16(3):307–15.
100. Romano S, Judd RM, Kim RJ, Kim HW, Klem I, Heitner J, et al. Association of feature-tracking cardiac magnetic resonance imaging left ventricular global longitudinal strain with all-cause mortality in patients with reduced left ventricular ejection fraction. Circulation. 2017;135(23):2313–5.
101. Romano S, Judd RM, Kim RJ, Kim HW, Klem I, Heitner JF, et al. Feature-tracking global longitudinal strain predicts death in a multicenter population of patients with ischemic and nonischemic dilated cardiomyopathy incremental to ejection fraction and late gadolinium enhancement. JACC Cardiovasc Imaging. 2018; https://doi.org/10.1016/j.jcmg.2017.10.024.
102. Riffel JH, Keller MG, Rost F, Arenja N, Andre F, Aus dem Siepen F, et al. Left ventricular long axis strain: a new prognosticator in non-ischemic dilated cardiomyopathy? J Cardiovasc Magn Reson. 2016;18(1):36.
103. Cui Y, Cao Y, Song J, Dong N, Kong X, Wang J, et al. Association between myocardial extracellular volume and strain analysis through cardiovascular magnetic resonance with his-

tological myocardial fibrosis in patients awaiting heart transplantation. J Cardiovasc Magn Reson. 2018;20(1):25.

104. Merlo M, Masè M, Vitrella G, Belgrano M, Faganello G, Di Giusto F, et al. Usefulness of addition of magnetic resonance imaging to echocardiographic imaging to predict left ventricular reverse remodeling in patients with non-ischemic cardiomyopathy. Am J Cardiol. 2018; https://doi.org/10.1016/j.amjcard.2018.04.017.
105. Bilchick KC, Dimaano V, Wu KC, Helm RH, Weiss RG, Lima JA, et al. Cardiac magnetic resonance assessment of dyssynchrony and myocardial scar predicts function class improvement following cardiac resynchronization therapy. JACC Cardiovasc Imaging. 2008;1(5):561–8.
106. Ponikowski P, Voors AA, Anker SD, Bueno H, Cleland JGF, Coats AJS, et al. 2016 ESC GUIDELINES for the diagnosis and treatment of acute and chronic heart failure: The Task Force for the diagnosis and treatment of acute and chronic heart failure of the European Society of Cardiology (ESC)Developed with the special contribution of the Heart Failure Association (HFA) of the ESC. Eur Heart J. 2016;37(27):2129–200.
107. Juilliere Y, Barbier G, Feldmann L, Grentzinger A, Danchin N, Cherrier F. Additional predictive value of both left and right ventricular ejection fractions on long-term survival in idiopathic dilated cardiomyopathy. Eur Heart J. 1997;18(2):276–80.
108. La Vecchia L, Paccanaro M, Bonanno C, Varotto L, Ometto R, Vincenzi M. Left ventricular versus biventricular dysfunction in idiopathic dilated cardiomyopathy. Am J Cardiol. 1999;83(1):120–2, A9.
109. Gulati A, Ismail TF, Jabbour A, Alpendurada F, Guha K, Ismail NA, et al. The prevalence and prognostic significance of right ventricular systolic dysfunction in nonischemic dilated cardiomyopathy. Circulation. 2013;128(15):1623–33.
110. Arenja N, Riffel JH, Halder M, Djiokou CN, Fritz T, Andre F, et al. The prognostic value of right ventricular long axis strain in non-ischaemic dilated cardiomyopathies using standard cardiac magnetic resonance imaging. Eur Radiol. 2017;27(9):3913–23.
111. Dini FL, Cortigiani L, Baldini U, Boni A, Nuti R, Barsotti L, et al. Prognostic value of left atrial enlargement in patients with idiopathic dilated cardiomyopathy and ischemic cardiomyopathy. Am J Cardiol. 2002;89(5):518–23.
112. Rossi A, Temporelli PL, Quintana M, Dini FL, Ghio S, Hillis GS, et al. Independent relationship of left atrial size and mortality in patients with heart failure: an individual patient meta-analysis of longitudinal data (MeRGE Heart Failure). Eur J Heart Fail. 2009;11(10):929–36.
113. Tsang MY, Barnes ME, Tsang TS. Left atrial volume: clinical value revisited. Curr Cardiol Rep. 2012;14(3):374–80.
114. Gulati A, Ismail TF, Jabbour A, Ismail NA, Morarji K, Ali A, et al. Clinical utility and prognostic value of left atrial volume assessment by cardiovascular magnetic resonance in non-ischaemic dilated cardiomyopathy. Eur J Heart Fail. 2013;15(6):660–70.
115. Moon J, Shim CY, Kim YJ, Park S, Kang SM, Chung N, et al. Left atrial volume as a predictor of left ventricular functional recovery in patients with dilated cardiomyopathy and absence of delayed enhancement in cardiac magnetic resonance. J Card Fail. 2016;22(4):265–71.
116. Amzulescu MS, Rousseau MF, Ahn SA, Boileau L, de Meester de Ravenstein C, Vancraeynest D, et al. Prognostic impact of hypertrabeculation and noncompaction phenotype in dilated cardiomyopathy: a CMR study. J Am Coll Cardiol Img. 2015;8(8):934–46.
117. Abunassar JG, Yam Y, Chen L, D'Mello N, Chow BJ. Usefulness of the Agatston score = 0 to exclude ischemic cardiomyopathy in patients with heart failure. Am J Cardiol. 2011;107(3):428–32.
118. Sousa PA, Bettencourt N, Dias Ferreira N, Carvalho M, Leite D, Ferreira W, et al. Role of cardiac multidetector computed tomography in the exclusion of ischemic etiology in heart failure patients. Rev Port Cardiol. 2014;33(10):629–36.
119. Raff GL, Gallagher MJ, O'Neill WW, Goldstein JA. Diagnostic accuracy of noninvasive coronary angiography using 64-slice spiral computed tomography. J Am Coll Cardiol. 2005;46(3):552–7.

120. Andreini D, Pontone G, Pepi M, Ballerini G, Bartorelli AL, Magini A, et al. Diagnostic accuracy of multidetector computed tomography coronary angiography in patients with dilated cardiomyopathy. J Am Coll Cardiol. 2007;49(20):2044–50.
121. Ghostine S, Caussin C, Habis M, Habib Y, Clement C, Sigal-Cinqualbre A, et al. Non-invasive diagnosis of ischaemic heart failure using 64-slice computed tomography. Eur Heart J. 2008;29(17):2133–40.
122. Bhatti S, Hakeem A, Yousuf MA, Al-Khalidi HR, Mazur W, Shizukuda Y. Diagnostic performance of computed tomography angiography for differentiating ischemic vs nonischemic cardiomyopathy. J Nucl Cardiol. 2011;18(3):407–20.
123. Mowatt G, Cook JA, Hillis GS, Walker S, Fraser C, Jia X, et al. 64-Slice computed tomography angiography in the diagnosis and assessment of coronary artery disease: systematic review and meta-analysis. Heart. 2008;94(11):1386–93.
124. de Graaf FR, Schuijf JD, van Velzen JE, Boogers MJ, Kroft LJ, de Roos A, et al. Diagnostic accuracy of 320-row multidetector computed tomography coronary angiography to noninvasively assess in-stent restenosis. Invest Radiol. 2010;45(6):331–40.
125. Guo SL, Guo YM, Zhai YN, Ma B, Wang P, Yang KH. Diagnostic accuracy of first generation dual-source computed tomography in the assessment of coronary artery disease: a meta-analysis from 24 studies. Int J Cardiovasc Imaging. 2011;27(6):755–71.
126. Juergens KU, Grude M, Maintz D, Fallenberg EM, Wichter T, Heindel W, et al. Multi-detector row CT of left ventricular function with dedicated analysis software versus MR imaging: initial experience. Radiology. 2004;230(2):403–10.
127. Lessick J, Mutlak D, Rispler S, Ghersin E, Dragu R, Litmanovich D, et al. Comparison of multidetector computed tomography versus echocardiography for assessing regional left ventricular function. Am J Cardiol. 2005;96(7):1011–5.
128. Yamamuro M, Tadamura E, Kubo S, Toyoda H, Nishina T, Ohba M, et al. Cardiac functional analysis with multi-detector row CT and segmental reconstruction algorithm: comparison with echocardiography, SPECT, and MR imaging. Radiology. 2005;234(2):381–90.
129. Burianova L, Riedlbauchova L, Lefflerova K, Marek T, Lupinek P, Kautznerova D, et al. Assessment of left ventricular function in non-dilated and dilated hearts: comparison of contrast-enhanced 2-dimensional echocardiography with multi-detector row CT angiography. Acta Cardiol. 2009;64(6):787–94.
130. Kang DK, Schoepf UJ, Bastarrika G, Nance JW Jr, Abro JA, Ruzsics B. Dual-energy computed tomography for integrative imaging of coronary artery disease: principles and clinical applications. Semin Ultrasound CT MR. 2010;31(4):276–91.
131. Ko SM, Choi JW, Song MG, Shin JK, Chee HK, Chung HW, et al. Myocardial perfusion imaging using adenosine-induced stress dual-energy computed tomography of the heart: comparison with cardiac magnetic resonance imaging and conventional coronary angiography. Eur Radiol. 2011;21(1):26–35.
132. Wang R, Yu W, Wang Y, He Y, Yang L, Bi T, et al. Incremental value of dual-energy CT to coronary CT angiography for the detection of significant coronary stenosis: comparison with quantitative coronary angiography and single photon emission computed tomography. Int J Cardiovasc Imaging. 2011;27(5):647–56.
133. Ko SM, Park JH, Hwang HK, Song MG. Direct comparison of stress- and rest-dual-energy computed tomography for detection of myocardial perfusion defect. Int J Cardiovasc Imaging. 2014;30(Suppl 1):41–53.
134. Osawa K, Miyoshi T, Koyama Y, Hashimoto K, Sato S, Nakamura K, et al. Additional diagnostic value of first-pass myocardial perfusion imaging without stress when combined with 64-row detector coronary CT angiography in patients with coronary artery disease. Heart. 2014;100(13):1008–15.
135. Varga-Szemes A, Meinel FG, De Cecco CN, Fuller SR, Bayer RR II, Schoepf UJ. CT myocardial perfusion imaging. AJR Am J Roentgenol. 2015;204(3):487–97.
136. Zhao L, Ma X, Feuchtner GM, Zhang C, Fan Z. Quantification of myocardial delayed enhancement and wall thickness in hypertrophic cardiomyopathy: multidetector computed tomography versus magnetic resonance imaging. Eur J Radiol. 2014;83(10):1778–85.

137. Nieman K, Shapiro MD, Ferencik M, Nomura CH, Abbara S, Hoffmann U, et al. Reperfused myocardial infarction: contrast-enhanced 64-Section CT in comparison to MR imaging. Radiology. 2008;247(1):49–56.
138. Wichmann JL, Arbaciauskaite R, Kerl JM, Frellesen C, Bodelle B, Lehnert T, et al. Evaluation of monoenergetic late iodine enhancement dual-energy computed tomography for imaging of chronic myocardial infarction. Eur Radiol. 2014;24(6):1211–8.
139. Esposito A, Palmisano A, Antunes S, Maccabelli G, Colantoni C, Rancoita PMV, et al. Cardiac CT with delayed enhancement in the characterization of ventricular tachycardia structural substrate: relationship between CT-segmented scar and electro-anatomic mapping. J Am Coll Cardiol Img. 2016;9(7):822–32.
140. Cerny V, Kuchynka P, Marek J, Lambert L, Masek M, Palecek T, et al. Utility of cardiac CT for evaluating delayed contrast enhancement in dilated cardiomyopathy. Herz. 2017;42(8):776–80.
141. Nacif MS, Kawel N, Lee JJ, Chen X, Yao J, Zavodni A, et al. Interstitial myocardial fibrosis assessed as extracellular volume fraction with low-radiation-dose cardiac CT. Radiology. 2012;264(3):876–83.
142. Nacif MS, Liu Y, Yao J, Liu S, Sibley CT, Summers RM, et al. 3D left ventricular extracellular volume fraction by low-radiation dose cardiac CT: assessment of interstitial myocardial fibrosis. J Cardiovasc Comput Tomogr. 2013;7(1):51–7.
143. Wichmann JL, Hu X, Kerl JM, Schulz B, Bodelle B, Frellesen C, et al. Non-linear blending of dual-energy CT data improves depiction of late iodine enhancement in chronic myocardial infarction. Int J Cardiovasc Imaging. 2014;30(6):1145–50.
144. Chang S, Han K, Youn JC, Im DJ, Kim JY, Suh YJ, et al. Utility of dual-energy CT-based monochromatic imaging in the assessment of myocardial delayed enhancement in patients with cardiomyopathy. Radiology. 2018;287(2):442–51.
145. Wolk MJ, Bailey SR, Doherty JU, Douglas PS, Hendel RC, Kramer CM, et al. ACCF/AHA/ASE/ASNC/HFSA/HRS/SCAI/SCCT/SCMR/STS 2013 multimodality appropriate use criteria for the detection and risk assessment of stable ischemic heart disease: a report of the American College of Cardiology Foundation Appropriate Use Criteria Task Force, American Heart Association, American Society of Echocardiography, American Society of Nuclear Cardiology, Heart Failure Society of America, Heart Rhythm Society, Society for Cardiovascular Angiography and Interventions, Society of Cardiovascular Computed Tomography, Society for Cardiovascular Magnetic Resonance, and Society of Thoracic Surgeons. J Am Coll Cardiol. 2014;63(4):380–406.
146. Garbi M, Edvardsen T, Bax J, Petersen SE, McDonagh T, Filippatos G, et al. EACVI appropriateness criteria for the use of cardiovascular imaging in heart failure derived from European National Imaging Societies voting. Eur Heart J Cardiovasc Imaging. 2016;17(7):711–21.

9

Endomyocardial Biopsy

Rossana Bussani, Furio Silvestri, Andrea Perkan,
Piero Gentile, and Gianfranco Sinagra

Abbreviations and Acronyms

CMR	Cardiac magnetic resonance
CS	Cardiac sarcoidosis
DCM	Dilated cardiomyopathy
EMB	Endomyocardial biopsy
HSM	Hypersensitivity myocarditis
LV	Left ventricular
LVEDD	Left ventricular end-diastolic diameter
LVEDVi	Left ventricular end-diastolic volume index
LVEF	Left ventricular ejection fraction
PCR	Polymerase chain reaction
PET	Positron emission tomography
RV	Right ventricular

R. Bussani · F. Silvestri
Department of Pathology, Azienda Sanitaria Universitaria Integrata, University of Trieste (ASUITS), Trieste, Italy
e-mail: bussani@units.it

A. Perkan (✉) · P. Gentile
Cardiovascular Department, Azienda Sanitaria Universitaria Integrata, University of Trieste (ASUITS), Trieste, Italy
e-mail: andrea.perkan@asuits.sanita.fvg.it

G. Sinagra
Cardiovascular Department, Azienda Sanitaria Universitaria Integrata, Trieste, Italy
e-mail: gianfranco.sinagra@asuits.sanita.fvg.it

9.1 Introduction

Endomyocardial biopsy (EMB) is a useful diagnostic tool for the investigation and treatment of myocardial diseases. The introduction of the transvascular endomyocardial bioptome by Konno and Sakakibara in 1962 [1] has been an important breakthrough in the EMB and in the in vivo diagnosis of heart muscle diseases. EMB has spread in subsequent years due to the availability of new and better devices, to the improved skill of the operators and to the development of new and more sophisticated methods of diagnosis.

In the first years, opinions on the use and on the usefulness of EMB in myocardial diseases were conflicting. Ferrans and Roberts [2], as early as 1978, concluded that in patients with suspected dilated cardiomyopathy (DCM), the technique is "informative" but of limited "diagnostic value". In spite of recurrent variations of opinions on the use and usefulness of EMB in myocardial diseases, its expansion gave the cardiologist the possibility of increasing the understanding about the histology of heart muscle disease, with an important role in the diagnosis of acute myocarditis.

The main use of EMB is the routine surveillance for rejection of a transplanted heart, but this scenario is outside the scope of this report.

9.2 Technique

Early EMBs were usually performed from the right ventricle (RV) and subsequently also from the left ventricle (LV). Although there are no clear recommendations, in our experience an approach based on the clinical question is preferred [3, 4], also considering the procedural feasibility in the individual patient (e.g. presence of left ventricular thrombosis, aortic valvular prosthesis or intra-aortic balloon pump).

In the largest head-to-head comparison study, complication rates for LV (0.33%) and RV (0.45%) EMB were comparable [5]. Actual techniques enable to perform multiple drawings of tissue samples from both ventricles with low incidence of procedural complications, but this is mostly dependent by the expertise of the operator.

Fluoroscopy is the most useful imaging modality and is often sufficient, but two-dimensional and three-dimensional echocardiography are increasingly being used to accurately direct biopsy forceps and reduce the likelihood of perforation or recurrent biopsy of the same area [6].

For the RV EMB, the right internal jugular vein is the most common access route. Alternative approaches include femoral vein, using longer bioptomes, and subclavian and brachial veins. Once in the right atrium, anticlockwise rotation might be needed to traverse the tricuspid valve, and then clockwise rotation will bring the tip with the open jaws into contact with the ventricular septum, the preferred site for EMB because of safety problems (direction of rotation should be reversed if approaching from the femoral vein). Going on in the ventricular chamber with open jaws reduces the perforation risk because it uses a greater contact surface. Confirmation of positioning on the septum can be made using contrast injection by the long sheath. Resistance can be appreciated by the operator and only gentle forward pressure is required. Ventricular ectopy or non-sustained ventricular tachycardia is common while the bioptome is in contact with the ventricular myocardium. The forceps should be closed and pulled away from the heart carefully, at which point a small amount of tension might be felt as the sample is removed [6]. The LV can be reached in two ways, in a retrograde direction from the aorta or via trans-septal puncture (uncommon). Currently, the typical approach for EMB is still via the femoral artery, but transradial access is increasingly adopted, particularly in patients with a significant bleeding risk. General advice about steering the bioptome is as for the right ventricle. Crossing the aortic valve is performed in the routine way, using a pigtail catheter into the long sheath to enter the LV. A ventriculography in the left anterior oblique projection should allow positioning of the sheath in the midcavity so that the bioptome forceps can open free of the ventricular wall. Before the procedure i.v. heparin is given to target an activated clotting time of 250–300 s to reduce the risk of embolism [6]. Technique for sampling the myocardium itself is as per RV EMB, with particular care to avoid damaging mitral valve apparatus. The sheath should be aspirated and flushed between each sample as the risk and consequence of air or tissue embolism is ostensibly higher than in the RV [7]. The median number of bioptic samples per patient is 4 (minimum–maximum, 1–6).

False-negative results are possible, particularly with multifocal or microfocal localized diseases (Table 9.1) [8]. Conflicting data exist regarding the benefit of cardiac magnetic resonance (CMR)-guided targeting of areas of late gadolinium enhancement [6]. An analysis of 540 patients undergoing CMR and EMB demonstrated no additional diagnostic yield when targeting areas of late gadolinium enhancement [3, 7].

Table 9.1 Indications and pitfalls of endomyocardial biopsy

Indications for endomyocardial biopsy	Pitfalls of endomyocardial biopsy
• Suspected myocarditis in patients with high-risk syndromes (cardiogenic shock, refractory heart failure or left ventricular dysfunction with LVEF <40% despite conventional therapy, persistent life-threatening ventricular arrhythmias) • Suspected giant cell myocarditis or eosinophilic myocarditis • Suspected cardiac sarcoidosis[a] • Suspected end-stage HCM • Suspected infiltrative cardiomyopathy[b] • Out-of-hospital cardiac arrest without significant coronary artery disease • Monitoring cardiac transplant rejection status • Histological diagnosis of cardiac tumors[c]	Diagnostic accuracy of EMB depends on: • Expertise of operator who performs the procedure • Timing of the procedure related to beginning of patient symptoms • Biopsy site (RV or LV) • Number of bioptic samples • Expertise of pathologist who analyses the samples • Patchy diseases

[a]In cardiac sarcoidosis (CS), the EMB has low sensitivity due to the focal nature of the disease, revealing non-caseating granulomas in less than 25% of patients with CS [30]

[b]In cardiac amyloidosis, the role of EMB has been resized by the recent implementation of non-invasive diagnostic technique as CMR, positron emission tomography (PET) and single-photon emission computed tomography (SPECT)

[c]Following characterization of a cardiac tumour, our multidisciplinary care team, which include cardiologists, radiologists, oncologists and cardiac surgeons, sit down together to develop an individualized treatment plan in order to achieve the optimal outcome. In general, patients with a primary cardiac tumour require surgical resection

9.3 Complications

EMB is invariably characterized by a mild, but not negligible, rate of major complications (around 1%) even when performed by experienced operators [3, 5, 9]. Complications include vasovagal syncope, vascular damage, pneumothorax, supraventricular and ventricular arrhythmias, heart block, damage to the tricuspid valve, ventricular perforation, pericardial tamponade, coronary-cameral fistula formation, bleeding complications and pulmonary and systemic embolism [6]. The risks of EMB likely vary with the experience of the operator, clinical status of the patient, presence or absence of left bundle branch block, access site and possibly bioptome. An echocardiographic control and a low dose of heparin are useful to minimize the risk of systemic embolism during LV EMB [10].

The death associated with EMB is possible and can be the result of perforation with pericardial tamponade [11]. Patients with increased right ventricular systolic pressures, bleeding diathesis, recent receipt of heparin or right ventricular enlargement seem to be at higher risk in case of RV EMB.

9.4 Indications in DCM Scenarios

EMB is an invasive procedure, and for this reason it is fundamental a correct selection of patients to undergo this diagnostic technique. In addition to some particular clinical contexts as after heart transplantation or suspected infiltrative disorders with heart failure presentation such as amyloidosis, the most frequent indication to EMB is suspected acute myocarditis in patients with "major" symptoms (DCM with mildly dilated left ventricle, recent-onset heart failure with relevant left ventricular dysfunction, sustained ventricular arrhythmias) [Fig. 9.1; Case I–IV; Figs. 9.2, 9.3, 9.4 and 9.5] [4].

Myocarditis is an inflammatory process affecting the myocardium that can be caused by infectious agents like virus, bacteria, rickettsia, protozoa and fungi but can be caused also by other agents like toxins, medications and autoimmune phenomena. It is characterized by extreme variability in clinical presentation and ensuing evolution, including a presentation as DCM with severe systolic dysfunction. This variability necessitates patient-tailored diagnostic and therapeutic management in which the advanced and often costly testing and treatments are reserved for those with the most severe and threatening clinical presentation.

Histopathologic analysis of myocardial tissue samples collected with EMB is the only way to definitively diagnose myocarditis. International recommendations about EMB implementation in clinical practice are controversial. The American College of Cardiology/American Heart Association guidelines recommend EMB in patients with severe clinical presentation in terms of recent heart failure or life-threatening arrhythmias [10, 12]. Conversely, the position statement on the diagnosis and management of myocarditis by the European Society of Cardiology Working Group on Myocardial and Pericardial Diseases expanded the spectrum of EMB indications, recommending this test for all cases of clinically suspected myocarditis

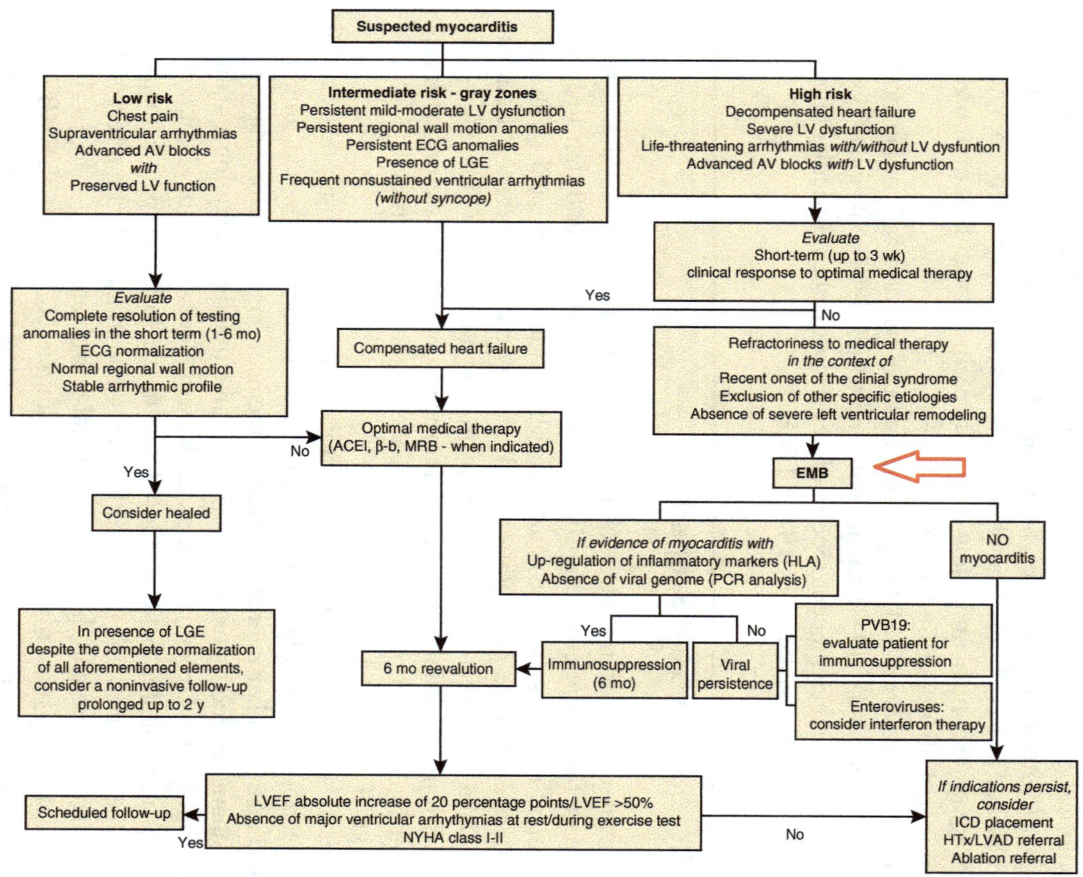

Fig. 9.1 Proposal for clinical management of patients with suspected myocarditis: the role of EMB. Modified from Sinagra G, et al. M. Myocarditis in Clinical Practice. Mayo Clin Proc. 2016 Sep;91(9):1256–66. *ACEI* angiotensin-converting enzyme inhibitor, *AV* atrioventricular, *b-b* b-blocker, *ECG* electrocardiographic, *EMB* endomyocardial biopsy, *HLA* HLA antigen, *HTx* heart transplant, *ICD* implantable cardioverter-defibrillator, *LGE* late gadolinium enhancement, *LV* left ventricular, *LVAD* LV assist device, *LVEF* LV ejection fraction, *MRB* mineralocorticoid receptor blocker, *NYHA* New York Heart Association, *PCR* polymerase chain reaction, *PVB19* parvovirus B19

regardless of the pattern and severity of clinical presentation [13]. In clinical practice, the value of EMB becomes crucial in detecting the specific histotype of the myocarditis and assessing the immunologic and virologic status of the myocardium through immunohistochemical and biomolecular PCR (polymerase chain reaction) analyses.

Hence, EMB should be performed for the in-depth evaluation of suspected myocarditis with recent-onset high-risk major clinical syndromes (heart failure and/or life-threatening arrhythmias, in particular when associated with severe left ventricular dysfunction), not responding to standard optimized medical therapy in the short term (from hours to 2 weeks after admission, on the basis of clinical status severity) [10]. The in-depth characterization of the myocardial substrate can provide the guide for a biopsy-driven therapeutic plan [14, 15]. Conversely, the value of EMB is questionable in patients presenting with low-risk syndromes and responding to standard care [8]. Finally, in the setting of intermediate-risk syndromes (presence of structural or functional abnormalities, such as mild-to-moderate ventricular dysfunction, persistent wall motion or ECG abnormalities, late gadolinium enhancement in the absence of severe left ventricular dysfunction and remodelling on cardiac magnetic resonance imaging or frequent non-sustained ventricular arrhythmias), EMB should be considered on a case-by-case basis according to the clinical status of the patient, the presence of extensive structured myocardial involvement and when findings on cardiac magnetic resonance imaging cannot be considered conclusive [4]. In particular, EMB could be useful in diagnosing cardiac sarcoidosis or giant cell myocarditis allowing to plan an appropriate therapeutic management [3, 16]. In this setting, unexplained heart failure of >3 months' duration associated with a dilated left ventricle and new ventricular arrhythmias, Mobitz type II second- or third-degree AV heart block, or failure to respond to usual care within 1–2 weeks can be the clinical presentation of cardiac sarcoidosis or idiopathic granulomatous myocarditis. EMB is reasonable in this clinical setting (class of recommendation 2a, level of evidence C) [10]. Interestingly, cardiac involvement is present in about 25% of patients with systemic sarcoidosis [17], but symptoms referable to cardiac sarcoidosis occur in only 5% of sarcoid patients [18, 19], and up to 50% of patients with granulomatous inflammation in the heart have no evidence of extracardiac disease. Patients with cardiac sarcoidosis sometimes may be distinguished from those with DCM by a high rate of heart block (8–67%) [4].

Suspected eosinophilic myocarditis can be another setting in which EMB can help to define the specific diagnosis. Eosinophilic myocarditis is associated with the hypereosinophilic syndrome and it typically evolves over weeks to months. The presentation is usually biventricular heart failure, although arrhythmias may lead to sudden death. Usually hypereosinophilia precedes or coincides with the onset of cardiac symptoms, but the eosinophilia may be delayed [20]. Eosinophilic myocarditis may also occur in the setting of hypersensitivity myocarditis (HSM), malignancy or parasite infection and early in the course of endocardial fibrosis. Early suspicion and recognition of HSM may lead to withdrawal of offending medications and administration of high dosage of corticosteroids. The hallmark histological findings of HSM include an interstitial infiltrate with prominent eosinophils with little myocyte necrosis; however, granulomatous myocarditis, or necrotizing eosinophilic myocarditis, may also be a manifestation of drug hypersensitivity [21] and may be distinguished from common forms of HSM only by EMB.

Moreover, the degree of fibrosis seen on EMB can be correlated with a poorer prognosis in terms of major adverse cardiovascular events (defined as cardiovascular death, an arrhythmic event and heart failure-related hospital admission) [22].

In conclusion, while in the past EMB was used more extensively in DCM patients also only for the detection of a histological typical pattern like cell involutive aspects and fibrosis, without a direct gain in terms of therapy, now the indications in DCM are limited to some selected cases (Table 9.1).

9.5 Diagnosis of Myocarditis

EMB, using standardized histopathological [23] and immunohistochemical diagnostic criteria, is the current gold standard by which a diagnosis of myocarditis is made. The Dallas criteria define active myocarditis as an inflammatory infiltrate of the myocardium with necrosis and/or degeneration of adjacent myocytes. The infiltrates are usually lymphocytic but might be neutrophilic or, occasionally, eosinophilic and almost always include macrophages [see Case I–IV]. "Borderline myocarditis" is the term used when the inflammatory infiltrate is too sparse or myocyte injury is not demonstrated [23]. The Dallas criteria are limited, however, by virtue of a high degree of interobserver variability in pathological interpretation and the inability to detect noncellular inflammatory processes and yield diagnostic information in only 10–20% of patients [24, 25]. Therefore, immunohistochemistry with the use of a large panel of monoclonal and polyclonal antibodies is now obligatory to differentiate the inflammatory components present and the immunological processes activated [13]. According to the WHO definition, active myocarditis is present with immunohistochemical detection of focal or diffuse mononuclear infiltrates (T lymphocytes and macrophages) using a cut-off of >14 cells per mm^2, in addition to increased expression of HLA class II molecules [26]. Molecular detection of viral genomic sequences in diseased myocardium is also feasible and, when coupled with immunohistochemical analysis, increases the diagnostic accuracy of EMB in addition to providing an aetiology and offering prognostic information [5, 27, 28]. Information about the safety of particular treatments can also be gleaned from data obtained via EMB. Detection of specific HLA markers on EMB tissue sections combined with the absence of infectious agents (PCR-negative for viral genome) suggests either primary or postinfectious immune-mediated myocarditis, at which point immunosuppression might be considered [29].

9.6 Examples of Endomyocardial Biopsy

9.6.1 Case I (J.D.)

EMB of patient (J.D., 30 years old, M) admitted with fulminant myocarditis with need of inotropes and intra-aortic balloon pump (IABP). Initial left ventricular ejection fraction (LVEF) 27%, left ventricular end-diastolic diameter (LVEDD) 56 mm and left ventricular end-diastolic volume index (LVEDVi) 39 mL/m^2. Discharged after 2 weeks with LVEF 65%. LVEF at 15 months of follow-up 62% (Fig. 9.2).

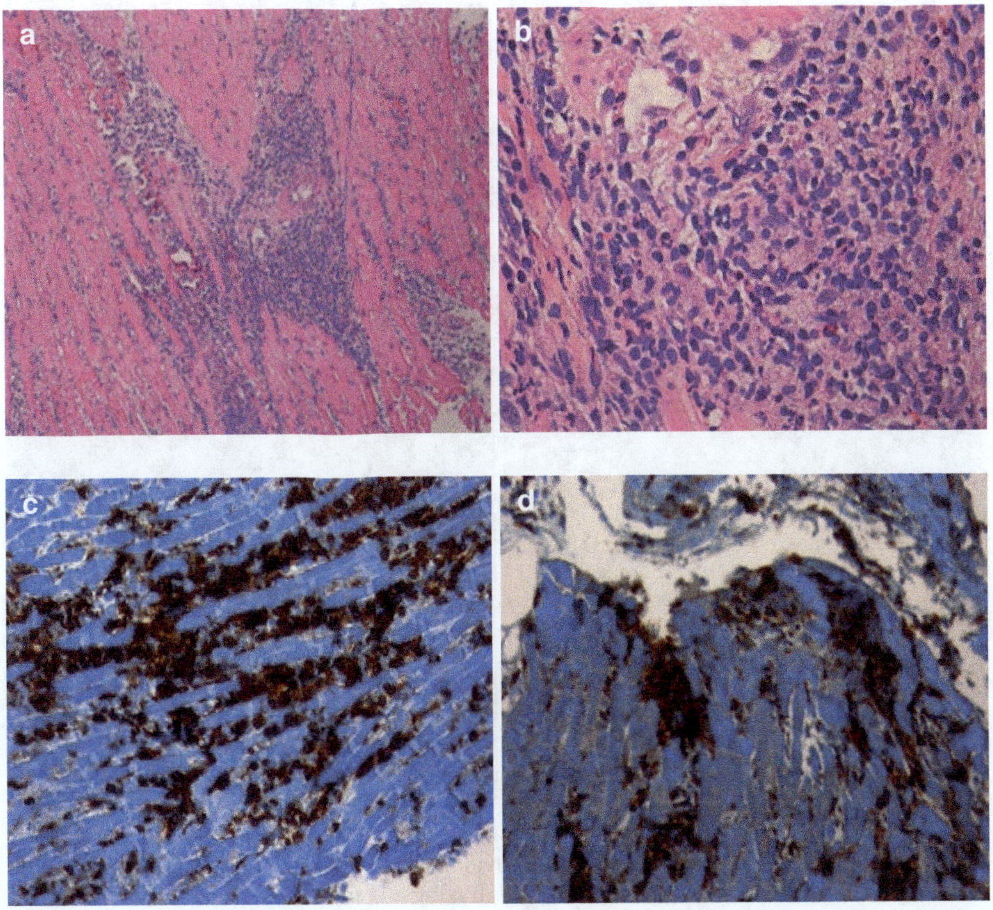

Fig. 9.2 (**a, b**) The haematoxylin-eosin (H&E) stain shows diffuse myocardial inflammatory infiltrates (lymphocytes, granulocytes, eosinophils) with some granulomatous pattern (**a**, H&E ×10; **b**, H&E ×40). (**c**) Myocardial interstitium with diffuse infiltrates of CD4-positive T cells (CD4 ×40). (**d**) High expression of HLA-DR by inflammatory elements (HLA-DR ×20)

9.6.2 Case II (C.P.)

EMB of patient (C.P., 52 years old, F) admitted with fulminant myocarditis with need of inotropes and non-invasive ventilation (NIV). Initial LVEF 36%, LVEDD 45 mm, LVEDVi 37 mL/m^2. Discharged after 2 weeks with LVEF 49%. LVEF at 2 years of follow-up 54% (Fig. 9.3).

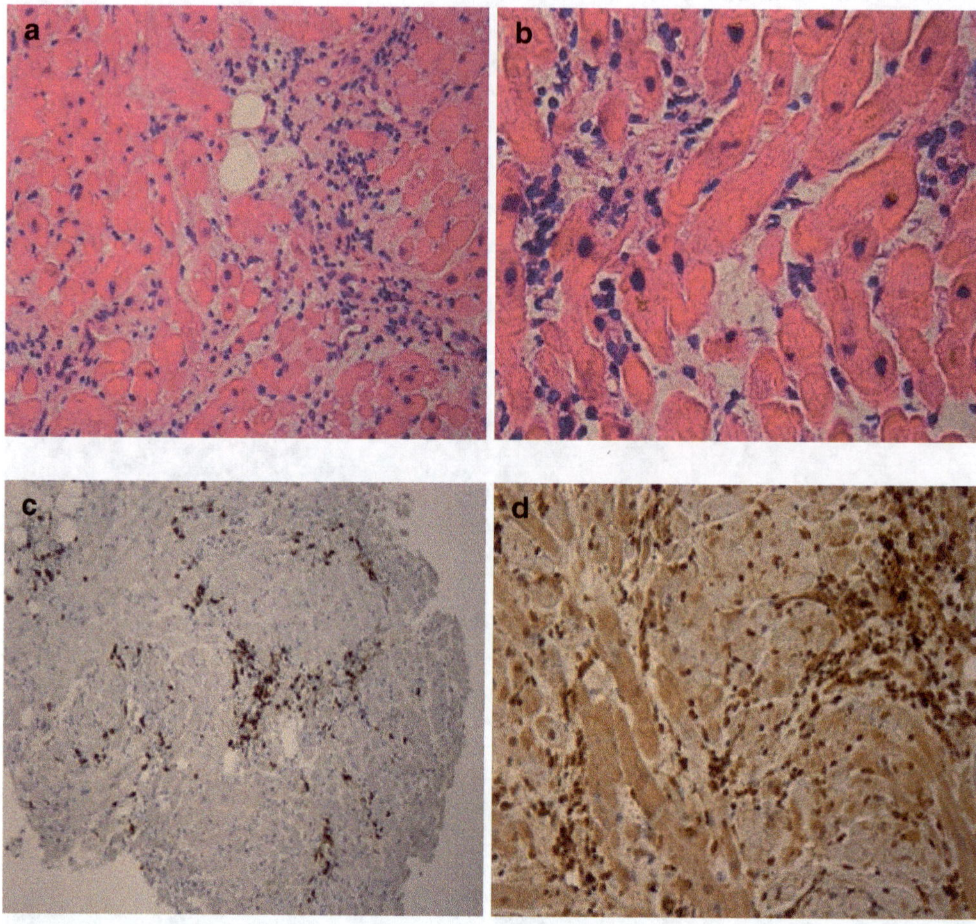

Fig. 9.3 (**a**, **b**) The haematoxylin-eosin (H&E) stain shows diffuse myocardial lympho-histiocytic infiltrates associated with myocyte degeneration, fraying and myocyte necrosis. The myocardial interstitium appears wide with abundant oedema and mild fibrosis (newly formed) (**a**, H&E ×20; **b**, H&E ×40). (**c**) Myocardial interstitium with diffuse infiltrates of CD8-positive suppressor cells (CD8 ×10). (**d**) High expression of HLA-DR by inflammatory elements, endothelium and myocytes (HLA-DR ×20)

9.6.3 Case III (C.S.)

EMB of patient (C.S., 51 years old, M) admitted with non-fulminant myocarditis. Initial LVEF 29%, LVEDD 62 mm, LVEDVi 80 mL/m^2. Discharged after 12 days with LVEF 28%, LVEDD 63 mm, LVEDVi 93 mL/m^2. LVEF at 3 years of follow-up 43% (Fig. 9.4).

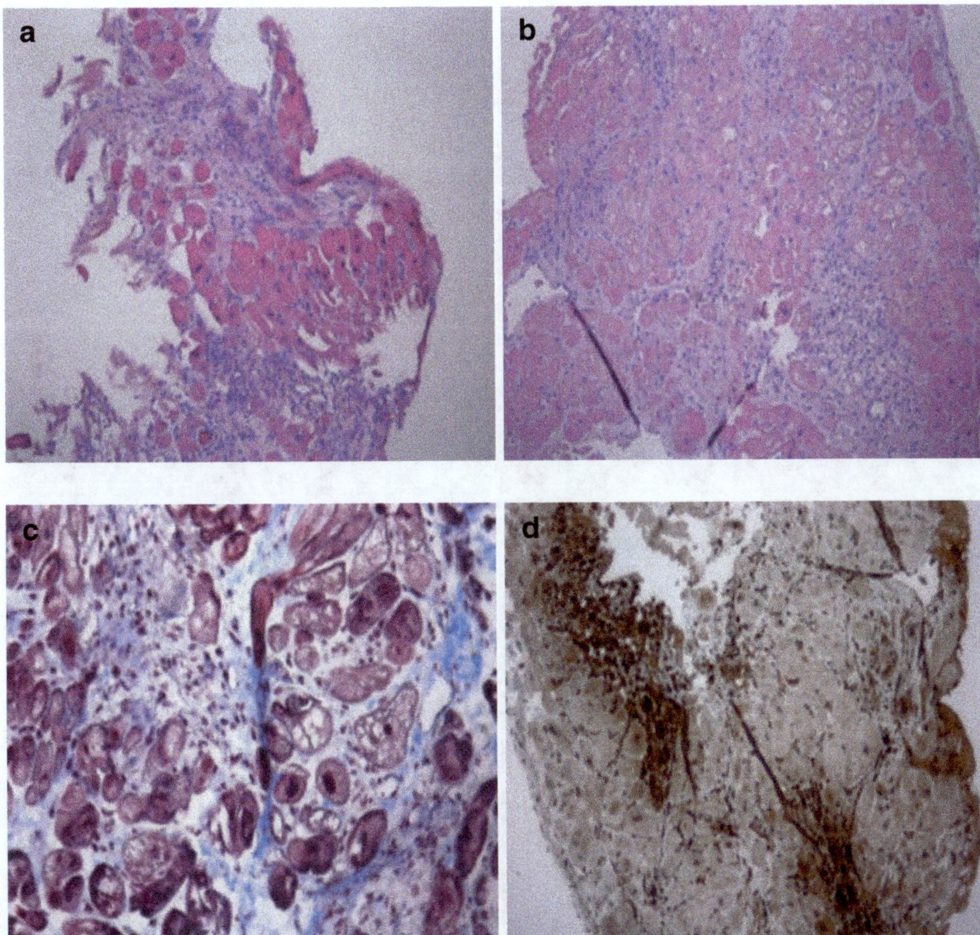

Fig. 9.4 (**a**, **b**) The haematoxylin-eosin (H&E) stain shows many myocardial lympho-histiocytic infiltrates, some of them localized in a wide fibrotic matrix. The EMB shows also cell involutive aspects (hypertrophic cells and/or cells with loss of contractile proteins) (**a**, H&E ×10; **b**, H&E ×10). (**c**) Mallory's trichrome stain shows interstitial fibrosis and severe involutive aspects of myocells (Mallory Trichrome ×20). (**d**) Diffuse myocardial lympho-histiocytic infiltrates (CD68 KP1 ×10)

9.6.4 Case IV (C.F.)

EMB of patient (C.F., 61 years old, M) admitted with non-fulminant myocarditis. Initial LVEF 27%, LVEDD 70 mm, LVEDVi 92 mL/m^2. Discharged after 21 days with LVEF 26%, LVEDD 71 mm, LVEDVi 97 mL/m^2. LVEF at 1 year of follow-up 49% (Fig. 9.5).

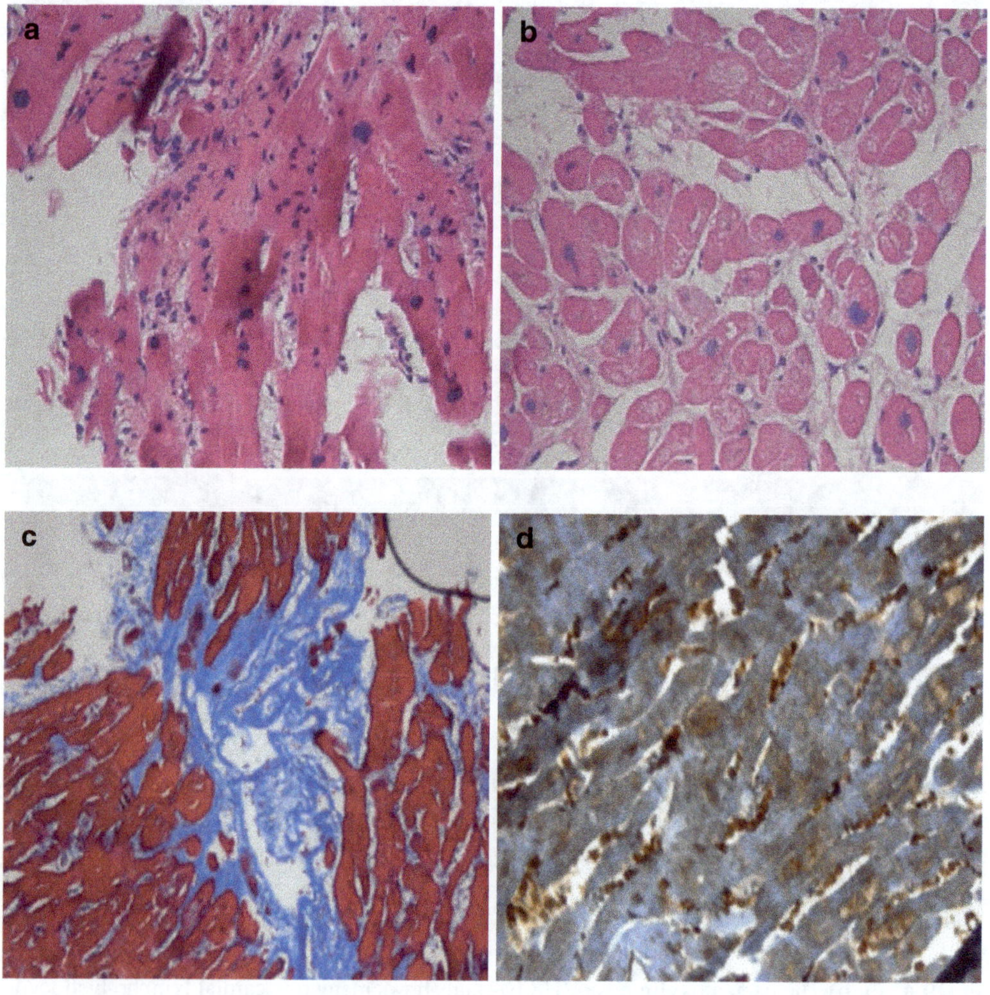

Fig. 9.5 (**a**) The haematoxylin-eosin (H&E) stain shows myocardial lympho-histiocytic infiltrate with replacement myocardial fibrosis (H&E ×20). (**b**) The EMB shows also hypertrophy, attenuation and involutive aspects of myocells with loss of contractile proteins (H&E ×20). (**c**) Mallory's trichrome stain shows interstitial and replacement fibrosis (Mallory trichrome ×10). (**d**) HLA-DR expression by interstitial inflammatory elements and by some myocells (HLA-DR ×20)

References

1. Sakakibara S, Konno S. Endomyocardial biopsy. Jpn Heart J. 1962;3:573–43.
2. Ferrans UJ, Roberts WC. Myocardial biopsy: a useful diagnostic procedure or only a research tool? Am J Cardiol. 1978;41:965–7.
3. Yilmaz A, Kindermann I, Kindermann M, Mahfoud F, Ukena C, Athanasiadis A, et al. Comparative evaluation of left and right ventricular endomyocardial biopsy: differences in complication rate and diagnostic performance. Circulation. 2010;122:900–9.
4. Sinagra G, Anzini M, Pereira NL, Bussani R, Finocchiaro G, Bartunek J, et al. Myocarditis in clinical practice. Mayo Clin Proc. 2016;91(9):1256–66.
5. Chimenti C, Frustaci A. Contribution and risks of left ventricular endomyocardial biopsy in patients with cardiomyopathies: a retrospective study over a 28-year period. Circulation. 2013;128:1531–41.
6. Francis R, Lewis C. Myocardial biopsy: techniques and indications. Heart. 2018;104(11):950–8.
7. Mahrholdt H, Goedecke C, Wagner A, Meinhardt G, Athanasiadis A, Vogelsberg H, et al. Cardiovascular magnetic resonance assessment of human myocarditis: a comparison to histology and molecular pathology. Circulation. 2004;109:1250–8.
8. Calabrese F, Thiene G. Myocarditis and inflammatory cardiomyopathy: microbiological and molecular biological aspects. Cardiovasc Res. 2003;60:11–25.
9. Bennett MK, Gilotra NA, Harrington C, Rao S, Dunn JM, Freitag TB, et al. Evaluation of the role of endomyocardial biopsy in 851 patients with unexplained heart failure from 2000-2009. Circ Heart Fail. 2013;6(4):676–84.
10. Cooper LT, Baughman KL, Feldman AM, Frustaci A, Jessup M, Kuhl U, et al. The role of endomyocardial biopsy in the management of cardiovascular disease: a scientific statement from the American Heart Association, the American College of Cardiology, and the European Society of Cardiology; endorsed by the Heart Failure Society of America and the Heart Failure Association of the European Society of Cardiology. Eur Heart J. 2007;28(24):3076–93.
11. Deckers JW, Hare JM, Baughman KL. Complications of transvenous right ventricular endomyocardial biopsy in adult patients with cardiomyopathy: a seven-year survey of 546 consecutive diagnostic procedures in a tertiary referral center. J Am Coll Cardiol. 1992;19:43–7.
12. Yancy CW, Jessup M, Bozkurt B, Butler J, Casey DE Jr, Colvin MM, et al. 2013 ACCF/AHA guideline for the management of heart failure: a report of the American College of Cardiology Foundation/American Heart Association task force on practice guidelines. Circulation. 2013;128(16):e240–327.
13. Caforio ALP, Pankuweit S, Arbustini E, Basso C, Gimeno-Blanes J, Felix SB, et al. Current state of knowledge on aetiology, diagnosis, management, and therapy of myocarditis: a position statement of the European Society of Cardiology Working Group on Myocardial and Pericardial Diseases. Eur Heart J. 2013;34(33):2636–48.
14. Wojnicz R, Nowalany-Kozielska E, Wojciechowska C, Wojciechowska C, Glanowska G, Wilczewski P, et al. Randomized, placebo-controlled study for immunosuppressive treatment of inflammatory dilated cardiomyopathy: two-year follow-up results. Circulation. 2001;104(1):39–45.
15. Frustaci A, Russo MA, Chimenti C. Randomized study on the efficacy of immunosuppressive therapy in patients with virus negative inflammatory cardiomyopathy: the TIMIC study. Eur Heart J. 2009;30(16):1995–2002.
16. Felker GM, Thompson RE, Hare JM, Glanowska G, Wilczewski P, Niklewski T, et al. Underlying causes and long-term survival in patients with initially unexplained cardiomyopathy. N Engl J Med. 2000;342(15):1077–84.
17. Silverman KJ, Hutchins GM, Bulkley BH. Cardiac sarcoid: a clinicopathologic study of 84 unselected patients with systemic sarcoidosis. Circulation. 1978;58:1204–11.
18. Okura Y, Dec GW, Hare JM, Berry GR, Tazelaar HD, Cooper LT. A multicentre registry comparison of cardiac sarcoidosis and idiopathic giantcell myocarditis. Circulation. 2000;102(18 Suppl II):II–788.

19. Sekiguchi M, Yazaki Y, Isobe M, Hiroe M. Cardiac sarcoidosis: diagnostic, prognostic, and therapeutic considerations. Cardiovasc Drugs Ther. 1996;10:495–510.
20. Morimoto S, Kato S, Hiramitsu S, Uemura A, Ohtsuki M, Kato Y, et al. Narrowing of the left ventricular cavity associated with transient ventricular wall thickening reduces stroke volume in patients with acute myocarditis. Circ J. 2003;67:490–4.
21. Daniels PR, Berry GJ, Tazelaar HD, Cooper LT. Giant cell myocarditis as a manifestation of drug hypersensitivity. Cardiovasc Pathol. 2000;9:287–91.
22. Mueller KA, Mueller II, Eppler D, Zuern CS, Seizer P, Kramer U, et al. Clinical and histopathological features of patients with systemic sclerosis undergoing endomyocardial biopsy. PLoS One. 2015;10:e0126707.
23. Aretz HT, Billingham ME, Edwards WD, Factor SM, Fallon JT, Fenoglio JJ Jr, et al. Myocarditis. A histopathologic definition and classification. Am J Cardiovasc Pathol. 1987;1:3–14.
24. Magnani JW, Dec GW. Myocarditis: current trends in diagnosis and treatment. Circulation. 2006;113:876–90.
25. Kindermann I, Barth C, Mahfoud F, Ukena C, Lenski M, Yilmaz A, et al. Update on myocarditis. J Am Coll Cardiol. 2012;59:779–92.
26. Richardson P, McKenna W, Bristow M, Maisch B, Mautner B, O'Connell J, et al. Report of the 1995 World Health Organization/International Society and Federation of Cardiology task force on the definition and classification of cardiomyopathies. Circulation. 1996;93:841–2.
27. Pollack A, Kontorovich AR, Fuster V, Dec GW. Viral myocarditis—diagnosis, treatment options, and current controversies. Nat Rev Cardiol. 2015;12(11):670–80.
28. Dennert R, Crijns HJ, Heymans S. Acute viral myocarditis. Eur Heart J. 2008;29:2073–82.
29. Leone O, Veinot JP, Angelini A, Baandrup UT, Basso C, Berry G, et al. 2011 consensus statement on endomyocardial biopsy from the Association for European Cardiovascular Pathology and the Society for Cardiovascular Pathology. Cardiovasc Pathol. 2012;21(4):245–74.
30. Birnie DH, Sauer WH, Bogun F, Cooper JM, Culver DA, Duvernoy CS, et al. HRS expert consensus statement on the diagnosis and management of arrhythmias associated with cardiac sarcoidosis. Heart Rhythm. 2014;11(7):1305–23.

10

Arrhythmias in Dilated Cardiomyopathy: Diagnosis and Treatment

Massimo Zecchin, Daniele Muser, Laura Vitali-Serdoz, Alessandra Buiatti, and Tullio Morgera

Abbreviations and Acronyms

AAD	Antiarrhythmic drugs
AATAC	Ablation vs. Amiodarone for Treatment of Atrial Fibrillation in Patients with Congestive Heart Failure and an Implanted ICD/CRTD
ACC	American College of Cardiology
AF	Atrial fibrillation
AHA	American Heart Association
AIC	Arrhythmia-induced cardiomyopathy

M. Zecchin (✉) · T. Morgera
Cardiovascular Department, Azienda Sanitaria Universitaria Integrata, University of Trieste (ASUITS), Trieste, Italy
e-mail: massimo.zecchin@asuits.sanita.fvg

D. Muser
Cardiac Electrophysiology, Cardiovascular Medicine Division, Hospital of the University of Pennsylvania, Philadelphia, PA, USA

Cardiothoracic Department, University Hospital of Udine, Udine, Italy
e-mail: daniele.muser@asuiud.sanita.fvg.it

L. Vitali-Serdoz
Division of Electrophysiology, Department of Cardiology, Klinikum Coburg, Coburg, Germany
e-mail: laura.vitali-serdoz@klinikum-fuerth.de

A. Buiatti
Cardiovascular Department, Azienda Sanitaria Universitaria Integrata, University of Trieste (ASUITS), Trieste, Italy

Klinik und Poliklinik für Innere Medizin I—Kardiologie, Klinikum rechts der Isar—Technische Universität München, Munich, Germany
e-mail: buiatti@mytum.de

ATP	Antitachycardia therapy
AV	Atrioventricular block
BBR	Bundle branch reentry
CA	Catheter ablation
CASTLE-AF	Catheter ablation vs. standard conventional treatment in patients with left ventricular dysfunction and atrial fibrillation
CMR	Cardiac magnetic resonance
DCM	Dilated cardiomyopathy
EAM	Electroanatomic mapping
ECG	Electrocardiogram
ES	Electrical storm
ESC	European Society of Cardiology
HF	Heart failure
HR	Hazard ratio
HRS	Heart Rhythm Society
ICD	Implantable cardioverter-defibrillator
LBBB	Left bundle branch block
LGE	Late gadolinium enhancement
LMNA	Lamin A/C
LVEF	Left ventricular ejection fraction
NS	Nonsustained
OR	Odds ratio
PJRT	Permanent junctional reciprocating tachycardia
RBBB	Right bundle branch block
RF	Radiofrequency
SCN5A	Sodium voltage-gated channel alpha subunit 5
SCD	Sudden cardiac death
SR	Sinus rhythm
VA	Ventricular arrhythmias
VEB	Ventricular ectopic beats
VT	Ventricular tachycardia

10.1 Burden and Kinds of Arrhythmias in Dilated Cardiomyopathy: Risk Stratification of Sudden Death

Patients with dilated cardiomyopathy (DCM) can develop a broad range of bradyrhythmias and tachyarrhythmias including sinus node dysfunction, various degrees of atrioventricular block, interventricular conduction delay, and atrial and ventricular arrhythmias.

Conduction system disease (sinus node dysfunction, various degrees of atrioventricular block (AV), interventricular conduction delay, and bundle branch block) can occur with all cardiomyopathies, particularly in some familial forms such as lamin A/C mutations (LMNA), mitochondrial diseases, storage disorders (Fabry disease), and infiltrative diseases (amyloidosis).

The arrhythmogenic substrate can be explained by an "irritable focus" resulting from myocardial fibrosis, high catecholamine levels, or stretching of myocardial fibers. In addition, the disruption of the link between the sarcolemma, the cytoskeleton, and the sarcomere can lead to modifications of ion channel function [1].

As the majority of dysfunctional ion channels are localized in the sarcolemma, disruption of the sarcolemma-sarcomere link could cause ion channel dysfunction; conversely, it is possible that the function of an ion channel caused by a gene mutation is primarily disturbed, leading to dysfunction of cytoskeletal protein binding partners and mechanical impairment with "secondary" DCM.

For example, in patients with DCM and sodium voltage-gated channel alpha subunit 5 (SCN5A) mutations, arrhythmias can be particularly frequent, including supraventricular arrhythmias (86%), sick sinus syndrome (33%), atrial fibrillation (AF) (60%), ventricular tachycardia (VT) (33%), and conduction disease (60%) [2]. Functional abnormalities in the sarcolemma, cytoskeleton, or sarcomere can occur secondarily to the SCN5A mutations, while desmosomal and other intercalated disk proteins could also play a role in the different phenotypes (arrhythmic and DCM) that result from SCN5A mutations.

10.1.1 Bradyrhythmias and Conduction Abnormalities

Conduction system diseases can occur with virtually all cardiomyopathies but is particularly prevalent in some familial forms of DCM such as the LMNA mutations and inflammatory, mitochondrial, storage, or infiltrative diseases [3]. Mutations of LMNA account for 6% of patients with DCM and [4] account for 33% of the DCMs with AV block [5]. In a large population with familial and sporadic DCM, conduction defects were present in 62% of patients with and only in 6% without LMNA mutations [6]. In these patients conduction abnormalities can occur even years before heart failure or left ventricular (LV) dysfunction, so the onset of AV conduction defects in middle age or earlier should prompt an evaluation for inflammatory or familial cardiomyopathy, and even in the presence of normal left ventricular function, a close follow-up is needed.

Left bundle branch block (LBBB) is present in 25–30% of patients with DCM; right bundle branch block (RBBB) is rare, accounting for less than 5% of patients [7, 8], while RBBB and AV block are the predominant features in sarcoidosis [9].

No clear data about the meaning of bradyrhythmias in patients with DCM have been reported, but LMNA defects, often present in these patients, are associated with a worse prognosis [6]. Some data suggest that an implantable cardiac defibrillator (ICD) should be considered in all patient candidates to pacemaker implantation even in the absence of left ventricular dysfunction or ventricular tachyarrhythmias [10].

The prognostic role of bundle branch blocks (particularly LBBB) is debated; patients with LBBB can have a higher risk of death from heart failure or heart transplantation [7], but its onset during follow-up, rather than its mere presence, seems to be more relevant for the risk stratification of all-cause mortality: Aleksova et al., analyzing 608 patients with DCM from our registry [8], observed that patients with baseline LBBB had a significantly higher mortality rate than those without LBBB at the univariate analysis, but after a multiple covariate adjustment, only new-onset LBBB was an independent predictor of all-cause mortality (HR 3.18, 95% CI:1.90–5.31, $P < 0.001$) at multivariable analysis.

10.1.2 Supraventricular Arrhythmias

Supraventricular arrhythmias can occur in patients with DCM, but their presence should prompt investigation for familial LMNA cardiomyopathy (present in 73% of patients with these gene carriers and only in 36% of patients without this gene defect) [6].

AV nodal reentry and accessory pathway-related tachycardia are usually unrelated to the DCM, while incessant atrial tachycardia can be the cause rather than the consequence of left ventricular dysfunction; however, in these patients diffuse fibrosis or alterations in the structure or LV function can be present also in the long-term follow-up, suggesting that, even after a successful treatment of arrhythmias, recovery can be incomplete due to a late treatment or the coexistence of a structural heart disease.

AF is present in about 10–15% of patients with DCM [11].

10.1.3 Ventricular Arrhythmias

Ventricular ectopic beats (VEB) and nonsustained ventricular arrhythmias (nsVA) are observed in about 40% of patients with DCM and reflect a particular arrhythmogenic substrate involving rapid nonsustained VT (nsVT) and/or frequent VEB, the latter occurring in up to 30% of cases [12]. However, the prognostic role of these arrhythmias is not clear, and conflicting data have been published in the last 30 years. Some studies [13–16] suggested a worse prognosis and a higher risk of Sudden Cardiac Death (SCD) in patients with nsVA. In others [17], nonsustained VT were predictors of SCD at univariate, but not at multivariable analysis, or were not predictive of SCD, maybe in light of the high incidence of nsVT in patients with DCM.

It was proposed that only the association of VA with other risk factors, as low left ventricular ejection fraction (LVEF), could help to identify patients at higher risk. Differently from other experiences, we observed that nsVT are associated with a higher risk only in patients without severe LV dysfunction ($LVEF > 0.35$) while in patients with $LVEF \leq 0.35$ they do not give any additional information [18].

In addition, we did not identify any specific characteristic VT that can be useful for the risk. However, an "arrhythmic pattern" at presentation, as defined by the presence of unexplained syncope, nsVT, ≥1000 VEB/24 h, or ≥50 ventricular couplets/24 h, was associated with a higher incidence of SCD, sustained VT, or ventricular fibrillation compared with other patients (30.3% vs. 17.6%, $P = 0.022$), independently from LVEF, with no difference in the total mortality [12].

10.1.4 Mechanisms

In heart failure, the mechanisms of atrial and ventricular tachyarrhythmias can be multiple.

According to old studies published decades ago, VEB and nonsustained VT in patients with DCM are initiated by a focal mechanism [19]. However, sustained VA are caused by reentry [20] in a significant amount of patients with DCM, as suggested also by the high rate and efficacy of antitachycardia therapy (ATP), unexpectedly similar to that found in patients with ischemic cardiomyopathy [21].

Bundle branch block reentry (BBR) VT is a form of sustained monomorphic VT that utilizes the conduction system as a reentry circuit, usually with anterograde propagation over the right bundle and retrograde conduction over the left bundle. Activation of the ventricles via the right bundle fibers produces VT that has a typical LBBB QRS morphology. More rarely, the reverse sequence of conduction can also occur, leading to an RBBB configuration. BBR VT are not uncommon in DCM. Rapid VT (>200 beats/min), often resulting in syncope or cardiac arrest, is the clinical presentation. Catheter ablation of the right bundle is highly effective in abolishing BBR VT, often (but not always) resulting in complete AV block (because of the preexistent LBBB, which sometimes is not complete). However, because of severe LV dysfunction, ICD and/or cardiac resynchronization therapy is required in most patients.

10.1.5 Risk Stratification of Sudden Cardiac Death

The assessment of SCD risk in patients with DCM has been a challenge for the last 30 years; nevertheless, both total mortality and SCD rate have been definitely reduced in the last three decades: [22] in the 1980s, SCD rate was up to 18% per year [13, 15], but it was only around 2–3% in patients medically evaluated in the early 2000 [17, 23]. According to the Trieste Cardiomyopathy Registry, including more than 1000 DCM patients with a mean follow-up of 10 years, the incidence of major cardiac events has fallen to less than 2% per year, while the incidence of SCD is less than 0.5% per year. This could have several explanations, including a better diagnostic definition, an earlier diagnosis, the widespread of beta-blockers and mineralocorticoid receptor antagonists (the only drugs significantly associated with a SCD reduction) and, finally, ICD and resynchronization therapy [24].

Because of the relatively low incidence of events, it is difficult to identify patients who could benefit more from ICD treatment and to demonstrate a significant mortality reduction in a not well-selected population. This could also explain why most trials evaluating patients with DCM failed to prove a statistically significant benefit of ICD even in the presence of SCD reduction. In addition, in some trials, patients with nonischemic cardiomyopathy (which is not always synonymous of DCM) of different etiologies and a non-negligible risk of non-arrhythmic death (due to pump failure or noncardiac events) were included [25].

Another important issue is the timing of risk stratification. Only 31% of the patients with LVEF ≤ 0.35 and NYHA class II–III at first presentation still have ICD indications 6 months after medical therapy implementation [26]. According to current European guidelines, at least 3 months of optimal medical treatment is required before considering ICD implantation [27].

Despite hundreds of publications and several parameters analyzed, the severity of left ventricular dysfunction is still the major predictor of arrhythmic events, and current guidelines for ICD implantation in patients with DCM rely solely on LVEF value (together with the New York Heart Association functional class) [27, 28].

However, the odds ratio (OR) for LVEF is only 2.86, with sensitivity and specificity of 71.1% and 50.5%, respectively [29], suggesting that many patients with severe LV dysfunction do not benefit from ICD implantation but also that many patients with LVEF ≥ 0.35 can be at risk of SCD.

In addition to LVEF, many other parameters have been evaluated. According to the meta-analysis by Goldberger et al., four groups of parameters were considered: autonomic parameters (heart rate variability, baroreflex sensitivity, heart rate turbulence), functional parameters (as LVEF, left ventricular dimensions), depolarization abnormalities (fragmented QRS, intraventricular delay, signal-averaged ECG), repolarization abnormalities (T wave alternans), and arrhythmic markers (spontaneous or induced arrhythmias) [29].

Taken individually, disturbances in autonomic function are poorly correlated with the risk of SCD, but also for other parameters, at best, the OR is generally between 2 and 4. T wave alternans was the most sensitive predictor, while electrophysiologic study (EPS) was the most specific. EPS has been thought to have no utility in predicting the risk of SCD, despite the presence of scars, and reentry has been considered the most frequent mechanism of sustained VT in DCM. However, Gatzoulis et al. recently found that the incidence of VT terminated by the ICD during a median follow-up of 42 months was 73% in patients with induction of sustained VA at EPS, compared with 18% in non-inducible patients [12].

Despite its utility for selecting patients to receive an ICD has yet to be demonstrated, late gadolinium enhancement (LGE) by cardiac magnetic resonance (CMR) can detect the presence, site, and extension of cardiac fibrosis. Recently, two meta-analyses involving approximately 3000 patients each were published. According to the analysis performed by Disertori et al. [30] in a population with both ischemic and nonischemic cardiomyopathy, a composite arrhythmic end point (SCD, aborted SCD, VT/VF, and appropriate ICD therapy) was reached in 23.9% of patients with a positive LGE test (annualized event rate of 8.6%) vs. 4.9% of patients with a negative LGE test (annualized event rate of 1.7%; $p < 0.0001$). The OR was 5.62, without finding any difference between ischemic and nonischemic patients. In the subgroup of patients with LVEF ≤0.30, the OR for the arrhythmic events increased to 9.56.

The CMR Guide (Cardiac Magnetic Resonance Guided Management of Mild-Moderate Left Ventricular Systolic Dysfunction) trial, which is currently randomizing ischemic and nonischemic patients with LVEF 36–50% and presence of LGE to either ICD or an implantable loop recorder, will help to identify the role of CMR for selection of candidates to ICD but is estimated to be completed in December 2020 [31].

Another promising tool for the risk stratification, at least in some subgroups of patients, is the genetic analysis. Some genetic defects have been associated both with LV dysfunction and high risk of SCD. In most cases, these defects can be suspected through some "red flags" as conduction defects or supraventricular arrhythmias sometimes preceding the occurrence of LV dysfunction [6, 32] or alteration in the ion channel gene SCN5A [2]. When associated to other risk factors as nsVT, LVEF < 0.45, non-missense mutation, and male sex, LMNA defects even in the absence of severe LV dysfunction represent a IIa recommendation to ICD implant according to both European and American guidelines [27, 28, 33]. In addition, in muscular dystrophies involving LMNA defects, an ICD is suggested as a IIb recommendation in the presence of conduction abnormalities and need of pacemaker implantation [27].

10.1.6 Role of Supraventricular and Ventricular Arrhythmias in Pathogenesis of DCM

10.1.6.1 Definition and Pathophysiology

Arrhythmias can initiate or aggravate acute heart failure (HF) in patients with preexisting heart disease. The arrhythmia-induced cardiomyopathy (AIC), known also as tachycardia-induced cardiomyopathy, is an important and potentially reversible cause of HF and DCM.

In 1949, Philips and Levine published the first description of HF induced by AF in patients without structural heart disease [34]. In the last decades, many reports underlined the role of arrhythmias in inducing HF or a DCM with a recovery of LV function after restoration of sinus rhythm or an adequate rate control.

Currently the AIC is defined on the basis of clinical criteria:

- Sustained heart rate >100/min
- Exclusion of other causes of HF
- Recovery (partial or complete) of LV function after achieving arrhythmia control (i.e., restoration of sinus rhythm or rate control)

Two forms of AIC can be identified: in the first form, "arrhythmia-induced" cardiomyopathy, the arrhythmia is the only identifiable cause of ventricular dysfunction, and in the second form, "arrhythmia-mediated," the arrhythmias aggravate ventricular dysfunction or worsens HF in subjects with underlying heart disease [35]. In patients with recent-onset HF and concomitant arrhythmias, a small LV end-diastolic diameter and mass index could indicate an AIC instead of a true DCM.

In animal models, the ventricular rapid pacing model demonstrated a more rapid reduction in LV function compared to the atrial pacing model, suggesting that myocardial electrical dyssynchrony plays an additional role accelerating the LV dysfunction [36].

In patients with AIC, the temporal relationship between occurrence of arrhythmias and development of LV remodeling, dysfunction and HF are not predictable. It is multifactorial, and there is no specific cutoff in heart rate determining a higher risk of developing AIC.

10.1.6.2 Specific Clinical Pictures

In adults, AF is the most common cause of AIC and is a concomitant arrhythmia in 10 up to 50% of patients in different cohort with HF [37]. Many mechanisms have been suggested as triggers for AIC during AF: loss of atrial contraction with concomitant irregular rhythm, resting tachycardia and inadequate exercise response affecting diastolic filling, and increasing left-sided filling pressure eventually leading to functional mitral regurgitation and mechano-electrical changes in the left atrium with a perpetuating cycle. The therapeutic options and strategies in patients with AF vary from a rate control (drugs or AV-node ablation with biventricular pacing) to a rhythm control strategy (amiodarone and cardioversion or ablation).

In adults a persistent atrial flutter can play a significant role in patients with suspected AIC, because rate control is more difficult to achieve, given less concealed AV-node conduction. In this subgroup of patients, a catheter ablation is the therapy of first choice.

Less often, a persistent supraventricular tachycardia can induce an AIC, and also in this subset, whenever possible, a catheter ablation can normalize LV function.

Another important subset of AIC includes patients with idiopathic VT or frequent VEB; also in this subset, many different mechanisms have been postulated as ventricular dyssynchrony (in particular in VEB arising from right or left ventricular outflow tract with LBBB morphology), abnormal ventricular filling, and modification of Ca^{++} handling. Moreover, some clinical characteristics have been identified in patients at high risk for AIC development: a high VEB burden (>24% or >26% per day is cutoff strongly related to AIC with recovery after VEB ablation) [38, 39], interpolated VEB, retrograde P waves, male sex, asymptomatic VEB, QRS duration, and LBBB morphology.

In children, supraventricular arrhythmias are the main trigger for AIC, in particular atrial ectopic tachycardia and permanent junctional reciprocating tachycardia (PJRT). Atrial tachycardias arising from foci near the sinus node are more difficult to identify, usually appearing in children without structural heart disease. The clinical course of PJRT is often incessant with an unlikely spontaneous resolution and a higher risk of AIC; also in this setting, the catheter ablation is the treatment of first choice. In children, ventricular arrhythmias are rarely identifiable as the cause of HF.

10.1.7 Management of Atrial Arrhythmias in Dilated Cardiomyopathy and Heart Failure

Congestive HF and AF often coexist and adversely affect each other with respect to management and prognosis. No specific data on patients with DCM exist. Generally HF predisposes to AF promoting atrial electrical and structural change, whereas conversely, AF is implicated in the development and/or exacerbation of LV dysfunction as discussed. AF has been demonstrated to increase the mortality risk 1.5- to 2-fold in both sexes and across a wide range of ages. The risk of patients with HF developing AF is 1.6-fold in males and 2.7-fold in females, and the prevalence of AF increases with HF severity, ranging from 5% in functional class I patients to ≈50% in class IV patients [40]. It is intuitive that maintenance of normal sinus rhythm (SR) should improve functional status and possibly reduce mortality in this population. Nevertheless, large randomized trials failed to demonstrate any significant mortality benefit of a pharmacologically based rhythm control strategy, even in patients with LV dysfunction when compared to a rate control strategy [41–43]. In-depth analysis of these trials, indeed, demonstrated that the use of antiarrhythmic drug therapy to restore SR was associated with a 49% increase in mortality rate. Therefore, pursuing SR by non-pharmacologic means can be justified, considering also that several studies have demonstrated the superiority of catheter ablation over medical therapy [44, 45]. Catheter ablation has demonstrated its superiority also compared to AV-node ablation and biventricular pacing and is associated with the reduction of inappropriate and appropriate ICD therapies and with improvement in LVEF in patients with DCM [46]. The multicenter randomized AATAC (Ablation vs. Amiodarone for Treatment of Atrial Fibrillation in Patients with Congestive Heart Failure and an Implanted ICD/CRTD) trial [40] first showed a mortality benefit of catheter ablation vs. amiodarone, albeit in a combined secondary end point. In the CASTLE-AF trial [47], catheter ablation reduced death or hospitalization for heart failure in patients with congestive HF and AF compared with those assigned to medical therapy. Freedom from AF was strongly associated with stroke-free survival.

Cure of AF does not necessary imply its complete elimination. A significant reduction in the amount of time in AF after catheter ablation may be sufficient for achieving clinical benefit in patients with congestive HF. Although available data suggest that the safety and efficacy of catheter ablation are very similar in patients with HF and in those with normal hearts [48], success rate and long-term outcomes are expected to be influenced by patient complexity and concomitant comorbidities. It is well known that HF is an independent predictor of recurrent arrhythmia after catheter ablation; however, other covariates (such as age, sex, diabetes mellitus, and hypertension) have shown an association with ablation outcome. Additional imaging-based variables to predict efficacy and risk of ablation (as left atrial strain by speckle-tracking echocardiography and CMR for left atrial fibrosis size) are currently under investigation.

10.1.8 Management of Ventricular Arrhythmias in Dilated Cardiomyopathy

The life expectancy of patients affected by DCM is progressively growing. As a consequence, recurrent VT and electrical storm (ES) represent an emerging problem mainly in patients with severely depressed LVEF in whom frequent ICD shocks have been associated with poor quality of life, repeated hospitalizations, and increased mortality. In this setting, catheter ablation (CA) has demonstrated to be superior to antiarrhythmic drugs (AAD) in reducing VT recurrences and ICD shocks even if a mortality benefit has never been convincingly proven [49, 50]. The management of VT in this setting is challenging because of the complexity of the substrate and the underlying HF. Outcomes after CA are generally poorer compared to those of post-infarct VT. However, the evolution of electroanatomic mapping (EAM) systems together with the integration of noninvasive imaging modalities has significantly improved ablation strategies and long-term outcomes.

10.1.9 Antiarrhythmic Drug Therapy of Ventricular Arrhythmias

Therapy with AADs is often used to prevent long-term recurrences. In a recent meta-analysis of randomized controlled trials, a 1.5-fold reduction of VAs leading to appropriate ICD shocks has been noted with AADs compared to control medical therapy in patients with structural heart disease [49]. However, there is a substantial lack of data on efficacy and safety of AADs in patients with DCM. In such population, the choice of a specific drug should always take into account a potential negative inotropic effect with the associated possibility of worsening of the hemodynamic status along with proarrhythmic effects (Table 10.1). Amiodarone is usually the drug of choice as its efficacy has been demonstrated in randomized controlled trials with an overall threefold reduction of the risk of recurrent VT compared to beta-blockers. Unfortunately, the use of amiodarone is burdened by a high prevalence of organ toxicity (i.e., thyroid disorders, hepatitis, pulmonary fibrosis). Furthermore, the long-term use of amiodarone has been associated with an increased risk of death [49, 51, 52]. Another commonly used class III AAD is sotalol. Albeit its use seems to be safe in patients with structural heart disease and HF, it has failed to demonstrate its superiority to other β-blockers in preventing recurrent ICD shocks [53–55]. Class I AADs should usually be avoided due to their significant negative inotropic effect and their potential proarrhythmic effect. Specifically, class IC drugs are contraindicated having been demonstrated to increase mortality in patients with structural heart disease [56]. Other class I AADs like mexiletine or procainamide may be used in adjunction to class III AADs or whether class III AADs cannot be administered. Adjuvant therapy with mexiletine has shown to reduce appropriate ICD therapies in case of amiodarone inefficacy [57]. However, it can worsen hemodynamic status in patients with severely reduced LVEF, and therefore its administration should be considered with caution. Procainamide is currently available only as an intravenous formulation in most countries, and there is some evidence suggesting high efficacy for acute termination of hemodynamically stable monomorphic VT even if it is generally avoided due to a significant risk of severe hypotension. No data concerning long-term oral administration are currently available.

Table 10.1 Antiarrhythmic medications for acute and long-term treatment of ventricular tachycardia in patients with structural heart disease

		Acute management	Long-term treatment	Desired plasma concentration
β-blockers	Propranolol	*Bolus*: 0.15 mg/kg IV over 10 min	10–40 mg orally three to four times a day	NA
	Metoprolol	*Bolus*: 2–5 mg IV every 5 min up to three doses in 15 min	25 mg orally twice a day up to 200 mg a day	NA
	Esmolol	*Bolus*: 300–500 mg/kg IV for 1 min *Infusion*: 25–50 mg/kg/min up to a maximum dose of 250 mg/kg/min (titration every 5–10 min)	Not recommended	NA
Class III agents	Amiodarone	*Bolus*: 150 mg IV over 10 min, up to total 2.2 g in 24 h *Infusion*: 1 mg/min for 6 h and then 0.5 mg/min for 18 h	*Oral load*: 800 mg orally twice a day until 10 g total *Maintenance dose*: 200–400 mg orally daily	1.0–2.5 μg/mL No efficacy proven for plasma concentrations <0.5 μg/mL Serious toxicity risk for plasma concentrations >2.5 μg/mL
	Sotalol	Not recommended	80 mg orally twice a day, up to 160 mg twice a day (serious side effects >320 mg/day)	1–3 μg/mL (not of great value, usually monitored by QT prolongation with indication to reduction/discontinuation if prolongation >15–20%)
Class I agents	Procainamide	*Bolus*: 10 mg/kg IV over 20 min *Infusion*: up to 2–3 g/24 h	3–6 g orally daily fractionated in ≥3 administrations	4–12 μg/mL
	Lidocaine	*Bolus*: 1.0–1.5 mg/kg IV, repeat dose of 0.5–0.75 mg/kg IV up to a total dose of 3 mg/kg *Infusion*: 20 μg/kg/min IV	Not recommended	2–6 μg/mL
	Mexiletine	Not recommended	200 mg orally three times a day, up to 400 mg orally three times a day	0.6–1.7 μg/mL

10.1.10 Catheter Ablation of Ventricular Arrhythmias

Current American Heart Association/American College of Cardiology/Heart Rhythm Society guidelines recommend CA in patients with sustained monomorphic VT refractory to AAD therapy, including patients with ES not due to a transient or reversible cause [28]. Radiofrequency CA has proven to be highly effective in controlling VT compared to AADs. However, a clear mortality benefit related to CA has never been reproduced [50, 58–60]. Outcomes after CA of VT in the setting of DCM are heterogeneous and generally poorer compared to ischemic cardiomyopathy (Table 10.2). Technically, comprehensive substrate-based ablation approaches

Table 10.2 Principal studies assessing the role of VT ablation in dilated cardiomyopathy

Study	Number of patients	Age	Baseline LVEF (%)	Epicardial procedures (%)	Amiodarone at time of procedure (%)	VT recurrence, %	Follow-up, months
Hsia et al. 2003 [61]	19	61 ± 16	34 ± 11	0	63	58	22 ± 12
Soejima et al. 2004 [20]	28	54 ± 14	30 ± 11	29	43	36	9 ± 9
Cano et al. 2009 [62]	22	56 ± 13	30 ± 13	100	59	29	18 ± 7
Nakahara et al. 2010 [63]	16	59 ± 11	27 ± 12	75	88	50	15 ± 13
Schmidt et al. 2010 [64]	16	57 ± 11	32 ± 8	94	69	47	12 (median)
Arya et al. 2010 [65]	13	57 ± 18	33 ± 9	24	–	38	23 (median)
Haqqani et al. 2011 [66]	31	59 ± 12	30 ± 14	45	74	32	20 ± 28
Piers et al. 2013 [67]	45	60 ± 16	44 ± 14	64	42	53	24 (median)
Dinov et al. 2014 [68]	63	59 ± 13	34 ± 11	30	33	59	12
Oloriz et al. 2014 [69]	87	–	–	74	–	51	18 (median)
Dinov et al. 2015 [70]	102	59 ± 15	33 ± 12	28	–	56	24
Tung et al. 2015 [59]	966	–	–	–	–	32	12
Yu et al. 2015 [71]	73	–	–	–	–	60	6
Muser et al. 2016 [58]	282	59 ± 15	36 ± 13	38	59	31	48 (median)

are related to better outcomes with long-term recurrence rates as low as 30% in experienced centers [58, 72].

Patients with advanced HF or ES are a high-risk group in which recurrent VT may simply represent a marker of worsening HF status, with limited possibility for achieving long-lasting arrhythmia control. In this setting, even if not able to directly improve survival, CA can still result in improved quality of life by reducing the number of ICD therapies and the need for AADs. In a large series of 193 patients, acute hemodynamic decompensation (AHD) occurred in 11% of subjects and was significantly related to increased mortality at follow-up (50% mortality after a mean follow-up of 21 months vs. 11%) [73]. In the same study, logistic regression analysis identified eight predictors of AHD which formed the PAINESD risk score, namely, chronic obstructive pulmonary disease (five points), age >60 years (three points), general anesthesia (four points), ischemic cardiomyopathy (six points), NYHA functional class III or IV (six points), ejection fraction <25% (three points), presentation with VT storm (five points), and diabetes mellitus (three points) (Fig. 10.1) [73]. The predictive value of this score in identifying patients at high risk of adverse procedural outcomes has been subsequently validated in independent studies and, more recently, in a large international multicenter VT ablation registry [74]. It has been recently reported how patients undergoing VT ablation and considered at high risk on the basis of PAINESD score (PAINESD ≥15) showed a substantial mortality benefit if treated with preemptive mechanical hemodynamic support (MHS) highlighting its potential role as bedside tool to select patients who may

***PAINESD* RISK SCORE**

VARIABLE	SCORE
Pulmonary disease [chronic obstructive] – COPD	5
Age >60 years	3
***A**nesthesia [general]*	*4*
Ischemic cardiomyopathy	6
NYHA class III or IV	6
Ejection fraction <25%	3
Storm [VT]	5
Diabetes mellitus	3

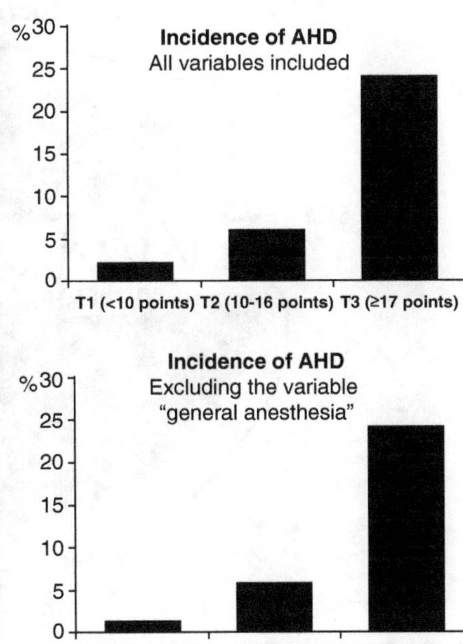

Fig. 10.1 Schematic representation of the PAINESD risk score to predict acute hemodynamic decompensation (AHD) during catheter ablation of ventricular tachycardia in patients with structural heart disease (Reproduced with permission from Santangeli et al. [73])

mostly benefit by advanced HF management and prophylactic implantation of a MHS device to reduce the risk of AHD and improve post-procedural outcomes.

10.1.11 Characteristics of the Arrhythmogenic Substrate and Its Impact on Catheter Ablation Approach

The electrophysiologic substrate of sustained VT in the setting of structural heart disease is usually represented by scar-related reentry, and the destruction of this substrate can potentially prevent VT (Fig. 10.2). The EAM substrate typically involves the basal perivalvular region of the LV and the interventricular septum with a high prevalence of midmyocardial or subepicardial substrates. Two typical scar patterns (anteroseptal and inferolateral) are found in up to 90% of patients with DCM and VT [66, 76]. Two VT morphologies are usually seen in presence of anteroseptal substrate: RBBB with inferior axis and positive concordance throughout the precordial leads or LBBB with inferior axis and early (≤V3) precordial transition (Figs. 10.3 and 10.4) [76]. Occasionally, VT arising from the septum may also present a characteristic precordial transition pattern break in V2 with a predominant R wave in V1 and V3 but an abrupt loss of the R wave in lead V2 due to an exit close to the anterior interventricular sulcus (opposite to lead V2) [66, 77]. A predominant inferolateral substrate can instead be identified in about half of the

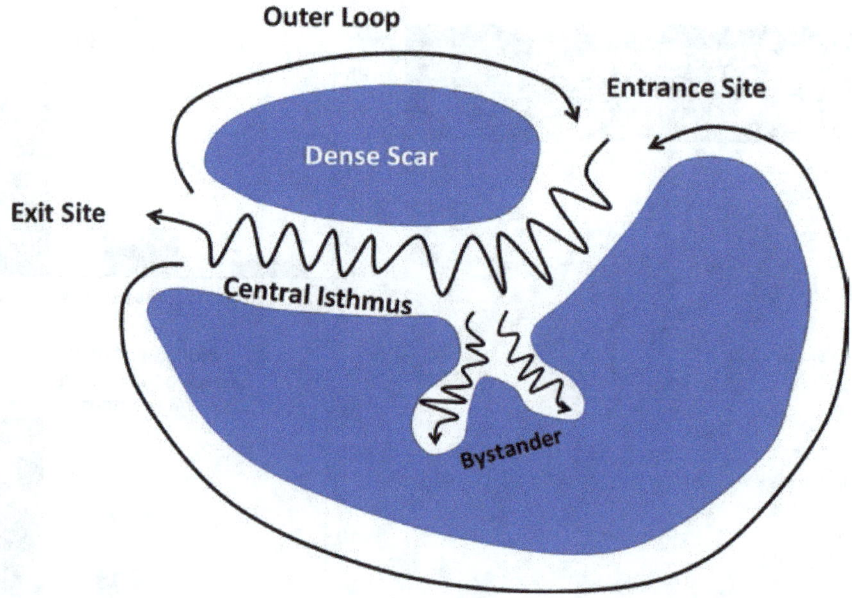

Fig. 10.2 Classic figure-of-eight reentry circuit as described by Stevenson et al. [75]. Blue regions represent areas of dense scar not excitable during tachycardia. The activation wave front propagates around two lines of conduction block sharing a central common isthmus. Bystander pathways can be attached to any point in the circuit and represent areas of tissue activated by the wave front but not playing an active role in the reentrant circuit

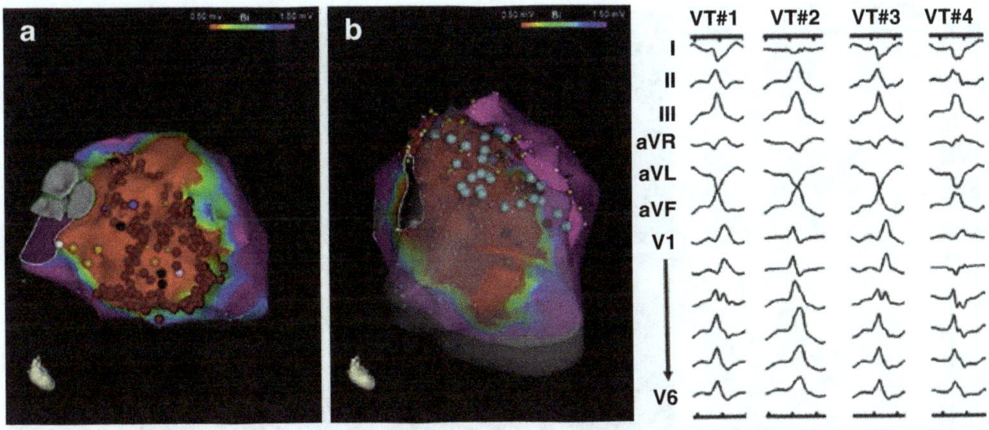

Fig. 10.3 Endocardial bipolar electroanatomic maps of a patient with multiple ventricular tachycardias (VT) arising from the interventricular septum who underwent extensive ablation from both the left ventricular (**a**, red dots) and right ventricular (**b**, light blue overlaid on LV septum) side of the septum

patients, and, in the majority of them (about 60%), the critical VT sites are located on the epicardium. These patients typically present VTs of RBBB morphology with right superior axis and late (≥V5) precordial transition (Fig. 10.5) [76]. The distinction between these two patterns is of great clinical value in terms of both procedural planning and outcomes. In patients with a predominant anteroseptal substrate, an epicardial approach is largely unnecessary, and the complex local anatomy (i.e., proximity to coronary vessels, presence of epicardial fat) usually limits the possibility to perform CA. Conversely, an epicardial approach is often required to achieve VT control in patients with a predominant inferolateral pattern. Even if epicardial coronary vessels and the phrenic nerve may obstacle epicardial CA in patients with inferolateral substrate, these patients typically have a more favorable outcome (75% vs. 25% VT-free survival at 1.5-year follow-up) and a lower need for redo procedures (7% vs. 59%) compared to patients with anteroseptal substrate [69]. In patients with septal VTs, the intramural location of the substrate can be difficult to address and may require sequential LV and right ventricular (RV) CA as well as the use of high RF energy potentially leading to collateral injury of the conduction system. A series of different approaches like bipolar RF ablation, high-intensity focused ultrasound, retractable needle ablation, and intracoronary ethanol ablation have been described to overcome the aforementioned limits, but none of them is currently available in routine clinical practice.

A variety of criteria can be used to address the need for epicardial mapping/ablation: (1) a 12-lead ECG of the VT suggesting an epicardial origin; (2) evidence of epicardial substrate on imaging studies (i.e., magnetic resonance, intracardiac echocardiography); (3) a unipolar voltage abnormality (<8.3 mV) in the presence of no or minimal bipolar (<1.5 mV) abnormality; and finally, failure of endocardial ablation (either early VT recurrence or persistent inducibility of clinical VT). Epicardial ablation approach is usually associated with a higher incidence of complications;

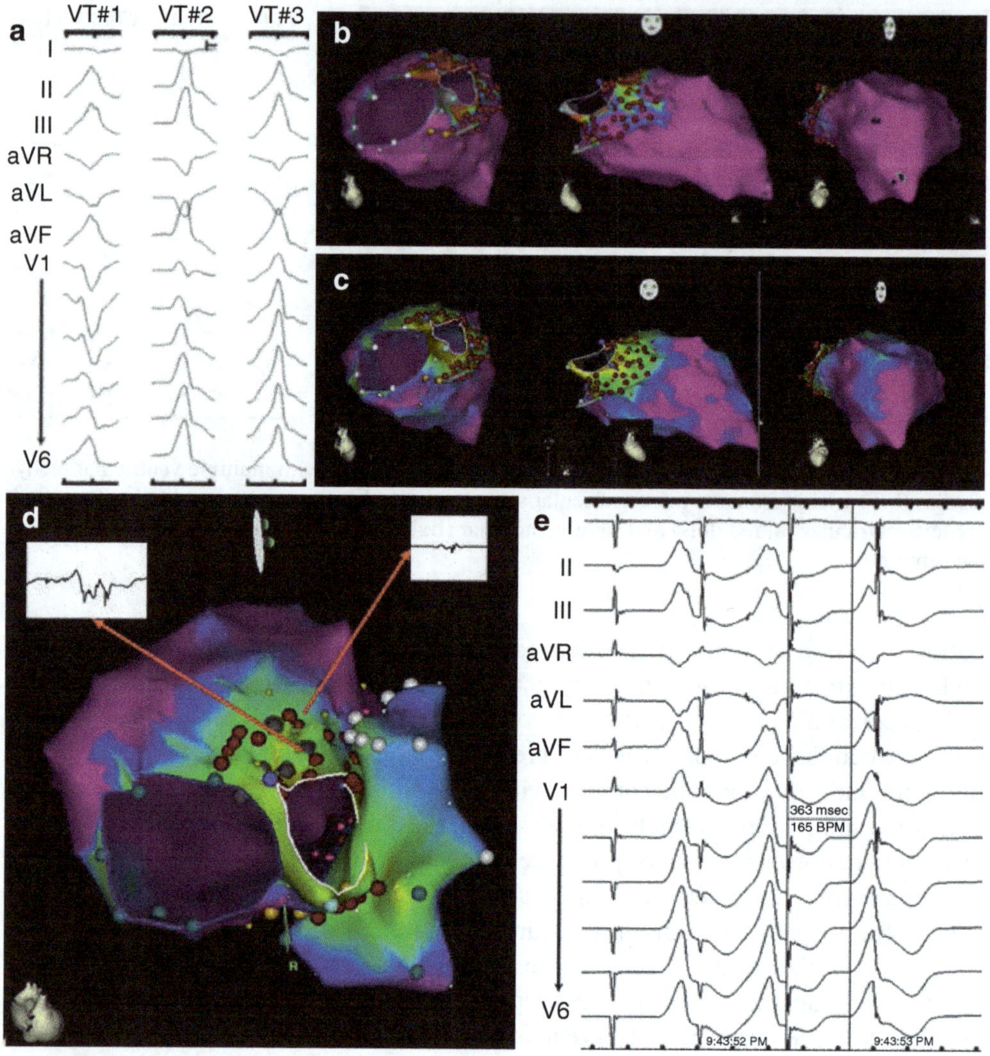

Fig. 10.4 Example of a 60-year-old lady with idiopathic dilated cardiomyopathy and left ventricular (LV) ejection fraction of 30% presenting with multiple ventricular tachycardias (VT) with both left bundle and right bundle branch morphology and inferior axis (**a**) consistent with an origin from the interventricular septum. Electroanatomic voltage mapping showed the presence of a small bipolar (**b**) and a larger unipolar (**c**) voltage abnormality involving the anterior septum. Extensive septal substrate ablation was performed from both the right and left side of the septum (**b–d**, red dots) targeting sites showing late potentials (**d**, red arrow) and long stim to QRS (**e**)

moreover, in a substantial proportion of cases (about 30%), even if critical VT sites are found on the epicardial surface, CA cannot be safely performed due to close proximity of epicardial coronary vessels and left phrenic nerve or presence of epicardial fat. Several ECG features have been correlated to epicardial VT origin like wide QRS complexes (shortest RS complex in precordial leads ≥121 ms), slow initial upstroke of the QRS complex "pseudo delta wave" ≥34 ms, intrinsicoid deflection time ≥85 ms, and maximum deflection index (shortest QRS onset to maximum precordial deflection/QRS duration) ≥0.55 (Fig. 10.6) [78].

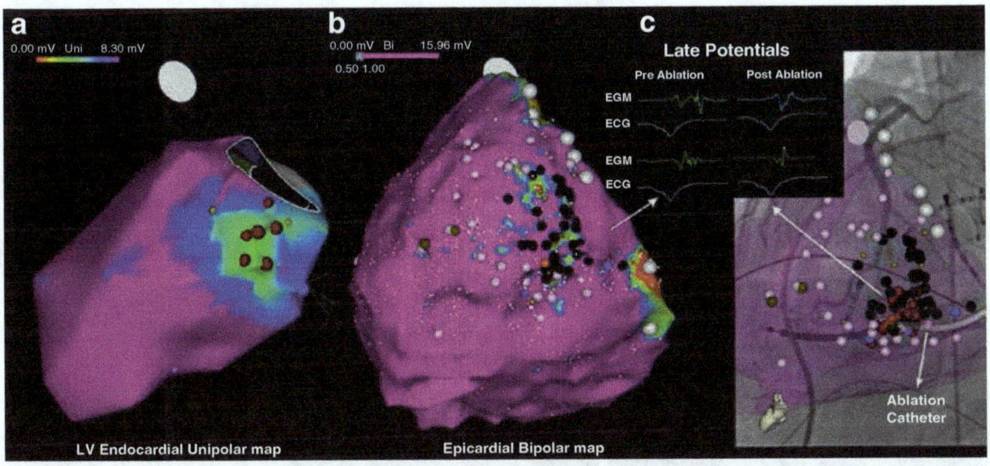

Fig. 10.5 Example of endocardial (**a**) and epicardial (**b** and **c**) substrate modification in a patient with minimal endocardial substrate and typical inferolateral epicardial substrate. Black dots (**b** and **c**) indicate abnormal electrograms. Coronary angiography was performed to confirm safe distance of the ablation sites on the epicardium from the major coronary vessels (Reproduced with permission from Muser et al. [58])

10.1.12 Role of ICD in DCM

Since the beginning of this century, many studies evaluated the role of ICD for primary prevention of SD in patients with DCM. Despite a striking reduction of SD was evident in most cases, total mortality was not significantly reduced in all trials with the exception of the COMPANION study, comparing resynchronization therapy (CRT-P) only with resynchronization therapy + ICD (CRT-D).

Mortality rate in nonischemic heart disease is lower than in ischemic heart disease (5.4% per year vs. 11.3% per year, respectively) [79], and this could partially explain why the absolute mortality reduction in patients with LV dysfunction of nonischemic origin is less evident [79]. In addition, nonischemic heart disease is not a synonymous of DCM: in unselected population with "nonischemic" HF, patients with other etiologies (hypertension, valvular heart disease, unrecognized myocarditis) have been included. The risk of death for other reasons (HF or noncardiac causes) can be not negligible, especially in older patients with other comorbidities, so the benefit of ICD could have been weakened by the competing risk due to other causes of death. Therefore, it is not surprising that in nonischemic patients, a significant effect on total mortality can be observed only in patients less likely to die for reasons different from SD (as young patients without severe heart failure symptoms) [25].

Nevertheless, the 2015 European Society of Cardiology (ESC) [27] Ventricular Arrhythmia Guidelines and the 2016 ESC Heart Failure Guidelines [80] give a 1B recommendation, while the 2017 AHA/ACC/HRS Guidelines give a 1A recommendation for ICD implantation for primary prevention in patients with nonischemic etiology [28].

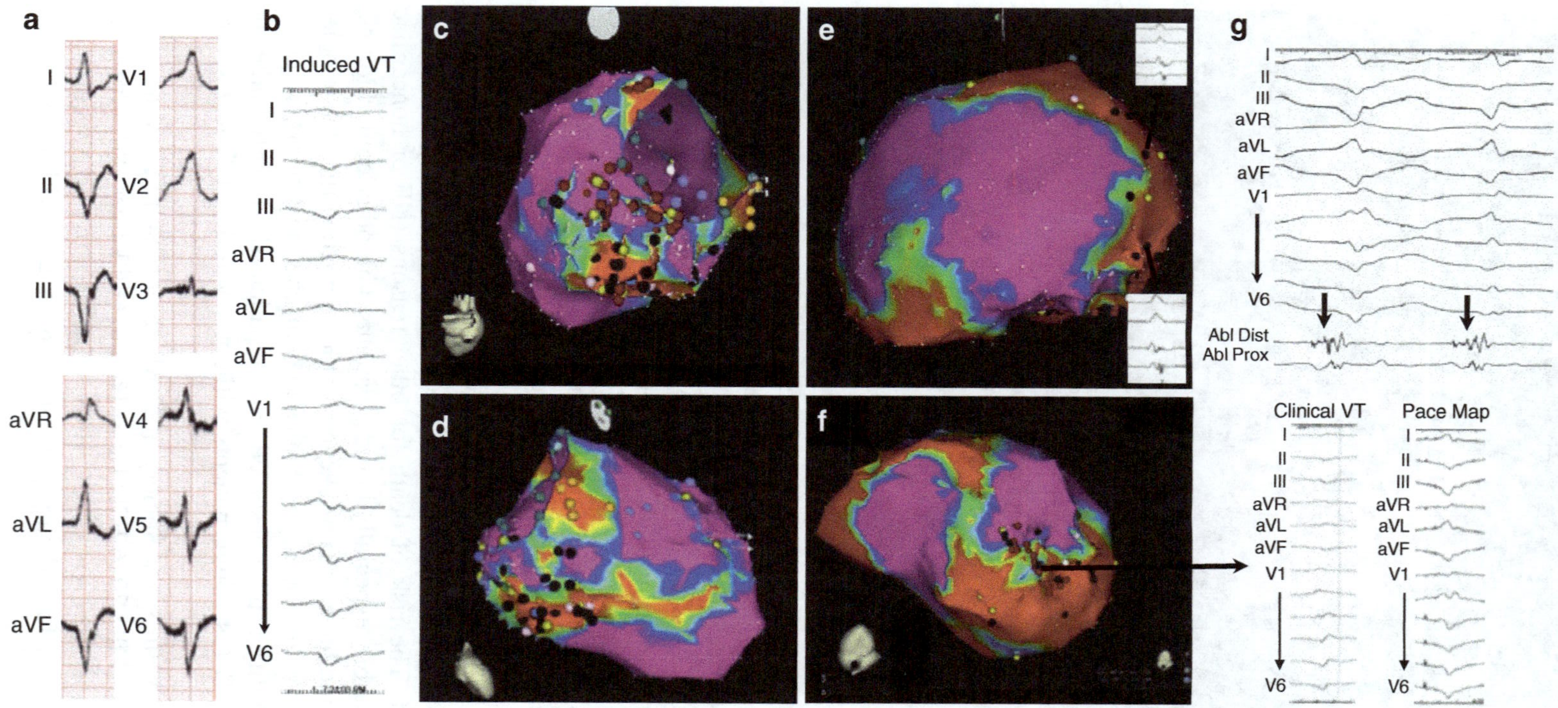

Fig. 10.6 Example of a 50-year-old man with mildly dilated cardiomyopathy and left ventricular (LV) ejection fraction of 40% presenting with recurrent ventricular tachycardia (VT) despite antiarrhythmic drug therapy with amiodarone and mexiletine. Baseline 12-lead ECG (**a**) shows a VT with right bundle branch block morphology and left superior axis consistent with an origin from the inferolateral LV. The clinical VT was easily inducible at the beginning of the procedure with programmed ventricular stimulation (**b**) and was still inducible after extensive endocardial LV ablation (**c–d**, red dots) performed at sites showing local abnormal ventricular activity (LAVA) (**c–d**, black dots). Epicardial mapping (**e**) demonstrated a large voltage abnormality involving the basal lateral LV wall with presence of LAVA (black dots). A good pace mapping site was identified in the inferolateral mid-wall (**f**). Mid-diastolic activity was recorded at this during VT (**g**, red arrows). Radiofrequency ablation here resulted in termination of the clinical VT which was no longer inducible

References

1. Towbin JA, Lorts A. Arrhythmias and dilated cardiomyopathy common pathogenetic pathways? J Am Coll Cardiol. 2011;57(21):2169–71.
2. McNair WP, Sinagra G, Taylor MR, Di Lenarda A, Ferguson DA, Salcedo EE, et al. SCN5A mutations associate with arrhythmic dilated cardiomyopathy and commonly localize to the voltage-sensing mechanism. J Am Coll Cardiol. 2011;57(21):2160–8.
3. Rapezzi C, Arbustini E, Caforio AL, Charron P, Gimeno-Blanes J, Heliö T, et al. Diagnostic work-up in cardiomyopathies: bridging the gap between clinical phenotypes and final diagnosis. A position statement from the ESC Working Group on Myocardial and Pericardial Diseases. Eur Heart J. 2013;34(19):1448–58.
4. Hershberger RE, Hedges DJ, Morales A. Dilated cardiomyopathy: the complexity of a diverse genetic architecture. Nat Rev Cardiol. 2013;10(9):531–47.
5. Arbustini E, Pilotto A, Repetto A, Grasso M, Negri A, Diegoli M, et al. Autosomal dominant dilated cardiomyopathy with atrioventricular block: a lamin A/C defect-related disease. J Am Coll Cardiol. 2002;39(6):981–90.
6. Taylor MR, Fain PR, Sinagra G, Robinson ML, Robertson AD, Carniel E, et al. Natural history of dilated cardiomyopathy due to lamin A/C gene mutations. J Am Coll Cardiol. 2003;41(5):771–80.
7. Brembilla-Perrot B, Alla F, Suty-Selton C, Huttin O, Blangy H, Sadoul N, et al. Nonischemic dilated cardiomyopathy: results of noninvasive and invasive evaluation in 310 patients and clinical significance of bundle branch block. Pacing Clin Electrophysiol. 2008;31(11):1383–90.
8. Aleksova A, Carriere C, Zecchin M, Barbati G, Vitrella G, Di Lenarda A, et al. New-onset left bundle branch block independently predicts long-term mortality in patients with idiopathic dilated cardiomyopathy: data from the Trieste Heart Muscle Disease Registry. Europace. 2014;16(10):1450–9.
9. Sekiguchi M, Hasegawa A, Hiroe M, Morimoto S, Nishikawa T. Inclusion of electric disturbance type cardiomyopathy in the classification of cardiomyopathy: a current review. J Cardiol. 2008;51(2):81–8.
10. Meune C, Van Berlo JH, Anselme F, Bonne G, Pinto YM, Duboc D. Primary prevention of sudden death in patients with lamin A/C gene mutations. N Engl J Med. 2006;354(2):209–10.
11. Aleksova A, Merlo M, Zecchin M, Sabbadini G, Barbati G, Vitrella G, et al. Impact of atrial fibrillation on outcome of patients with idiopathic dilated cardiomyopathy: data from the Heart Muscle Disease Registry of Trieste. Clin Med Res. 2010;8(3–4):142–9.
12. Spezzacatene A, Sinagra G, Merlo M, Barbati G, Graw SL, Brun F, et al. Arrhythmogenic phenotype in dilated cardiomyopathy: natural history and predictors of life-threatening arrhythmias. J Am Heart Assoc. 2015;4(10):e002149.
13. Holmes J, Kubo SH, Cody RJ, Kligfield P. Arrhythmias in ischemic and nonischemic dilated cardiomyopathy: prediction of mortality by ambulatory electrocardiography. Am J Cardiol. 1985;55(1):146–51.
14. Doval HC, Nul DR, Grancelli HO, Varini SD, Soifer S, Corrado G, et al. Nonsustained ventricular tachycardia in severe heart failure. Independent marker of increased mortality due to sudden death. GESICA-GEMA Investigators. Circulation. 1996;94(12):3198–203.
15. Meinertz T, Hofmann T, Kasper W, Treese N, Bechtold H, Stienen U, et al. Significance of ventricular arrhythmias in idiopathic dilated cardiomyopathy. Am J Cardiol. 1984;53(7):902–7.
16. Singh SN, Fisher SG, Carson PE, Fletcher RD. Prevalence and significance of nonsustained ventricular tachycardia in patients with premature ventricular contractions and heart failure treated with vasodilator therapy. Department of Veterans Affairs CHF STAT Investigators. J Am Coll Cardiol. 1998;32(4):942–7.
17. Grimm W, Christ M, Bach J, Müller HH, Maisch B. Noninvasive arrhythmia risk stratification in idiopathic dilated cardiomyopathy: results of the Marburg Cardiomyopathy Study. Circulation. 2003;108(23):2883–91.

18. Zecchin M, Di Lenarda A, Gregori D, Merlo M, Pivetta A, Vitrella G, et al. Are nonsustained ventricular tachycardias predictive of major arrhythmias in patients with dilated cardiomyopathy on optimal medical treatment? Pacing Clin Electrophysiol. 2008;31(3):290–9.
19. Pogwizd SM, McKenzie JP, Cain ME. Mechanisms underlying spontaneous and induced ventricular arrhythmias in patients with idiopathic dilated cardiomyopathy. Circulation. 1998;98(22):2404–14.
20. Soejima K, Stevenson WG, Sapp JL, Selwyn AP, Couper G, Epstein LM. Endocardial and epicardial radiofrequency ablation of ventricular tachycardia associated with dilated cardiomyopathy: the importance of low-voltage scars. J Am Coll Cardiol. 2004;43(10):1834–42.
21. Streitner F, Kuschyk J, Dietrich C, Mahl E, Streitner I, Doesch C, et al. Comparison of ventricular tachyarrhythmia characteristics in patients with idiopathic dilated or ischemic cardiomyopathy and defibrillators implanted for primary prevention. Clin Cardiol. 2011;34(10):604–9.
22. Merlo M, Pivetta A, Pinamonti B, Stolfo D, Zecchin M, Barbati G, et al. Long-term prognostic impact of therapeutic strategies in patients with idiopathic dilated cardiomyopathy: changing mortality over the last 30 years. Eur J Heart Fail. 2014;16(3):317–24.
23. Strickberger SA, Hummel JD, Bartlett TG, Frumin HI, Schuger CD, Beau SL, et al. Amiodarone versus implantable cardioverter-defibrillator: randomized trial in patients with nonischemic dilated cardiomyopathy and asymptomatic nonsustained ventricular tachycardia–AMIOVIRT. J Am Coll Cardiol. 2003;41(10):1707–12.
24. Merlo M, Gentile P, Naso P, Sinagra G. The natural history of dilated cardiomyopathy: how has it changed? J Cardiovasc Med (Hagerstown). 2017;18(Suppl 1):e161–e5.
25. Køber L, Thune JJ, Nielsen JC, Haarbo J, Videbæk L, Korup E, et al. Defibrillator implantation in patients with nonischemic systolic heart failure. N Engl J Med. 2016;375(13):1221–30.
26. Zecchin M, Merlo M, Pivetta A, Barbati G, Lutman C, Gregori D, et al. How can optimization of medical treatment avoid unnecessary implantable cardioverter-defibrillator implantations in patients with idiopathic dilated cardiomyopathy presenting with "SCD-HeFT criteria?". Am J Cardiol. 2012;109(5):729–35.
27. Priori SG, Blomström-Lundqvist C. 2015 European Society of Cardiology Guidelines for the management of patients with ventricular arrhythmias and the prevention of sudden cardiac death summarized by co-chairs. Eur Heart J. 2015;36(41):2757–9.
28. Al-Khatib SM, Stevenson WG, Ackerman MJ, Bryant WJ, Callans DJ, Curtis AB, et al. 2017 AHA/ACC/HRS guideline for management of patients with ventricular arrhythmias and the prevention of sudden cardiac death: executive summary: a report of the American College of Cardiology/American Heart Association Task Force on Clinical Practice Guidelines and the Heart Rhythm Society. Circulation. 2017;15(10):e190–252.
29. Goldberger JJ, Subačius H, Patel T, Cunnane R, Kadish AH. Sudden cardiac death risk stratification in patients with nonischemic dilated cardiomyopathy. J Am Coll Cardiol. 2014;63(18):1879–89.
30. Disertori M, Rigoni M, Pace N, Casolo G, Masè M, Gonzini L, et al. Myocardial fibrosis assessment by LGE is a powerful predictor of ventricular tachyarrhythmias in ischemic and nonischemic LV dysfunction: a meta-analysis. JACC Cardiovasc Imaging. 2016;9(9):1046–55.
31. Arbustini E, Disertori M, Narula J. Primary prevention of sudden arrhythmic death in dilated cardiomyopathy current guidelines and risk stratification. JACC Heart Fail. 2017;5(1):39–43.
32. Bécane HM, Bonne G, Varnous S, Muchir A, Ortega V, Hammouda EH, et al. High incidence of sudden death with conduction system and myocardial disease due to lamins A and C gene mutation. Pacing Clin Electrophysiol. 2000;23(11 Pt 1):1661–6.
33. van Rijsingen IA, Arbustini E, Elliott PM, Mogensen J, Hermans-van Ast JF, van der Kooi AJ, et al. Risk factors for malignant ventricular arrhythmias in lamin a/c mutation carriers a European cohort study. J Am Coll Cardiol. 2012;59(5):493–500.
34. Phillips E, Levine SA. Auricular fibrillation without other evidence of heart disease; a cause of reversible heart failure. Am J Med. 1949;7(4):478–89.
35. Fenelon G, Wijns W, Andries E, Brugada P. Tachycardiomyopathy: mechanisms and clinical implications. Pacing Clin Electrophysiol. 1996;19(1):95–106.

36. Gopinathannair R, Etheridge SP, Marchlinski FE, Spinale FG, Lakkireddy D, Olshansky B. Arrhythmia-induced cardiomyopathies: mechanisms, recognition, and management. J Am Coll Cardiol. 2015;66(15):1714–28.
37. Ellison KE, Stevenson WG, Sweeney MO, Epstein LM, Maisel WH. Management of arrhythmias in heart failure. Congest Heart Fail. 2003;9(2):91–9.
38. Baman TS, Lange DC, Ilg KJ, Gupta SK, Liu TY, Alguire C, et al. Relationship between burden of premature ventricular complexes and left ventricular function. Heart Rhythm. 2010;7(7):865–9.
39. Ban JE, Park HC, Park JS, Nagamoto Y, Choi JI, Lim HE, et al. Electrocardiographic and electrophysiological characteristics of premature ventricular complexes associated with left ventricular dysfunction in patients without structural heart disease. Europace. 2013;15(5):735–41.
40. Di Biase L, Mohanty P, Mohanty S, Santangeli P, Trivedi C, Lakkireddy D, et al. Ablation versus amiodarone for treatment of persistent atrial fibrillation in patients with congestive heart failure and an implanted device: results from the AATAC multicenter randomized trial. Circulation. 2016;133(17):1637–44.
41. Roy D, Talajic M, Nattel S, Wyse DG, Dorian P, Lee KL, et al. Rhythm control versus rate control for atrial fibrillation and heart failure. N Engl J Med. 2008;358(25):2667–77.
42. Van Gelder IC, Hagens VE, Bosker HA, Kingma JH, Kamp O, Kingma T, et al. A comparison of rate control and rhythm control in patients with recurrent persistent atrial fibrillation. N Engl J Med. 2002;347(23):1834–40.
43. Wyse DG, Waldo AL, DiMarco JP, Domanski MJ, Rosenberg Y, Schron EB, et al. A comparison of rate control and rhythm control in patients with atrial fibrillation. N Engl J Med. 2002;347(23):1825–33.
44. Pappone C, Augello G, Sala S, Gugliotta F, Vicedomini G, Gulletta S, et al. A randomized trial of circumferential pulmonary vein ablation versus antiarrhythmic drug therapy in paroxysmal atrial fibrillation: the APAF Study. J Am Coll Cardiol. 2006;48(11):2340–7.
45. Jais P, Cauchemez B, Macle L, Daoud E, Khairy P, Subbiah R, et al. Catheter ablation versus antiarrhythmic drugs for atrial fibrillation: the A4 study. Circulation. 2008;118(24):2498–505.
46. Kosiuk J, Nedios S, Darma A, Rolf S, Richter S, Arya A, et al. Impact of single atrial fibrillation catheter ablation on implantable cardioverter defibrillator therapies in patients with ischaemic and non-ischaemic cardiomyopathies. Europace. 2014;16(9):1322–6.
47. Marrouche NF, Brachmann J, Andresen D, Siebels J, Boersma L, Jordaens L, et al. Catheter ablation for atrial fibrillation with heart failure. N Engl J Med. 2018;378(5):417–27.
48. Bunch TJ, May HT, Bair TL, Jacobs V, Crandall BG, Cutler M, et al. Five-year outcomes of catheter ablation in patients with atrial fibrillation and left ventricular systolic dysfunction. J Cardiovasc Electrophysiol. 2015;26(4):363–70.
49. Santangeli P, Muser D, Maeda S, Filtz A, Zado ES, Frankel DS, et al. Comparative effectiveness of antiarrhythmic drugs and catheter ablation for the prevention of recurrent ventricular tachycardia in patients with implantable cardioverter-defibrillators: a systematic review and meta-analysis of randomized controlled trials. Heart Rhythm. 2016;13(7):1552–9.
50. Sapp JL, Parkash R, Tang AS. Ventricular tachycardia ablation versus antiarrhythmic-drug escalation. N Engl J Med. 2016;375(15):1499–500.
51. Packer DL, Prutkin JM, Hellkamp AS, Mitchell LB, Bernstein RC, Wood F, et al. Impact of implantable cardioverter-defibrillator, amiodarone, and placebo on the mode of death in stable patients with heart failure: analysis from the sudden cardiac death in heart failure trial. Circulation. 2009;120(22):2170–6.
52. Saksena S, Slee A, Waldo AL, Freemantle N, Reynolds M, Rosenberg Y, et al. Cardiovascular outcomes in the AFFIRM Trial (Atrial Fibrillation Follow-Up Investigation of Rhythm Management). An assessment of individual antiarrhythmic drug therapies compared with rate control with propensity score-matched analyses. J Am Coll Cardiol. 2011;58(19):1975–85.
53. Connolly SJ, Dorian P, Roberts RS, Gent M, Bailin S, Fain ES, et al. Comparison of beta-blockers, amiodarone plus beta-blockers, or sotalol for prevention of shocks from implantable cardioverter defibrillators: the OPTIC Study: a randomized trial. JAMA. 2006;295(2):165–71.

54. Pacifico A, Hohnloser SH, Williams JH, Tao B, Saksena S, Henry PD, et al. Prevention of implantable-defibrillator shocks by treatment with sotalol. d,l-Sotalol Implantable Cardioverter-Defibrillator Study Group. N Engl J Med. 1999;340(24):1855–62.
55. Kettering K, Mewis C, Dörnberger V, Vonthein R, Bosch RF, Kühlkamp V. Efficacy of metoprolol and sotalol in the prevention of recurrences of sustained ventricular tachyarrhythmias in patients with an implantable cardioverter defibrillator. Pacing Clin Electrophysiol. 2002;25(11):1571–6.
56. Investigators CASTC. Preliminary report: effect of encainide and flecainide on mortality in a randomized trial of arrhythmia suppression after myocardial infarction. N Engl J Med. 1989;321(6):406–12.
57. Gao D, Van Herendael H, Alshengeiti L, Dorian P, Mangat I, Korley V, et al. Mexiletine as an adjunctive therapy to amiodarone reduces the frequency of ventricular tachyarrhythmia events in patients with an implantable defibrillator. J Cardiovasc Pharmacol. 2013;62(2):199–204.
58. Muser D, Santangeli P, Castro SA, Pathak RK, Liang JJ, Hayashi T, et al. Long-term outcome after catheter ablation of ventricular tachycardia in patients with nonischemic dilated cardiomyopathy. Circ Arrhythm Electrophysiol. 2016;9(10). pii: e004328.
59. Tung R, Vaseghi M, Frankel DS, Vergara P, Di Biase L, Nagashima K, et al. Freedom from recurrent ventricular tachycardia after catheter ablation is associated with improved survival in patients with structural heart disease: an International VT Ablation Center Collaborative Group study. Heart Rhythm. 2015;12(9):1997–2007.
60. Muser D, Mendelson T, Fahed J, Liang JJ, Castro SA, Zado E, et al. Impact of timing of recurrence following catheter ablation of scar-related ventricular tachycardia on subsequent mortality. Pacing Clin Electrophysiol. 2017;40(9):1010–6.
61. Hsia HH, Callans DJ, Marchlinski FE. Characterization of endocardial electrophysiological substrate in patients with nonischemic cardiomyopathy and monomorphic ventricular tachycardia. Circulation. 2003;108(6):704–10.
62. Cano O, Hutchinson M, Lin D, Garcia F, Zado E, Bala R, et al. Electroanatomic substrate and ablation outcome for suspected epicardial ventricular tachycardia in left ventricular nonischemic cardiomyopathy. J Am Coll Cardiol. 2009;54(9):799–808.
63. Nakahara S, Tung R, Ramirez RJ, Michowitz Y, Vaseghi M, Buch E, et al. Characterization of the arrhythmogenic substrate in ischemic and nonischemic cardiomyopathy implications for catheter ablation of hemodynamically unstable ventricular tachycardia. J Am Coll Cardiol. 2010;55(21):2355–65.
64. Schmidt B, Chun KR, Baensch D, Antz M, Koektuerk B, Tilz RR, et al. Catheter ablation for ventricular tachycardia after failed endocardial ablation: epicardial substrate or inappropriate endocardial ablation? Heart Rhythm. 2010;7(12):1746–52.
65. Arya A, Bode K, Piorkowski C, Bollmann A, Sommer P, Gaspar T, et al. Catheter ablation of electrical storm due to monomorphic ventricular tachycardia in patients with nonischemic cardiomyopathy: acute results and its effect on long-term survival. Pacing Clin Electrophysiol. 2010;33(12):1504–9.
66. Haqqani HM, Tschabrunn CM, Tzou WS, Dixit S, Cooper JM, Riley MP, et al. Isolated septal substrate for ventricular tachycardia in nonischemic dilated cardiomyopathy: incidence, characterization, and implications. Heart Rhythm. 2011;8(8):1169–76.
67. Piers SR, Leong DP, van Huls van Taxis CF, Tayyebi M, Trines SA, Pijnappels DA, et al. Outcome of ventricular tachycardia ablation in patients with nonischemic cardiomyopathy: the impact of noninducibility. Circ Arrhythm Electrophysiol. 2013;6(3):513–21.
68. Dinov B, Fiedler L, Schönbauer R, Bollmann A, Rolf S, Piorkowski C, et al. Outcomes in catheter ablation of ventricular tachycardia in dilated nonischemic cardiomyopathy compared with ischemic cardiomyopathy. Circulation. 2014;129:728–36.
69. Oloriz T, Silberbauer J, Maccabelli G, Mizuno H, Baratto F, Kirubakaran S, et al. Catheter ablation of ventricular arrhythmia in nonischemic cardiomyopathy: anteroseptal versus inferolateral scar sub-types. Circ Arrhythm Electrophysiol. 2014;7(3):414–23.
70. Dinov B, Arya A, Schratter A, Schirripa V, Fiedler L, Sommer P, et al. Catheter ablation of ventricular tachycardia and mortality in patients with nonischemic dilated cardiomyopathy:

can noninducibility after ablation be a predictor for reduced mortality? Circ Arrhythm Electrophysiol. 2015;8(3):598–605.
71. Yu R, Ma S, Tung R, Stevens S, Macias C, Bradfield J, et al. Catheter ablation of scar-based ventricular tachycardia: relationship of procedure duration to outcomes and hospital mortality. Heart Rhythm. 2015;12(1):86–94.
72. Gökoğlan Y, Mohanty S, Gianni C, Santangeli P, Trivedi C, Güneş MF, et al. Scar homogenization versus limited-substrate ablation in patients with nonischemic cardiomyopathy and ventricular tachycardia. J Am Coll Cardiol. 2016;68(18):1990–8.
73. Santangeli P, Muser D, Zado ES, Magnani S, Khetpal S, Hutchinson MD, et al. Acute hemodynamic decompensation during catheter ablation of scar-related ventricular tachycardia: incidence, predictors, and impact on mortality. Circ Arrhythm Electrophysiol. 2015;8(1):68–75.
74. Muser D, Liang JJ, Castro SA, Hayashi T, Enriquez A, Troutman GS, et al. Outcomes with prophylactic use of percutaneous left ventricular assist devices in high-risk patients undergoing catheter ablation of scar-related ventricular tachycardia: a propensity-matched analysis. Heart Rhythm. 2018;15(10):1500–6.
75. Stevenson WG, Khan H, Sager P, Saxon LA, Middlekauff HR, Natterson PD, et al. Identification of reentry circuit sites during catheter mapping and radiofrequency ablation of ventricular tachycardia late after myocardial infarction. Circulation. 1993;88(4 Pt 1):1647–70.
76. Piers SR, Tao Q, van Huls van Taxis CF, Schalij MJ, van der Geest RJ, Zeppenfeld K. Contrast-enhanced MRI-derived scar patterns and associated ventricular tachycardias in nonischemic cardiomyopathy: implications for the ablation strategy. Circ Arrhythm Electrophysiol. 2013;6(5):875–83.
77. Hayashi T, Santangeli P, Pathak RK, Muser D, Liang JJ, Castro SA, et al. Outcomes of catheter ablation of idiopathic outflow tract ventricular arrhythmias with an R wave pattern break in lead V2: a distinct clinical entity. J Cardiovasc Electrophysiol. 2017;28(5):504–14.
78. Berruezo A, Mont L, Nava S, Chueca E, Bartholomay E, Brugada J. Electrocardiographic recognition of the epicardial origin of ventricular tachycardias. Circulation. 2004;109(15):1842–7.
79. Shun-Shin MJ, Zheng SL, Cole GD, Howard JP, Whinnett ZI, Francis DP. Implantable cardioverter defibrillators for primary prevention of death in left ventricular dysfunction with and without ischaemic heart disease: a meta-analysis of 8567 patients in the 11 trials. Eur Heart J. 2017;38(22):1738–46.
80. Ponikowski P, Voors AA, Anker SD, Bueno H, Cleland JGF, Coats AJS, et al. 2016 ESC Guidelines for the diagnosis and treatment of acute and chronic heart failure: The Task Force for the diagnosis and treatment of acute and chronic heart failure of the European Society of Cardiology (ESC) Developed with the special contribution of the Heart Failure Association (HFA) of the ESC. Eur Heart J. 2016;37(27):2129–200.

11

Regenerative Medicine and Biomarkers for Dilated Cardiomyopathy

Pierluigi Lesizza, Aneta Aleksova, Benedetta Ortis, Antonio Paolo Beltrami, Mauro Giacca, and Gianfranco Sinagra

Abbreviations and Acronyms

BMMNC	Bone marrow mononuclear cell
BNP	Brain natriuretic peptide
BUN	Blood urea nitrogen
CM	Cardiomyocyte
CPC	Cardiac progenitor cell
DCM	Dilated cardiomyopathy
ESC	Embryonic stem cell
Gal-3	Galectin-3
GDF-15	Growth and differentiation factor-15
GFR	Glomerular filtration rate
Hb	Haemoglobin
HF	Heart failure
hs-TnT	High-sensitivity troponin T
IL-1β	Interleukin-1β
iPSC	Induced pluripotent stem cell

P. Lesizza (✉) · A. Aleksova · B. Ortis
Cardiovascular Department, Azienda Sanitaria Universitaria Integrata, University of Trieste (ASUITS), Trieste, Italy

A. P. Beltrami
Pathology Department, School of Medicine, University of Udine, Udine, Italy
e-mail: antonio.beltrami@uniud.it

M. Giacca
Molecular Medicine Laboratory, International Centre for Genetic Engineering and Biotechnology (ICGEB), Trieste, Italy
e-mail: giacca@icgeb.org

G. Sinagra
Cardiovascular Department, Azienda Sanitaria Universitaria Integrata, Trieste, Italy
e-mail: gianfranco.sinagra@asuits.sanita.fvg.it

KCCQ	Kansas City Cardiomyopathy Questionnaire
KIM-1	Kidney injury molecule-1
LGE	Late gadolinium enhancement
LVAD	Left ventricular assist device
LVEF	Left ventricle ejection fraction
LVRR	Left ventricular reverse remodelling
MACE	Major adverse cardiac event
MLHFQ	Minnesota Living with Heart Failure Questionnaire
MRI	Magnetic resonance imaging
NPs	Natriuretic peptides
NT-proBNP	N-terminal pro-BNP
NYHA	New York Heart Association
SHFM	Seattle Heart Failure Model
sST2	Soluble ST2
TGF	Transforming growth factor
Tns	Troponins
WRF	Worsening renal function

Dilated cardiomyopathy (DCM) is associated with the loss of cardiomyocytes (CMs) and with the replacement of lost CMs by non-contractile fibrous tissue.

In the past years, the inability of the heart to repair itself after damage has led to the conclusion that CMs are unable to proliferate. More recently, however, it was discovered that CMs conserve a very low proliferation rate throughout adult life [1–3]. Consequently, many strategies to enhance endogenous CM proliferation and achieve myocardial repair have been developed.

11.1 Strategies for Heart Regeneration

Strategies for heart regeneration and repair may be divided into two broad groups, based on either cell or gene therapy (Fig. 11.1).

11.1.1 Cell Therapy

Several populations of putative cardiac progenitor cells, bone marrow-derived stem cells and pluripotent stem cells have been identified in the last two decades. Generally, cardiac progenitor cells are very rare in heart tissue and heterogeneous in nature, but all identified populations have been originally reported to be able to differentiate in vitro in various cell lines, among which CMs [4]. Cardiac progenitor cells and bone marrow-derived stem cells were thought to be able to engraft in damaged tissue and proliferate and differentiate in mature CMs [5]. Based on these original findings, administration of cardiac progenitor cells or bone marrow-derived stem cells has been extensively investigated in clinical trials for the treatment of ischaemic cardiomyopathy [5, 6] and DCM (see below). The negative outcome of

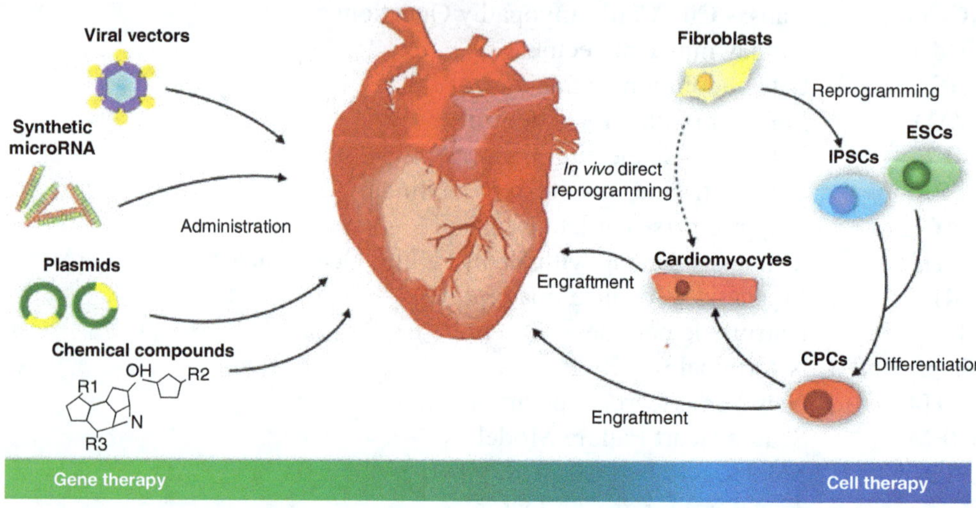

Fig. 11.1 Schematic representation of the strategies to enhance myocardial regeneration. On the left, strategies based on gene therapy, involving the administration of viral vectors, plasmids or synthetic RNA molecules (messenger RNA or microRNA) or the interference with specific genes using chemical compounds or microRNAs. On the right, strategies based on cell therapy, such as in vitro cardiomyocytes production from ESCs, IPSCs or CPCs and following engraftment of obtained cardiomyocytes or in vivo direct reprogramming of fibroblasts

these trials and a proper re-evaluation of the results obtained in experimental animals eventually led to the conclusion that none of these so-called stem cell populations efficiently engraft in heart tissue, proliferate and differentiate into functional CMs. The marginal beneficial effects of cell administration are mainly due to their paracrine anti-apoptotic and pro-angiogenic effect, limited by their very short persistence in vivo [7].

Another cell-based strategy involves the production and in vitro expansion of CMs from human embryonic stem cells or iPSCs [8]. The treatment in culture of these cells with an appropriate cocktail of growth factors leads to the production of relatively pure CM populations that can be injected directly as a cell suspension in the heart or grow and engraft into 3D synthetic matrices creating heart tissue patches. A major limitation in the clinical application of embryonic stem cell- and iPSC-derived CMs relates to the relative difficulty in expanding and differentiating these cells in large numbers and to the high cost needed for the their production and characterization [9]. In addition, CMs administered as a cell suspension poorly couple with native CMs, thus asynchronously contracting and potentially being arrhythmogenic [10]. The use of cardiac patches is also limited by the poor electromechanical coupling with native heart tissue and by the need of a very high amount of CMs to produce a sufficiently large cardiac patch. Improvement in these technologies is however expected in the next years; for example, Shadrin et al. [11] recently reported the production of a patch with clinically relevant dimensions (4 × 4 cm).

An additional cell-based strategy is in vivo cell reprogramming. Treatment of fibroblasts in heart tissue with a cocktail of growth factors may directly induce their transdifferentiation in CMs. This strategy has been already applied with success in animal models, and clinical trials are awaited to confirm their efficacy in humans [12]. Principal limitations of this strategy are the low yield of conversion of fibroblasts to CMs and the need to use viral vectors as administration tools, which is fraught with low efficiency in vivo.

11.1.2 Gene Therapy

Gene therapy strategies aim at enhancing endogenous CM proliferation by the administration of genes encoding for proteins or non-coding RNAs. The discovery of new genes with therapeutic potential in this field mirrors the study of the mechanisms that regulate CM proliferation during embryonic and foetal development and the mechanism that induce CM withdrawal from proliferative state after birth [13]. With this approach, a protein, neuregulin-1 [14], and an intracellular signal transmission pathway, the Hippo pathway [15], have been identified as fundamental regulators of CM differentiation and proliferation during embryogenesis. Overexpression of neuregulin receptor ErbB2 and deactivation of the suppressive Hippo pathway have both been proven effective in animal models of myocardial infarction and may reach the clinical scenario as potential new therapies in a few years [13, 16].

In the field of gene therapy, microRNAs have been extensively studied as potential tools to induce heart regeneration due to their ability to control complex cellular processes such as proliferation, apoptosis, differentiation, migration and metabolism. Several microRNAs have been identified as regulators of CM proliferation (e.g. miR-1, miR-499, miR-133, miR-29a, miR-15 family as proliferation inhibitors and miR-17/92, miR-302/367, miR-199a-3p and miR-590-3p as proliferation activators) [17]. Some of the miRNAs have been characterized in preclinical models as potential therapeutic tools for heart regeneration, especially after myocardial infarction. Also in this case, clinical studies are warranted in the incoming years.

11.2 Regenerative Approaches in Dilated Cardiomyopathy

In the field of regenerative medicine, much effort has been put on the study of new therapies for ischaemic cardiomyopathy, whereas attempts to find new therapies in DCM have instead been limited [18, 19].

DCM has lagged behind in the field of regenerative medicine mostly because of its lower prevalence in comparison with ischaemic heart disease. Preclinical models of DCM are more difficult to obtain being DCM the final common phenotype of multiple pathophysiological processes, some of which even poorly understood. Moreover, the presence of regenerating cells and the extension of regenerated tissue are much easier to identify in ischaemic heart disease models, in which the necrotic tissue and scar are even macroscopically well-defined, than in DCM models, in which loss of CMs and fibrosis is diffuse. As a consequence, only a few preclinical studies have been conducted in models of DCM with a definite aetiology (i.e. anthracycline-induced cardiomyopathy [20] and chagasic cardiomyopathy [21]).

Despite the scarce preclinical experience in DCM, a few clinical trials have been conducted to assess the effect of putative stem cell administration in non-ischaemic DCM.

The DCM branch of MiHeart trial has been the first, and to date only, multicentre, double-blinded, placebo-controlled phase I–II trial testing the efficacy of bone marrow-derived mononuclear cells (BMMNCs) in patients affected by non-ischaemic DCM [22]. Subjects enrolled had a previous diagnosis of heart failure, heart failure symptoms for at least 1 year, a diagnosis of non-ischaemic DCM according to the World Health Organization criteria, LVEF <35% and NYHA class III or IV and were on optimal medical therapy for at least 4 weeks before randomization and throughout the study. One hundred sixteen patients were enrolled and randomized (1:1) to intracoronary injection of BMMNCs or placebo injection. The treatment proved safe, but at 12 months of follow-up, there were no statistically significant differences with regard to LVEF, MLHFQ score, 6-min walk test, VO2 max or NYHA classification. Thus, the investigators concluded that BMMNCs do not have a beneficial effect in the setting of DCM. This is most likely related to the wrong assumption that the administered cells had a true regenerative potential.

Other smaller studies have been conducted to assess the efficacy of stem cell treatment in the setting of DCM.

The first proof-of-concept study in this field was TOPCARE-DCM, a cohort study enrolling 33 patients affected by DCM with LVEF ≤40% and NYHA class I–III [23]. All patients underwent intracoronary infusion of BMMNCs, and investigators reported a mean improvement in LVEF at 3 months of 3.2% as assessed by echocardiography. It has to be underlined that this is a single-centre, nonrandomized, prospective cohort study.

Vrtovec et al. reported in three different studies [24–26] that treatment with CD34+ cells led to significant improvement in global ejection fraction and in 1-year mortality. Nevertheless, all these studies enrolled a small cohort of patients, were performed at a single centre, were not double-blind nor placebo-controlled and were not powered to test for mortality.

The Autologous Bone Marrow Cells in DCM (ABCD) trial enrolled 84 patients with non-ischaemic DCM, LVEF ≤35% and NYHA class ≥II that were randomized to intracoronary infusion of BMMNCs or optimal medical therapy [27]. At 3-year follow-up investigators reported a mean improvement in ejection fraction of 5.9% in the treated group with a significant difference between treated and control group in LVEF, left ventricle end-diastolic volume and KCCQ functional status and clinical summary score.

The INTRACELL study randomized 30 patients affected by non-ischaemic DCM, LVEF ≤35% and NYHA class III or IV to intramyocardial injection of BMMNCs or optimal medical therapy, but at follow-up there was no improvement in LVEF [28].

The IMPACT-DCM/Catheter-DCM enrolled both patients affected by ischaemic and non-ischaemic DCM (29 patients with non-ischaemic DCM) and randomized them to transendocardial injections with BMMNCs enriched in mesenchymal stromal cells and M2-like macrophages or to optimal medical therapy [29]. After 1 year of follow-up, there were no significant differences between control and treated group in terms of LVEF and functional status.

Taken together, the data from these experimentations, most of which were small, single-centre and non-blinded, indicate that the eventual benefit provided by administration of bone marrow mononuclear cells is marginal at best and most likely related to the paracrine effect of these cells rather than to their regenerative potential [30].

As a consequence, regenerative approaches to heal the heart, both in the ischaemic and non-ischaemic settings, are now moving from stem cell therapies to gene therapy, which presents with a much more relevant preclinical background, holding high promise, even though still far from extensive clinical application.

11.3 Biomarkers and Dilated Cardiomyopathy

Idiopathic DCM is a primary myocardial disease characterized by progressive left ventricular o biventricular dilatation and dysfunction, presenting with different degrees of HF, ranging from asymptomatic dysfunction to advanced HF with refractory symptoms, which often requires heart transplantation. Patients with idiopathic DCM are younger than those with ischaemic cardiomyopathy, have fewer comorbidities and have a longer life expectancy. For this reason, prognostic assessment is particularly important for these patients.

In the last years, the advances in the comprehension of HF pathophysiology led to the identification of several molecules that act as biomarkers and are representative of HF complex biological mechanisms, such as inflammation, oxidative stress and neurohormonal activation. Biomarkers may help clinicians in diagnosing, assessing severity and especially predicting prognosis of HF. The term biomarker was defined in 2001 by the Biomarkers Definition Working Group of the National Institutes of Health [31] as "a characteristic that is objectively measured and evaluated as an indicator of normal biological processes, pathogenic processes, or pharmacologic responses to a therapeutic intervention". Focusing on laboratory biomarkers, Prof. Braunwald identified seven main categories, corresponding to an equal number of pathobiological processes occurring in HF: myocardial stretch, inflammation, matrix remodelling, myocyte injury, renal dysfunction, neurohumoral activation and oxidative stress [32].

The most widely used biomarkers in patients suffering from HF are natriuretic peptides. BNP and NT-proBNP are secreted in response to the stretching of atrial and ventricular walls and are recommended tools for the diagnosis of HF, according to the latest ESC guidelines [33]. Accordingly, the evaluation of their plasmatic concentration on hospital admission is predictive of outcome in patients with acute HF, and their increase despite optimized therapy in chronic HF predicts morbidity and mortality [34]. Moreover, in the setting of acute decompensated HF, the occurrence of WRF with a significant decrease of BNP is a marker of adequate decongestion and favourable outcome [35]. Few studies investigated the role of natriuretic peptides in the peculiar setting of idiopathic DCM. BNP was correlated to clinical severity of HF and congestion [36], and NT-proBNP correlated with LVEF, NYHA class and mortality [37], identifying patients with a more severe HF, and it was the best predictor of long-term LVRR, which by itself is a predictor of favourable outcomes [38].

Inflammation and matrix remodelling, expressed as fibrosis, are two pathobiological processes involved in systolic and diastolic dysfunction, leading to cardiac remodelling and overt heart failure. Gal-3 is a lectin secreted by activated macrophages that favours the development of cardiac fibrosis via fibroblast stimulation [39] and represents the link between inflammation and fibrosis. Gal-3 already showed to have a prognostic role in patients affected by HF: the higher the levels, the more severe the cardiac fibrosis and left ventricular remodelling [40]. In the setting of chronic HF, values of plasmatic Gal-3 above 17.8 ng/mL predict an unfavourable outcome in terms of hospitalization and mortality [41, 42]. However, Gal-3 is not a heart-specific biomarker and is abundantly expressed in many organs and tissues, and its values are influenced also by comorbid conditions such as diabetes and renal or liver dysfunction [40]. With specific regard to idiopathic DCM, Besler et al. showed that Gal-3 myocardial expression directly correlates with the extent of histologically assessed cardiac fibrosis [43]. Additionally, in this peculiar setting, Gal-3 maintains its predictive power. Indeed, in two independent studies, Gal-3 was compared with LGE presence at cardiac MRI in idiopathic DCM patients. Gal-3 plasma levels represented the extent of fibrosis at MRI [44], and both Gal-3 and LGE presence significantly predicted MACEs in DCM, especially when the two are combined [45]. Another biomarker of inflammation and fibrosis is sST2, a member of the interleukin (IL)-1 receptor-like family, that is secreted in response to myocardial strain and IL1 stimulation [46]. sST2, acting as a decoy receptor, reduces the cardioprotective effects of IL-33. High sST2 values are predictors of short- and long-term mortality in chronic HF [47]. Ky et al. demonstrated that patients with sST2 higher than 36.6 ng/mL have a three times higher risk of death or cardiac transplantation than those with lower values [48]. When compared to other biomarkers, sST2 is superior to Gal-3 and NT-proBNP in risk stratification [39], being the best predictor of cardiovascular mortality. These results are particularly interesting, because sST2 levels are not significantly influenced by other conditions, such as renal dysfunction or obesity [49]. Moreover, the increase over time of sST2 levels is predictive of disease progression in HF [50] and could identify patients with a more severe fibrosis. Lupon et al. developed the ST2-R2 score to predict reverse remodelling in HF with systolic dysfunction; patients with sST2 values above 48 ng/mL will unlikely experience LVRR [51]. These findings are confirmed in idiopathic DCM stable patients: Wojciechowska et al. demonstrated that sST2 correlates with all-cause mortality and the combined outcome of death, cardiac transplantation and LVAD implantation, in particular when assessing serial changes in sST2 values [52].

Besides Gal-3 and sST2, the inflammatory and fibrotic processes are also mirrored by elevation of interleukin and growth factor levels, which can therefore be employed as useful biomarkers for prognostic stratification. The activation of the inflammasome drives the inflammatory response that promotes cardiac remodelling and heart failure [53]. This process can be detected dosing circulating interleukins. In idiopathic DCM patients, IL-1β showed to be a highly significant long-term predictor of death or cardiac transplantation [54].

GDF-15 belongs to the TGF family and is involved in inflammation, fibrosis and ventricular remodelling [55]. In idiopathic DCM patients, it correlates with symptoms severity, BNP and sST2 levels and grade of systolic dysfunction. Stojkovic et al. demonstrated that GDF-15 is able to predict not only all-cause mortality, but also arrhythmic deaths, which are a not negligible cause of mortality in idiopathic DCM patients. GDF-15 levels above 884 pg/mL conferred a two times higher risk of arrhythmic death or resuscitated cardiac arrest and a three times higher risk of all-cause mortality, predicting the outcome with a higher accuracy than ST2 [56].

Troponins are well-known markers of myocardial injury. In the setting of HF, high values of troponin I or T predict a worse grade of left ventricular dysfunction and a higher risk of death [40]. In a study by Kawahara et al., hs-TnT value above 0.01 ng/mL reflected the degree of myocardial damage and was an independent predictor of mortality, especially when combined with left ventricular dysfunction. The result was conserved even in the cohort of patients with chronic HF caused by idiopathic DCM patients [57].

Besides laboratory biomarkers, also clinical variables are important in defining prognosis in HF in clinically stable idiopathic DCM patients. Aleksova et al. demonstrated that anaemia, defined as haemoglobin concentration lower than 13 g/dL in men and 12 g/dL in women, was a predictor of unfavourable outcomes. Moreover, the new onset of anaemia was as well an independent predictor of poor outcome, leading to a doubled risk of death or heart transplantation [58].

Renal failure is as well-known prognostically relevant complication occurring in HF patients. Consistently, creatinine, BUN and estimated GFR are independent predictors of prognosis [40]. However, WRF occurs frequently during uptitration of diuretic treatment in case of clinical congestion and is not necessarily related to poor outcomes [35]. In idiopathic DCM, renal failure occurs in 20% of patients during the first 8 years after diagnosis, up to 50% at 20-year follow-up [59]. In these patients, a GFR between 30 and 60 mL/min/1.73 m^2 nearly triplicates the risk for cardiac events [60]. NGAL and KIM-1 are useful biomarkers in early detection of WRF, even before the decline in GFR. When used in HF patients, they are also predictors of all-cause mortality and hospital admission [61].

In clinical practice, biomarkers are widely used to better characterize patients with HF and are useful tools in predicting prognosis (Fig. 11.2). The wide spectrum of pathophysiological processes explored by the amount of available biomarkers and the specific characteristics of each one make them advantageous especially when used in combination. The additive value of a multimarker approach in HF has been largely investigated in literature. Pascual-Figal et al. stratified acutely decompensated HF patients using sST2, NT-proBNP and hs-TnT: patients with all three biomarkers elevated had 50% of risk of death, compared to 0% of risk in those with none elevated [62]. Ky et al. identified eight biomarkers ameliorating risk

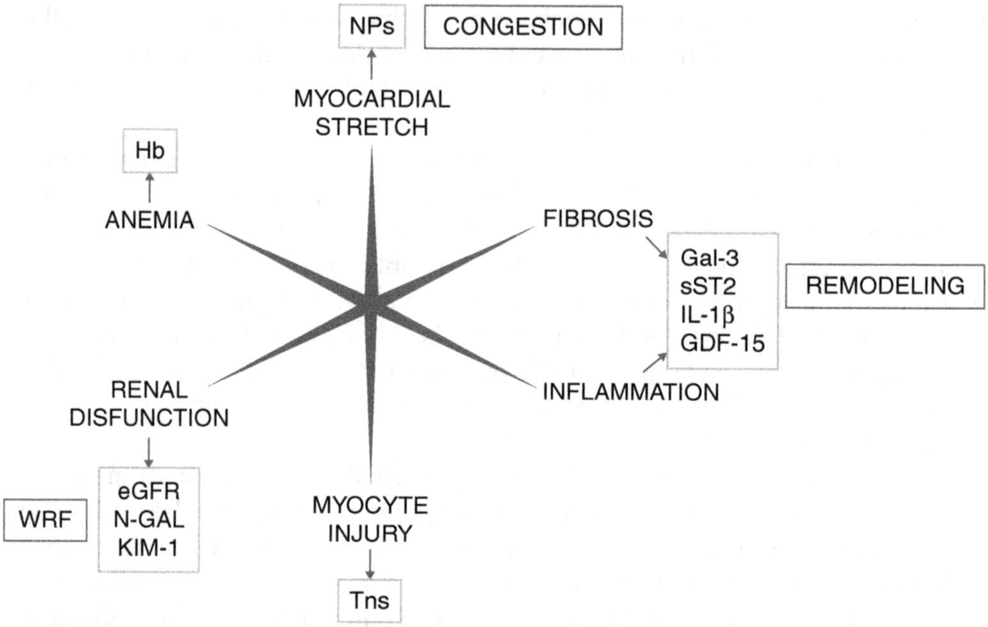

Fig. 11.2 Overview of biomarker classification and their significance in DCM

stratification in addition to the SHFM, a validated risk score in HF patients. They identified three classes of risk: low, intermediate and high; the latter two had, respectively, 4.7- and 13.3-fold increase of risk of adverse outcomes [63]. Lupon et al. developed a risk calculator (BCN Bio-HF) incorporating NT-proBNP, hs-TnT, sST2 and clinical variables; when biomarkers levels were added, a better risk classification in individual prediction of death was achieved [64].

In conclusion, a multimarker strategy is able to characterize every patient identifying those with more fibrotic, inflammatory or ischaemic elements. Multimarker strategy gives a deeper insight in HF pathophysiology and, above all, is needed for a tailored diagnostic and therapeutic strategy based on each patient's characteristics.

References

1. Bergmann O, Bhardwaj RD, Bernard S, Zdunek S, Barnabé-Heider F, Walsh S, et al. Evidence for cardiomyocyte renewal in humans. Science. 2009;324(5923):98–102. https://doi.org/10.1126/science.1164680.
2. Bergmann O, Zdunek S, Felker A, Salehpour M, Alkass K, Bernard S, et al. Dynamics of cell generation and turnover in the human heart. Cell. 2015;161(7):1566–75. https://doi.org/10.1016/j.cell.2015.05.026.
3. Senyo SE, Steinhauser ML, Pizzimenti CL, Yang VK, Cai L, Wang M, et al. Mammalian heart renewal by pre-existing cardiomyocytes. Nature. 2013;493(7432):433–6. https://doi.org/10.1038/nature11682.
4. Santini MP, Forte E, Harvey RP, Kovacic JC. Developmental origin and lineage plasticity of endogenous cardiac stem cells. Development. 2016;143(8):1242–58. https://doi.org/10.1242/dev.111591.

5. Bolli R, Chugh AR, D'Amario D, Loughran JH, Stoddard MF, Ikram S, et al. Cardiac stem cells in patients with ischaemic cardiomyopathy (SCIPIO): initial results of a randomised phase 1 trial. Lancet. 2011;378(9806):1847–57. https://doi.org/10.1016/S0140-6736(11)61590-0.
6. Keith MC, Bolli R. "String theory" of c-kit(pos) cardiac cells: a new paradigm regarding the nature of these cells that may reconcile apparently discrepant results. Circ Res. 2015;116(7):1216–30. https://doi.org/10.1161/CIRCRESAHA.116.305557.
7. Lin Z, Pu WT. Strategies for cardiac regeneration and repair. Sci Transl Med. 2014;6(239):239rv1. https://doi.org/10.1126/scitranslmed.3006681.
8. Takahashi K, Yamanaka S. Induction of pluripotent stem cells from mouse embryonic and adult fibroblast cultures by defined factors. Cell. 2006;126(4):663–76. https://doi.org/10.1016/j.cell.2006.07.024.
9. Laflamme MA, Murry CE. Heart regeneration. Nature. 2011;473(7347):326–35. https://doi.org/10.1038/nature10147.
10. Chong JJ, Yang X, Don CW, Minami E, Liu YW, Weyers JJ, et al. Human embryonic-stem-cell-derived cardiomyocytes regenerate non-human primate hearts. Nature. 2014;510(7504):273–7. https://doi.org/10.1038/nature13233.
11. Shadrin IY, Allen BW, Qian Y, Jackman CP, Carlson AL, et al. Cardiopatch platform enables maturation and scale-up of human pluripotent stem cell-derived engineered heart tissues. Nat Commun. 2017;8(1):1825. https://doi.org/10.1038/s41467-017-01946-x.
12. Srivastava D, DeWitt N. In vivo cellular reprogramming: the next generation. Cell. 2016;166(6):1386–96. https://doi.org/10.1016/j.cell.2016.08.055.
13. Uygur A, Lee RT. Mechanisms of cardiac regeneration. Dev Cell. 2016;36(4):362–74. https://doi.org/10.1016/j.devcel.2016.01.018.
14. Polizzotti BD, Ganapathy B, Walsh S, Choudhury S, Ammanamanchi N, Bennett DG, et al. Neuregulin stimulation of cardiomyocyte regeneration in mice and human myocardium reveals a therapeutic window. Sci Transl Med. 2015;7(281):281ra45. https://doi.org/10.1126/scitranslmed.aaa5171.
15. Heallen T, Zhang M, Wang J, Bonilla-Claudio M, Klysik E, Johnson RL, et al. Hippo pathway inhibits Wnt signaling to restrain cardiomyocyte proliferation and heart size. Science. 2011;332(6028):458–61. https://doi.org/10.1126/science.1199010.
16. D'Uva G, Aharonov A, Lauriola M, Kain D, Yahalom-Ronen Y, Carvalho S, et al. ERBB2 triggers mammalian heart regeneration by promoting cardiomyocyte dedifferentiation and proliferation. Nat Cell Biol. 2015;17(5):627–38. https://doi.org/10.1038/ncb3149.
17. Giacca M, Zacchigna S. Harnessing the microRNA pathway for cardiac regeneration. J Mol Cell Cardiol. 2015;89(Pt A):68–74. https://doi.org/10.1016/j.yjmcc.2015.09.017.
18. McNally EM, Mestroni L. Dilated cardiomyopathy: genetic determinants and mechanisms. Circ Res. 2017;121(7):731–48. https://doi.org/10.1161/CIRCRESAHA.
19. Bolli R, Ghafghazi S. Current status of cell therapy for non-ischaemic cardiomyopathy: a brief overview. Eur Heart J. 2015;36(42):2905–8. https://doi.org/10.1093/eurheartj/ehv454.
20. Psaltis PJ, Carbone A, Nelson AJ, Lau DH, Jantzen T, Manavis J, et al. Reparative effects of allogeneic mesenchymal precursor cells delivered transendocardially in experimental nonischemic cardiomyopathy. JACC Cardiovasc Interv. 2010;3(9):974–83. https://doi.org/10.1016/j.jcin.2010.05.016.
21. Guarita-Souza LC, Carvalho KA, Woitowicz V, Rebelatto C, Senegaglia A, Hansen P, et al. Simultaneous autologous transplantation of cocultured mesenchymal stem cells and skeletal myoblasts improves ventricular function in a murine model of Chagas disease. Circulation. 2006;114(1 Suppl):I120–4. https://doi.org/10.1161/CIRCULATIONAHA.105.000646.
22. Martino H, Brofman P, Greco O, Bueno R, Bodanese L, Clausell N, et al.; Dilated Cardiomyopathy Arm of the MiHeart Study Investigators. Multicentre, randomized, double-blind trial of intracoronary autologous mononuclear bone marrow cell injection in non-ischaemic dilated cardiomyopathy (the dilated cardiomyopathy arm of the MiHeart study). Eur Heart J. 2015;36(42):2898–904. https://doi.org/10.1093/eurheartj/ehv477.
23. Fischer-Rasokat U, Assmus B, Seeger FH, Honold J, Leistner D, Fichtlscherer S, et al. A pilot trial to assess potential effects of selective intracoronary bone marrow-derived progeni-

tor cell infusion in patients with nonischemic dilated cardiomyopathy: final 1-year results of the transplantation of progenitor cells and functional regeneration enhancement pilot trial in patients with nonischemic dilated cardiomyopathy. Circ Heart Fail. 2009;2(5):417–23. https://doi.org/10.1161/CIRCHEARTFAILURE.109.855023.

24. Vrtovec B, Poglajen G, Sever M, Lezaic L, Domanovic D, Cernelc P, et al. Effects of intracoronary stem cell transplantation in patients with dilated cardiomyopathy. J Card Fail. 2011;17(4):272–81. https://doi.org/10.1016/j.cardfail.2010.11.007.
25. Vrtovec B, Poglajen G, Lezaic L, Sever M, Domanovic D, Cernelc P, et al. Effects of intracoronary CD34+ stem cell transplantation in nonischemic dilated cardiomyopathy patients: 5-year follow-up. Circ Res. 2013;112(1):165–73. https://doi.org/10.1161/CIRCRESAHA.112.276519.
26. Vrtovec B, Poglajen G, Lezaic L, Sever M, Socan A, Domanovic D, et al. Comparison of transendocardial and intracoronary CD34+ cell transplantation in patients with nonischemic dilated cardiomyopathy. Circulation. 2013;128(11 Suppl 1):S42–9. https://doi.org/10.1161/CIRCULATIONAHA.112.000230.
27. Seth S, Bhargava B, Narang R, Ray R, Mohanty S, Gulati G, et al. The ABCD (autologous bone marrow cells in dilated cardiomyopathy) trial a long-term follow-up study. J Am Coll Cardiol. 2010;55(15):1643–4. https://doi.org/10.1016/j.jacc.2009.11.070.
28. Sant'Anna RT, Fracasso J, Valle FH, Castro I, Nardi NB, et al. Direct intramyocardial transthoracic transplantation of bone marrow mononuclear cells for non-ischemic dilated cardiomyopathy: INTRACELL, a prospective randomized controlled trial. Rev Bras Cir Cardiovasc. 2014;29(3):437–47. https://doi.org/10.5935/1678-9741.20140091.
29. Henry TD, Traverse JH, Hammon BL, East CA, Bruckner B, Remmers AE, et al. Safety and efficacy of ixmyelocel-T: an expanded, autologous multi-cellular therapy, in dilated cardiomyopathy. Circ Res. 2014;115(8):730–7. https://doi.org/10.1161/CIRCRESAHA.115.304554.
30. Menasché P. Cell therapy trials for heart regeneration—lessons learned and future directions. Nat Rev Cardiol. 2018;15(11):659–71. https://doi.org/10.1038/s41569-018-0013-0.
31. Biomarkers Definition Working Group. Biomarkers and surrogate endpoints: preferred definitions and conceptual framework. Clin Pharmacol Ther. 2001;69:89–95. https://doi.org/10.1067/mcp.2001.113989.
32. Braunwald E. Biomarkers in heart failure. N Engl J Med. 2008;358:2148–59. https://doi.org/10.1056/NEJMra0800239.
33. Ponikowski P, Voors AA, Anker SD, Bueno H, Cleland JGF, Coats AJS, et al. 2016 ESC guidelines for the diagnosis and treatment of acute and chronic heart failure: the task force for the diagnosis and treatment of acute and chronic heart failure of the European Society of Cardiology (ESC). Eur Heart J. 2016;37:2129–200. https://doi.org/10.1093/eurheartj/ehw128.
34. Phreaner N, Shah K, Maisel A. Natriuretic peptides and biomarkers in the diagnosis of heart failure. In: Jagadesh G, Balakumar P, Maung UK, editors. Pathophysiology and pharmacotherapy of cardiovascular disease. Switzerland: Springer International Publishing AG; 2015. https://doi.org/10.1007/978-3-319-15961-4_12.
35. Stolfo D, Stenner E, Merlo M, Porto AG, Moras C, Barbati G, et al. Prognostic impact of BNP variations in patients admitted for acute decompensated heart failure with in hospital worsening renal function. Heart Lung Circ. 2017;26(3):226–34. https://doi.org/10.1016/j.hlc.2016.06.1205.
36. Amorim S, Campelo M, Moura B, Martins E, Rodrigues J, Barroso I, et al. The role of biomarkers in dilated cardiomyopathy: assessment of clinical severity and reverse remodeling. Rev Port Cardiol. 2017;36(10):709–16. https://doi.org/10.1016/j.repc.2017.02.015.
37. Bielecka-Dabrowa A, von Haehling S, Aronow WS, Ahmed MI, Rysz J, Banach M. Heart failure biomarkers in patients with dilated cardiomyopathy. Int J Cardiol. 2013;168(3):2404–10. https://doi.org/10.1016/j.ijcard.2013.01.157.
38. Merlo M, Pyxaras SA, Pinamonti B, Barbati G, Di Lenarda A, Sinagra G. Prevalence and prognostic significance of left ventricular reverse remodeling in dilated cardiomyopathy receiving tailored medical treatment. J Am Coll Cardiol. 2011;57:1468–76. https://doi.org/10.1016/j.jacc.2010.11.030.

39. Bayes-Genis A, de Antonio M, Vila J, Peñafiel J, Galán A, Barallat J. Head-to-head comparison of 2 myocardial fibrosis biomarkers for long-term heart failure risk stratification: ST2 versus galectin-3. J Am Coll Cardiol. 2014;63(2):158–66. https://doi.org/10.1016/j.jacc.2013.07.087.
40. Correale M, Monaco I, Brunetti ND, Di Biase M, Metra M, Nodari S, et al. Redefining biomarkers for heart failure. Heart Fail Rev. 2018;23(2):237–53. https://doi.org/10.1007/s10741-018-9683-2.
41. Lok DJ, Van Der Meer P, de la Porte PW, Lipsic E, Van Wijngaarden J, Hillege HL, et al. Prognostic value of galectin-3, a novel marker of fibrosis, in patients with chronic heart failure: data from the DEAL-HF study. Clin Res Cardiol. 2010;99(5):323–8. https://doi.org/10.1007/s00392-010-0125-y.
42. Meijers WC, Januzzi JL, de Filippi C, Adourian AS, Shah SJ, van Veldhuisen DJ, et al. Elevated plasma galectin-3 is associated with near-term rehospitalization in heart failure: a pooled analysis of 3 clinical trials. Am Heart J. 2014;167(6):853–60.e4. https://doi.org/10.1016/j.ahj.2014.02.011.
43. Besler C, Lang D, Urban D, Rommel KP, von Roeder M, Fengler K, et al. Plasma and cardiac galectin-3 in patients with heart failure reflects both inflammation and fibrosis. Circ Heart Fail. 2017;10(3). pii: e003804. https://doi.org/10.1161/CIRCHEARTFAILURE.116.003804.
44. Vergaro G, Del Franco A, Giannoni A, Prontera C, Ripoli A, Barison A, et al. Galectin-3 and myocardial fibrosis in nonischemic dilated cardiomyopathy. Int J Cardiol. 2015;184:96–100. https://doi.org/10.1016/j.ijcard.2015.02.008.
45. Hu DJ, Xu J, Du W, Zhang JX, Zhong M, Zhou YN. Cardiac magnetic resonance and galectin-3 level as predictors of prognostic outcomes for non-ischemic cardyomyopathy patients. Int J Cardiovasc Imaging. 2016;32(12):1725–33. https://doi.org/10.1007/s10554-016-0958-1.
46. Kakkar R, Lee RT. The IL-33/ST2 pathway: therapeutic target and novel biomarker. Nat Rev Drug Discov. 2008;7(10):827–40. https://doi.org/10.1038/nrd2660.
47. Felker GM, Fiuzat M, Thompson V, Shaw LK, Neely ML, Adams KF, et al. Soluble ST2 in ambulatory patients with heart failure: association with functional capacity and long-term outcomes. Circ Heart Fail. 2013;6(6):1172–9. https://doi.org/10.1161/CIRCHEARTFAILURE.113.000207.
48. Ky B, French B, McCloskey K, Rame JE, McIntosh E, Shahi P, et al. High-sensitivity ST2 for prediction of adverse outcomes in chronic heart failure. Circ Heart Fail. 2011;4(2):180–7. https://doi.org/10.1161/CIRCHEARTFAILURE.110.958223.
49. Mallick A, Januzzi JL Jr. Biomarkers in acute heart failure. Rev Esp Cardiol (Engl Ed). 2015;68(6):514–25. https://doi.org/10.1016/j.rec.2015.02.009.
50. Wu AH, Wians F, Jaffe A. Biological variation of galectin-3 and soluble ST2 for chronic heart failure: implication on interpretation of test results. Am Heart J. 2013;165(6):995–9. https://doi.org/10.1016/j.ahj.2013.02.029.
51. Lupón J, Gaggin HK, de Antonio M, Domingo M, Galán A, Zamora E, et al. Biomarker-assist score for reverse remodelling prediction in heart failure: the ST2-R2 score. Int J Cardiol. 2015;184:337–43. https://doi.org/10.1016/j.ijcard.2015.02.019.
52. Wojciechowska C, Romuk E, Nowalany-Kozielska E, Jacheć W. Serum galectin-3 and ST2 as predictors of unfavourable outcome in stable dilated cardiomyopathy patients. Hellenic J Cardiol. 2017;58(5):350–9. https://doi.org/10.1016/j.hjc.2017.03.006.
53. Toldo S, Mezzaroma E, Mauro AG, Salloum F, Van Tassell BW, Abbate A. The inflammasome in myocardial injury and cardiac remodelling. Antioxid Redox Signal. 2015;22:1146–61. https://doi.org/10.1089/ars.2014.5989.
54. Aleksova A, Beltrami AP, Carriere C, Barbati G, Lesizza P, Perrieri-Montanino M, et al. Interleukin-1β levels predict long-term mortality and need for heart transplantation in ambulatory patients affected by idiopathic dilated cardiomyopathy. Oncotarget. 2017;8(15):25131–40. https://doi.org/10.18632/oncotarget.15349.
55. Nair N, Gongora E. Correlations of GDF-15 with sST2, MMPs, and worsening functional capacity in idiopathic dilated cardiomyopathy: can we gain new insights into the pathophysiology? J Circ Biomark. 2018;7:1–8. https://doi.org/10.1177/1849454417751735.

56. Stojkovic S, Kaider A, Koller L, Brekalo M, Wojta J, Diedrich A, et al. GDF-15 is a better complimentary marker for risk stratification of arrhythmic death in non-ischemic, dilated cardiomyopathy than soluble ST2. J Cell Mol Med. 2018;22(4):2422–9. https://doi.org/10.1111/jcmm.13540.
57. Kawahara C, Tsutamoto T, Nishiyama K, Yamaji M, Sakai H, Fujii M, et al. Prognostic role of high-sensitivity cardiac troponin T in patients with nonischemic dilated cardyomyopathy. Circ J. 2011;75(3):656–61. https://doi.org/10.1253/circj.CJ-10-0837.
58. Aleksova A, Barbati G, Merlo M, Stolfo D, Sabbadini G, Di Lenarda A, et al. Deleterious impact of mild anemia on survival of young adult patients (age 45 +− 14 years) with idiopathic dilated cardiomyopathy: data from the Trieste Cardiomyopathies Registry. Heart Lung. 2011;40(5):454–61. https://doi.org/10.1016/j.hrtlng.2010.06.001.
59. Tanaka K, Ito M, Kodama M, Maruyama H, Hoyano M, Mitsuma W, et al. Longitudinal change in renal function in patients with idiopathic dilated cardiomyopathy without renal insufficiency at initial diagnosis. Circ J. 2007;71(12):1927–31. https://doi.org/10.1253/circj.71.1927.
60. Ohshima K, Hirashiki A, Cheng XW, Hayashi M, Hayashi D, Okumura T, et al. Impact of mild to moderate renal dysfunction on left ventricular relaxation function and prognosis in ambulatory patients with nonischemic dilated cardiomyopathy. Int Heart J. 2011;52(6):366–71. https://doi.org/10.1536/ihj.52.366.
61. Latini R, Aleksova A, Masson S. Novel biomarkers and therapies in cardiorenal syndrome. Curr Opin Pharmacol. 2016;27:56–61. https://doi.org/10.1016/j.coph.2016.01.010.
62. Pascual-Figal DA, Manzano-Fernández S, Boronat M, Casas T, Garrido IP, Bonaque JC, et al. Soluble ST2, high-sensitivity troponin T and N-terminal pro-B-type natriuretic peptide: complementary role for risk stratification in acutely decompensated heart failure. Eur J Heart Fail. 2011;13(7):718–25. https://doi.org/10.1093/eurjhf/hfr047.
63. Ky B, French B, Levy WC, Sweitzer NK, Fang JC, Wu AH, et al. Multiple biomarkers for risk prediction in chronic heart failure. Circ Heart Fail. 2012;5(2):183–90. https://doi.org/10.1161/CIRCHEARTFAILURE.111.965020.
64. Lupòn J, De Antonio M, Vila J, Peñafiel J, Galán A, Zamora E, et al. Development of a novel heart failure risk tool: the Barcelona bio-heart failure risk calculator (BCN bio-HF calculator). PLoS One. 2014;9:e85466. https://doi.org/10.1371/journal.pone.0085466.

12

Prognostic Stratification and Importance of Follow-Up

Antonio Cannatà, Davide Stolfo, Marco Merlo, Cosimo Carriere, and Gianfranco Sinagra

Abbreviations and Acronyms

ACEi	Angiotensin-converting enzyme inhibitors
ARBs	Angiotensin receptor blockers
CMR	Cardiac magnetic resonance
CPET	Cardiopulmonary exercise test
CRT	Cardiac resynchronization therapy
DCM	Dilated cardiomyopathy
EMB	Endomyocardial biopsy
FMR	Functional mitral regurgitation
ICD	Implantable cardioverter-defibrillator
LGE	Late gadolinium enhancement
LMNA	Lamin A/C
LVEF	Left ventricular ejection fraction
LVRR	Left ventricular reverse remodeling
RAAS	Renin-angiotensin-aldosterone system
SCD	Sudden cardiac death
TTN	Titin

Dilated cardiomyopathy (DCM) is a particular phenotype of heart failure, frequently with a genetic background, which affects mostly relatively young patients with low comorbidity. Patients affected by DCM are usually in their third/fifth decade of life

A. Cannatà · D. Stolfo (✉) · C. Carriere
Cardiovascular Department, Azienda Sanitaria Universitaria Integrata, University of Trieste (ASUITS), Trieste, Italy
e-mail: Davide.stolfo@asuits.sanita.fvg.it

M. Merlo · G. Sinagra
Cardiovascular Department, Azienda Sanitaria Universitaria Integrata, Trieste, Italy
e-mail: gianfranco.sinagra@asuits.sanita.fvg.it

and more frequently males (male/female ratio 3:1) [1]. It is a relatively rare disease (prevalence approximately 1:250); however, it requires difficult choices in terms of clinical management, device treatment, and indication to heart transplantation, thus emphasizing the role of an accurate prognostic stratification [2].

The Heart Muscle Disease Registry of Trieste enrolled so far more than 1500 patients with DCM, followed for more than 10 years, and represents the largest monocentric registry for this type of disease. The information obtained from the analysis of those data is crucial to understand the cornerstones of the management of patients with DCM. Yet from the early 1990s, significant improvements in prognosis of DCM patients have been achieved. Indeed, the yearly incidence of adverse events, death, or heart transplantation has been dramatically reduced to less than 2% per year, the incidence of sudden cardiac death (SCD) less than 0.5% per year, and a survival free from transplantation more than 87% at 8 years of follow-up [3, 4]. All these achievements are mainly due to several milestones reached in the management of DCM patients. Earlier diagnosis, etiological characterization, optimized medical therapy, and timely device implantation have been the main goals in this fight [2].

12.1 Prognosis of DCM: The Milestones of the Management

In the last decades, prognosis of DCM has dramatically been improved. The data from the Heart Muscle Disease Registry of Trieste perfectly highlight the results over time. Once believed as an irreversible disease, DCM has rapidly become a more treatable condition thanks to the advancements made. Analyzing three decades of enrollment of the Heart Muscle Disease Registry of Trieste is possible to underline the milestones reached in the management of DCM patients. In the late 1980s, treatment of patients with DCM was mainly symptomatic. Approximately one third of patients were treated with renin-angiotensin-aldosterone system (RAAS) blockade, and less than 15% of patients were treated with beta-blockers [5]. Neurohormonal blockade was yet at the beginning, and only a minority of patients received optimized medical treatment. With time, in the 1990s, treatment with angiotensin-converting enzyme inhibitors (ACEi) or angiotensin receptor blockers (ARBs) and with beta-blockers became widespread. These improvements led to a significant shift upward of the survival curves, with a reduction of mortality of approximately 20% [5]. Finally, with the introduction of cardiac devices such as implantable cardioverter-defibrillator (ICD) and cardiac resynchronization therapy (CRT), the incidence of SCD and the occurrence of life-threatening arrhythmias have been dramatically reduced with parallel prognostic improvements [5]. Therefore, proper management of DCM patients follows the guidelines on HF and requires multidisciplinary cardiologic approach among clinicians, invasive cardiologist, electrophysiologist, and noninvasive imaging specialists in order to optimize medical and device treatment for those patients.

12.2 Etiological Characterization as an Important Prognostic Factor

Etiological characterization of DCM is the hinge of clinical management, fundamental to improve the outcome of the disease. Ideally, patients with nonischemic DCM should undergo each and every diagnostic test to rule out potentially reversible causes of left ventricular dysfunction, which may benefit from specific therapeutic intervention. Several noxae may lead to a clinical phenotype of DCM. Among the most common causes, tachyarrhythmias (either frequent ventricular ectopy, ventricular tachycardia, or atrial tachyarrhythmias), elevated catecholamine level, or exogenous toxins, such as alcohol or cocaine, may be a reversible cause of DCM. Furthermore, systemic inflammatory syndromes, such as systemic autoimmune disorders (e.g., Churg-Strauss syndrome, sarcoidosis), and a significant history of arterial hypertension are common reversible causes of DCM [2, 4].

Severe left ventricular dysfunction can also be secondary to inflammatory cardiomyopathy. In this scenario, prompt diagnosis and timely management of post-myocarditis DCM or acute myocarditis with severe left ventricular dysfunction have significant prognostic implications. In those patients, a comprehensive integrated approach, including third-level diagnostic tools, such as cardiac magnetic resonance (CMR) and endomyocardial biopsy (EMB) in selected cases, should be systematically performed given their prognostic significance. Indeed, as recently reported, patients with post-myocarditis DCM have better outcomes compared to those with genetically determined DCMs [6–8].

Thus, differentiating between idiopathic DCM, genetically determined disease, and DCM of specific etiologies plays a fundamental role in the management and prognostic stratification. In the latter cases, nearly all patients experience favorable left ventricular reverse remodeling (LVRR) when the initial noxa has been dismissed or treated [2, 4]. Therefore, prognostic stratification should include proper etiological characterization and third-level analysis, such as CMR, and should systematically be performed in each and every patient with DCM from unknown cause.

12.3 DCM as a Dynamic Disease: The Importance of Follow-Up

DCM has been considered for a long time as an invariably irreversible condition. The cumulative experience derived from referral centers revealed that almost 40% of DCM patients under optimal medical and device treatments experience a significant left ventricular reverse remodeling [2–4, 9]. Optimal management of DCM is largely based on conventional therapy of systolic heart failure, according to current guidelines [10]. ACE inhibitors/angiotensin receptor blockers, beta-blockers, and mineralocorticoid receptor antagonists remain the cornerstone of DCM therapy. In persistently symptomatic patients fulfilling specific criteria, ivabradine may be advocated on top of medical therapy [10]. Despite the striking results of the

PARADIGM-HF trial and the data on the long-term outcomes in patients treated with LCZ-696 [11, 12], no data are available on the sacubitril/valsartan in the specific subgroup of patients with DCM.

Device treatment represents nowadays one of the pillars of the management of DCM patients. On the one hand, cardiac resynchronization therapy (CRT) is able to reduce mortality and improve outcomes of patients with DCM. On the other hand, the role of ICD in nonischemic cardiomyopathies is still controversial, and the correction of mitral regurgitation with MitraClip®, although can contribute to LV reverse remodeling (LVRR), has limited evidences from large series of DCM patients [2, 13–15].

From our experience, DCM natural history is characterized by improvement of ventricular involvement within 2 years from optimization of therapy, followed by a subsequent period of stability. As previously described, a complete LVRR within 24 months from the onset of the disease has been recently demonstrated as an independent prognostic tool [16]. CRT has been proven to positively influence LVRR, possibly inducing a persistent normalization of LV size and dimension specifically in DCM [17–20]. Noteworthy, identification of early markers of LVRR is still foggy highlighting the difficulties in prognostic stratification of those patients. However, patients without left bundle branch block (LBBB) at ECG [16] or late gadolinium enhancement (LGE) at CMR [21] are the most likely candidates to a favorable evolution of the disease.

12.4 Left Ventricular Reverse Remodeling Beyond the Left Ventricle

Besides LVRR, it is important to define specific and earlier features for prognostic stratification in DCM patients. Genetic background seems to have an impact on the prognosis of patients with DCM. The improved efficiency of genetic testing allowed better characterization of pathogenic mutations and their prognostic role. Mutations in lamin A/C (LMNA) have distinct genotype-phenotype correlations, requiring therefore specific treatments. Cytoskeleton and Z-disk mutations are associated with lower probability of LVRR, whereas mutations in gene encoding for desmosomal proteins and titin (TTN) mutations tend to have higher rate of LVRR. However, clear evidences on these scenarios should be further investigated [22].

Noninvasive assessments provide critical information of natural history of DCM. Hemodynamic indexes measured at echocardiography, i.e., improvement of functional mitral regurgitation (FMR) and right ventricular function, seem to foretell amelioration of ventricular function and thus LVRR. Those two indexes emerged already at a short time point of 6 months and represent early therapeutic targets and upmost useful tools for prognostic stratification in DCM [13, 14, 23]. The presence and the severity of FMR convey important therapeutic (i.e., percutaneous repair of mitral valve) and prognostic implications [13, 23], and right ventricular (RV) dysfunction along with the estimation of pulmonary arterial pressure is essential in the stratification of the disease [13, 23]. Furthermore, left ventricular diastolic function and left atrial dimension should be systematically assessed for the estimation of left ventricular filling pressures and identification of restrictive filling pattern [24].

The definite identification of predictors of LVRR appears to be an important target for future researches, and the genetic background of LVRR appears to be the most interesting field to be explored. Therefore, echocardiographic evaluation of patients affected by DCM should be as much accurate as possible, beyond LV systolic function and dimensions, both at baseline and during follow-up. Newer noninvasive techniques assessing myocardial deformation (e.g., speckle-tracking echocardiography or CMR-derived strain) have greater sensitivity than Left Ventricular Ejection Fraction (LVEF) for identifying subclinical abnormalities of systolic function and may assume a role in the early detection of disease [2, 3, 25].

12.5 Prognostic Role of Cardiopulmonary Exercise Testing

DCM represents a specific model of HF characterized by relatively young patients with low comorbidity rate and a long asymptomatic history of disease, and these features may affect the traditional evaluation of symptomatic heart failure patients. In clinical management of DCM patients, this issue has always to be considered since it may influence the diagnostic and therapeutic workup. Cardiopulmonary exercise test (CPET), using peak of oxygen consumption, has driven the optimal timing for the selection of heart transplant candidates [26]. Due to the advances in knowledge of exercise impairment in HF, new indexes have been proposed, including the percentage of predicted peak VO_2, peak systolic blood pressure, and ventilatory efficiency, expressed as VE/VCO_2 slope [2, 3, 27–29]. Notably, patients affected by DCM perform better at CPET compared to other etiologies of HF due to their intrinsic characteristics; therefore the abovementioned markers need further future validation in DCM. Recently predicted $VO_2\%$ and VE/VCO_2 slope emerged as the strongest CPET predictors in a large cohort of DCM, with cutoffs of 60% and 29%, respectively [30]. Validation in prospective series is advocated, but it is clear that the etiology of HF is fundamental in interpreting the parameters of CPET for candidates to heart transplant [30].

12.6 Arrhythmic Risk Stratification

In the last years, ICDs dramatically reduced the risk of SCD and mortality in patients with reduced ejection fraction HF on optimal medical treatment [10]. However, in patients with nonischemic cardiomyopathies, the real benefits of ICD implantation appear disputable [15, 31, 32]. Although ICD implantation dropped the mortality rate in young and mildly symptomatic patients with DCM [5], ICD indication for primary prevention of SCD is largely based on the severity of systolic dysfunction [10, 33]. However, approximately 50% of SCD occur in patients without severely reduced LVEF [34]. Therefore, it appears crucial a more accurate characterization of the arrhythmic risk in DCM patients (Fig. 12.1) [35].

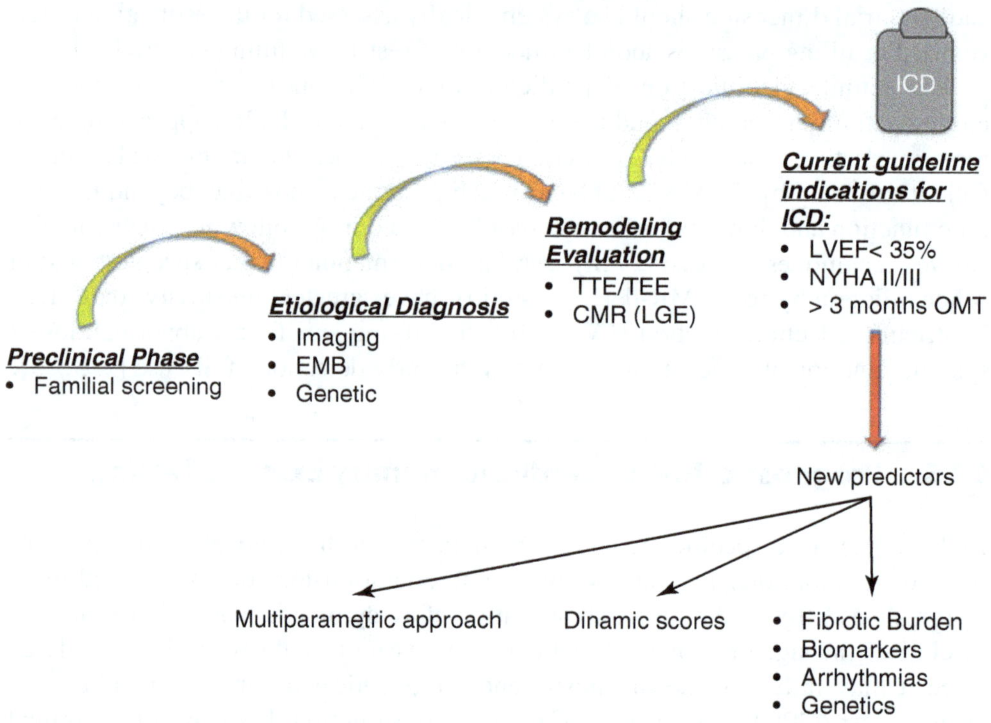

Fig. 12.1 Arrhythmic risk evaluation and the need for novel predictors in DCM. *CMR* cardiac magnetic resonance, *EMB* endomyocardial biopsy, *LGE* late gadolinium enhancement, *LVEF* left ventricular ejection fraction, *NYHA* New York Heart Association, *TEE* transesophageal echocardiogram, *TTE* transthoracic echocardiogram

Furthermore, early arrhythmic stratification in DCM patients may encase important prognostic features. Indeed, solely one third of cases on optimal medical therapy, admitted with the criteria for ICD implantation, maintain those criteria over a 6-month follow-up [19]. The occurrence of LVRR has important prognostic implications in particular in those candidates for ICD implantation in primary prevention. Accordingly, a wait-and-see period of about 3–9 months on optimal medical therapy is recommended before the ICD implantation [2, 10, 33]. However as showed by Losurdo et al., approximately 2% of patients with DCM die suddenly in the first 6 months after the diagnosis [36]. Unfortunately, there are not yet definitive predictors of early arrhythmic events. A severe LV dilatation at baseline with prolonged QRS duration and a long duration of symptoms seem to be useful tools in identifying high-risk patients [36]. Moreover the familial history of SCD, the history of probable cardiac syncope, or the presence of highly arrhythmic expression at Holter ECG monitoring could identify arrhythmogenic DCM at elevated risk of SCD [37]. Further data are required to confirm these findings. In the next future, techniques as CMR and specific genetic tests could help for better identification of patients at higher risk [2, 21, 38].

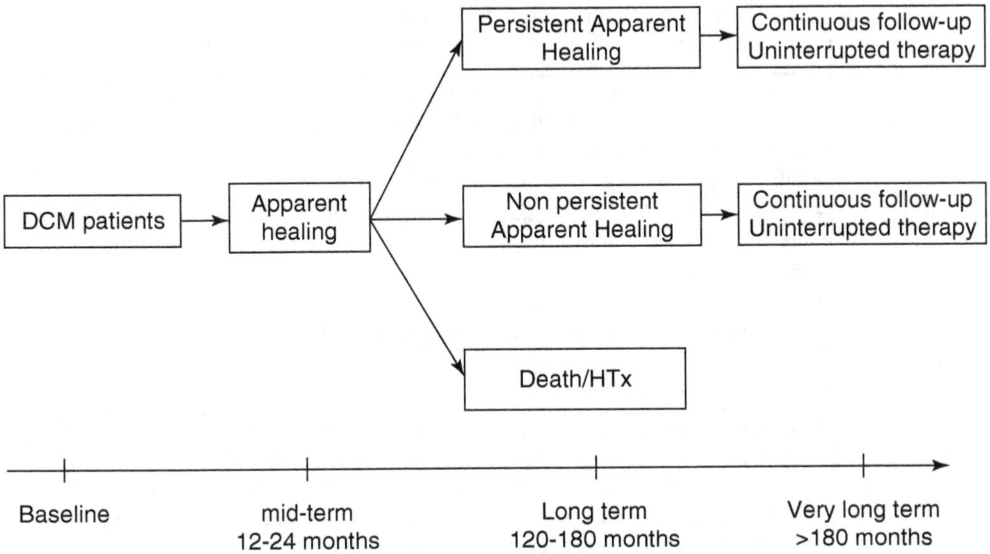

Fig. 12.2 Proposed follow-up time points to assess apparent healing. *DCM* dilated cardiomyopathy, *HTx* heart transplantation

12.7 The "Apparent Healing" Phenomenon

Approximately 15% of patients with DCM on optimal medical treatment normalize their LV size and function persistently over 10 years of follow-up. However, over a very long-term follow-up (15 years), a non-negligible percentage (5%) of patients with persistent "apparent healing" as a consequence of progressive deterioration of left ventricular function underwent CRT-ICD implantation, died for refractory heart failure, or needed cardiac transplantation [2, 3, 5, 39]. Therefore, at the current state of knowledge, the treatment should be continued lifelong and also in apparently stable/healed DCM patients (Fig. 12.2).

12.8 Uninterrupted Follow-Up and Continuous Reclassification of the Disease

Optimal treatment of patients with DCM has significantly increased the survival rates and has resulted in long periods of clinical stability. Data from the registries highlighted that from the sixth to eighth year of follow-up, a new progression of the disease may occur [2, 4, 39], indicating the pivotal role not only of an accurate and complete initial diagnosis but also of a continuous, individualized, and long-term follow-up evaluation in DCM patients (Table 12.1). In everyday clinical practice, DCM patients of more than 50–60 years of age and with duration of the disease of more than 10 years are more often seen. In those patients systematic reassessment of risk factors and continuous reclassification of the disease is mandatory (Fig. 12.3).

Table 12.1 Important time points in the natural history of DCM

Time	Evaluation
Baseline	• Complete evaluation (noninvasive and invasive, if necessary) in order to assess an etiological characterization, to decide timing of individualized follow-up and timing and type of therapeutic strategies • Administration of optimal medical treatment
3–9 months	• "Hemodynamic" reverse remodeling (improvement of mitral regurgitation; normalization of right ventricular systolic function; improvement of diastolic dysfunction) • Consider ICD/CRT-D implantation • Attention to the onset of negative prognostic factors[a]
24 months	• Left ventricular reverse remodeling completed • Attention to the onset of negative prognostic factors[a]
72–84 months	• Possible progression of the disease after stability induced by medical therapy • Reclassification of the disease in the presence of progression of the disease (attention to possible onset of possible causes of left ventricular dysfunction: hypertension; diabetes; ischemic heart disease; structural valve disease) • Attention to the onset of negative prognostic factors[a]
After 120 months	• Need of continuing follow-up and therapy lifelong in order to early detect signs of progression of the disease in the long term • Attention to the onset of negative prognostic factors[a]

CRT-D cardiac resynchronization therapy defibrillator, *ICD* implanted cardioverter-defibrillator
[a]*Negative prognostic factors*: atrial fibrillation; right ventricular dysfunction; left ventricular bundle branch block; functional mitral regurgitation

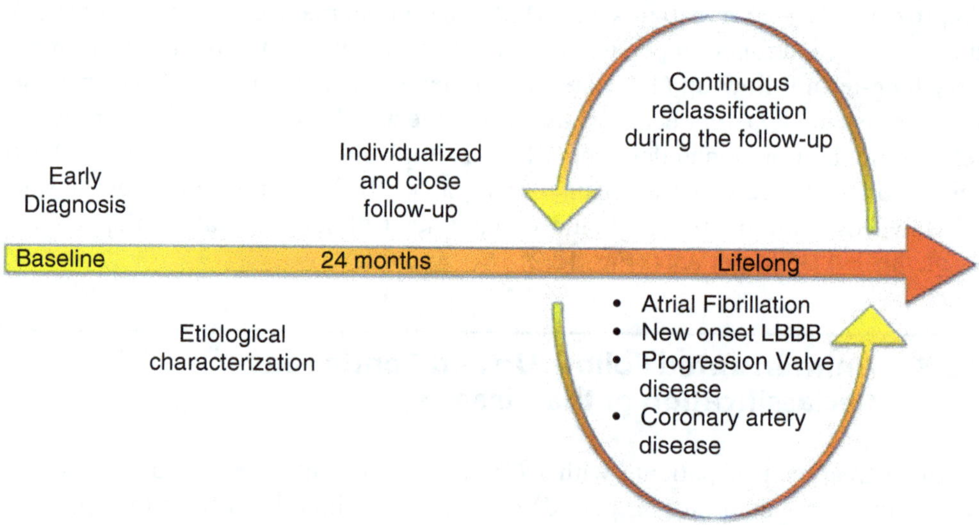

Fig. 12.3 Key point in DCM management. *LBBB* left bundle branch block

Abrupt deterioration of LV ejection fraction or progressive LV dilation as well as new onset of significant arrhythmic burden could be related to the progression of the disease but also to the development of coronary artery disease; hypertensive heart disease, structured valve disease, or acute myocarditis should be ruled out given their prognostic relevance in the natural history of the disease (Fig. 12.4) [2, 3].

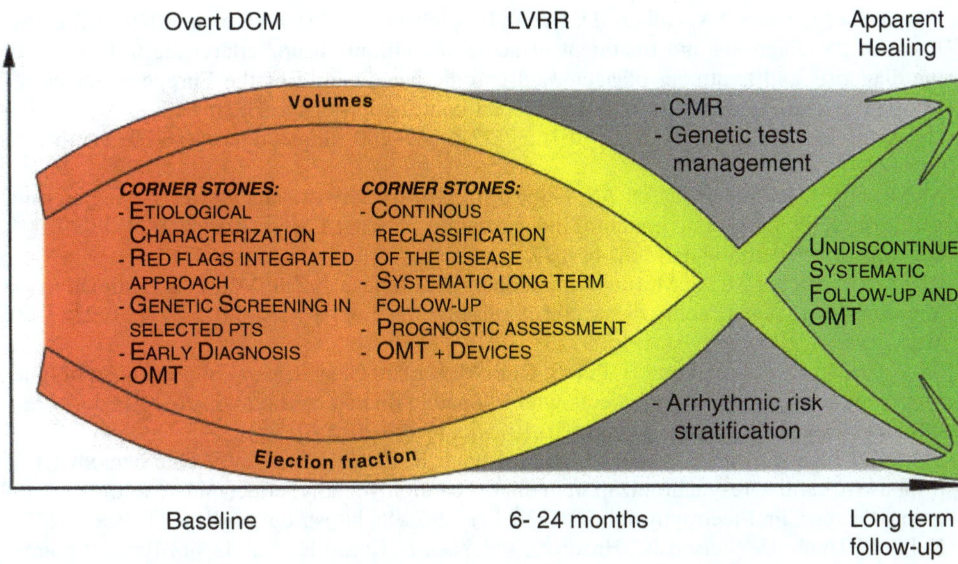

Fig. 12.4 The importance of follow-up in DCM patients [2]

References

1. Hershberger RE, Hedges DJ, Morales A. Dilated cardiomyopathy: the complexity of a diverse genetic architecture. Nat Rev Cardiol. 2013;10(9):531–47. https://doi.org/10.1038/nrcardio.2013.105.
2. Merlo M, Cannata A, Gobbo M, Stolfo D, Elliott PM, Sinagra G. Evolving concepts in dilated cardiomyopathy. Eur J Heart Fail. 2018;20(2):228–39. https://doi.org/10.1002/ejhf.1103.
3. Merlo M, Cannata A, Vitagliano A, Zambon E, Lardieri G, Sinagra G. Clinical management of dilated cardiomyopathy: current knowledge and future perspectives. Expert Rev Cardiovasc Ther. 2016;14(2):137–40. https://doi.org/10.1586/14779072.2016.1125292.
4. Merlo M, Gentile P, Naso P, Sinagra G. The natural history of dilated cardiomyopathy: how has it changed? J Cardiovasc Med (Hagerstown). 2017;18(Suppl 1):e161–e5. https://doi.org/10.2459/JCM.0000000000000459.
5. Merlo M, Pivetta A, Pinamonti B, Stolfo D, Zecchin M, Barbati G, et al. Long-term prognostic impact of therapeutic strategies in patients with idiopathic dilated cardiomyopathy: changing mortality over the last 30 years. Eur J Heart Fail. 2014;16(3):317–24. https://doi.org/10.1002/ejhf.16.
6. Anzini M, Merlo M, Sabbadini G, Barbati G, Finocchiaro G, Pinamonti B, et al. Long-term evolution and prognostic stratification of biopsy-proven active myocarditis. Circulation. 2013;128(22):2384–94. https://doi.org/10.1161/CIRCULATIONAHA.113.003092.
7. Sinagra G, Anzini M, Pereira NL, Bussani R, Finocchiaro G, Bartunek J, et al. Myocarditis in clinical practice. Mayo Clin Proc. 2016;91(9):1256–66. https://doi.org/10.1016/j.mayocp.2016.05.013.
8. Merlo M, Anzini M, Bussani R, Artico J, Barbati G, Stolfo D, et al. Characterization and long-term prognosis of postmyocarditic dilated cardiomyopathy compared with idiopathic dilated cardiomyopathy. Am J Cardiol. 2016;118(6):895–900. https://doi.org/10.1016/j.amjcard.2016.05.063.
9. Matsumura Y, Hoshikawa-Nagai E, Kubo T, Yamasaki N, Furuno T, Kitaoka H, et al. Left ventricular reverse remodeling in long-term (>12 years) survivors with idiopathic dilated cardiomyopathy. Am J Cardiol. 2013;111(1):106–10. https://doi.org/10.1016/j.amjcard.2012.08.056.

10. Ponikowski P, Voors AA, Anker SD, Bueno H, Cleland JG, Coats AJ, et al. 2016 ESC guidelines for the diagnosis and treatment of acute and chronic heart failure: the task force for the diagnosis and treatment of acute and chronic heart failure of the European Society of Cardiology (ESC) developed with the special contribution of the Heart Failure Association (HFA) of the ESC. Eur Heart J. 2016;37(27):2129–200. https://doi.org/10.1093/eurheartj/ehw128.
11. McMurray JJ, Packer M, Desai AS, Gong J, Lefkowitz MP, Rizkala AR, et al. Angiotensin-neprilysin inhibition versus enalapril in heart failure. N Engl J Med. 2014;371(11):993–1004. https://doi.org/10.1056/NEJMoa1409077.
12. Claggett B, Packer M, McMurray JJ, Swedberg K, Rouleau J, Zile MR, et al. Estimating the long-term treatment benefits of sacubitril-valsartan. N Engl J Med. 2015;373(23):2289–90. https://doi.org/10.1056/NEJMc1509753.
13. Stolfo D, Merlo M, Pinamonti B, Poli S, Gigli M, Barbati G, et al. Early improvement of functional mitral regurgitation in patients with idiopathic dilated cardiomyopathy. Am J Cardiol. 2015;115(8):1137–43. https://doi.org/10.1016/j.amjcard.2015.01.549.
14. Stolfo D, Tonet E, Barbati G, Gigli M, Pinamonti B, Zecchin M, et al. Acute hemodynamic response to cardiac resynchronization in dilated cardiomyopathy: effect on late mitral regurgitation. Pacing Clin Electrophysiol. 2015;38(11):1287–96. https://doi.org/10.1111/pace.12731.
15. Kober L, Thune JJ, Nielsen JC, Haarbo J, Videbaek L, Korup E, et al. Defibrillator implantation in patients with nonischemic systolic heart failure. N Engl J Med. 2016;375(13):1221–30. https://doi.org/10.1056/NEJMoa1608029.
16. Merlo M, Pyxaras SA, Pinamonti B, Barbati G, Di Lenarda A, Sinagra G. Prevalence and prognostic significance of left ventricular reverse remodeling in dilated cardiomyopathy receiving tailored medical treatment. J Am Coll Cardiol. 2011;57(13):1468–76. https://doi.org/10.1016/j.jacc.2010.11.030.
17. Serdoz LV, Daleffe E, Merlo M, Zecchin M, Barbati G, Pecora D, et al. Predictors for restoration of normal left ventricular function in response to cardiac resynchronization therapy measured at time of implantation. Am J Cardiol. 2011;108(1):75–80. https://doi.org/10.1016/j.amjcard.2011.02.347.
18. Verhaert D, Grimm RA, Puntawangkoon C, Wolski K, De S, Wilkoff BL, et al. Long-term reverse remodeling with cardiac resynchronization therapy: results of extended echocardiographic follow-up. J Am Coll Cardiol. 2010;55(17):1788–95. https://doi.org/10.1016/j.jacc.2010.01.022.
19. Zecchin M, Merlo M, Pivetta A, Barbati G, Lutman C, Gregori D, et al. How can optimization of medical treatment avoid unnecessary implantable cardioverter-defibrillator implantations in patients with idiopathic dilated cardiomyopathy presenting with "SCD-HeFT criteria?". Am J Cardiol. 2012;109(5):729–35. https://doi.org/10.1016/j.amjcard.2011.10.033.
20. Zecchin M, Proclemer A, Magnani S, Vitali-Serdoz L, Facchin D, Muser D, et al. Long-term outcome of 'super-responder' patients to cardiac resynchronization therapy. Europace. 2014;16(3):363–71. https://doi.org/10.1093/europace/eut339.
21. Masci PG, Doulaptsis C, Bertella E, Del Torto A, Symons R, Pontone G, et al. Incremental prognostic value of myocardial fibrosis in patients with non-ischemic cardiomyopathy without congestive heart failure. Circ Heart Fail. 2014;7(3):448–56. https://doi.org/10.1161/CIRCHEARTFAILURE.113.000996.
22. Dal Ferro M, Stolfo D, Altinier A, Gigli M, Perrieri M, Ramani F, et al. Association between mutation status and left ventricular reverse remodelling in dilated cardiomyopathy. Heart. 2017;103(21):1704–10. https://doi.org/10.1136/heartjnl-2016-311017.
23. Merlo M, Gobbo M, Stolfo D, Losurdo P, Ramani F, Barbati G, et al. The prognostic impact of the evolution of RV function in idiopathic DCM. JACC Cardiovasc Imaging. 2016;9(9):1034–42. https://doi.org/10.1016/j.jcmg.2016.01.027.
24. Lang RM, Badano LP, Mor-Avi V, Afilalo J, Armstrong A, Ernande L, et al. Recommendations for cardiac chamber quantification by echocardiography in adults: an update from the American

Society of Echocardiography and the European Association of Cardiovascular Imaging. J Am Soc Echocardiogr. 2015;28(1):1–39 e14. https://doi.org/10.1016/j.echo.2014.10.003.
25. Japp AG, Gulati A, Cook SA, Cowie MR, Prasad SK. The diagnosis and evaluation of dilated cardiomyopathy. J Am Coll Cardiol. 2016;67(25):2996–3010. https://doi.org/10.1016/j.jacc.2016.03.590.
26. Mancini DM, Eisen H, Kussmaul W, Mull R, Edmunds LH Jr, Wilson JR. Value of peak exercise oxygen consumption for optimal timing of cardiac transplantation in ambulatory patients with heart failure. Circulation. 1991;83(3):778–86.
27. Ingle L, Rigby AS, Sloan R, Carroll S, Goode KM, Cleland JG, et al. Development of a composite model derived from cardiopulmonary exercise tests to predict mortality risk in patients with mild-to-moderate heart failure. Heart. 2014;100(10):781–6. https://doi.org/10.1136/heartjnl-2013-304614.
28. Jefferies JL, Towbin JA. Dilated cardiomyopathy. Lancet. 2010;375(9716):752–62. https://doi.org/10.1016/S0140-6736(09)62023-7.
29. Stelken AM, Younis LT, Jennison SH, Miller DD, Miller LW, Shaw LJ, et al. Prognostic value of cardiopulmonary exercise testing using percent achieved of predicted peak oxygen uptake for patients with ischemic and dilated cardiomyopathy. J Am Coll Cardiol. 1996;27(2):345–52.
30. Sinagra G, Iorio A, Merlo M, Cannata A, Stolfo D, Zambon E, et al. Prognostic value of cardiopulmonary exercise testing in idiopathic dilated cardiomyopathy. Int J Cardiol. 2016;223:596–603. https://doi.org/10.1016/j.ijcard.2016.07.232.
31. Kadish A. Prophylactic defibrillator implantation—toward an evidence-based approach. N Engl J Med. 2005;352(3):285–7. https://doi.org/10.1056/NEJMe048351.
32. Kadish A, Dyer A, Daubert JP, Quigg R, Estes NA, Anderson KP, et al. Prophylactic defibrillator implantation in patients with nonischemic dilated cardiomyopathy. N Engl J Med. 2004;350(21):2151–8. https://doi.org/10.1056/NEJMoa033088.
33. Pinto YM, Elliott PM, Arbustini E, Adler Y, Anastasakis A, Bohm M, et al. Proposal for a revised definition of dilated cardiomyopathy, hypokinetic non-dilated cardiomyopathy, and its implications for clinical practice: a position statement of the ESC working group on myocardial and pericardial diseases. Eur Heart J. 2016;37(23):1850–8. https://doi.org/10.1093/eurheartj/ehv727.
34. Wellens HJ, Schwartz PJ, Lindemans FW, Buxton AE, Goldberger JJ, Hohnloser SH, et al. Risk stratification for sudden cardiac death: current status and challenges for the future. Eur Heart J. 2014;35(25):1642–51. https://doi.org/10.1093/eurheartj/ehu176.
35. Goldberger JJ, Subacius H, Patel T, Cunnane R, Kadish AH. Sudden cardiac death risk stratification in patients with nonischemic dilated cardiomyopathy. J Am Coll Cardiol. 2014;63(18):1879–89. https://doi.org/10.1016/j.jacc.2013.12.021.
36. Losurdo P, Stolfo D, Merlo M, Barbati G, Gobbo M, Gigli M, et al. Early arrhythmic events in idiopathic dilated cardiomyopathy. JACC Clin Electrophysiol. 2016;2(5):535–43. https://doi.org/10.1016/j.jacep.2016.05.002.
37. Spezzacatene A, Sinagra G, Merlo M, Barbati G, Graw SL, Brun F, et al. Arrhythmogenic phenotype in dilated cardiomyopathy: natural history and predictors of life-threatening arrhythmias. J Am Heart Assoc. 2015;4(10):e002149. https://doi.org/10.1161/JAHA.115.002149.
38. Gulati A, Jabbour A, Ismail TF, Guha K, Khwaja J, Raza S, et al. Association of fibrosis with mortality and sudden cardiac death in patients with nonischemic dilated cardiomyopathy. JAMA. 2013;309(9):896–908. https://doi.org/10.1001/jama.2013.1363.
39. Merlo M, Stolfo D, Anzini M, Negri F, Pinamonti B, Barbati G, et al. Persistent recovery of normal left ventricular function and dimension in idiopathic dilated cardiomyopathy during long-term follow-up: does real healing exist? J Am Heart Assoc. 2015;4(1):e001504. https://doi.org/10.1161/JAHA.114.000570.

13

Current Management and Treatment

Alessandro Altinier, Alessia Paldino, Marta Gigli,
Aniello Pappalardo, and Gianfranco Sinagra

Abbreviations and Acronyms

ACEi	Angiotensin-converting enzyme inhibitor
AF	Atrial fibrillation
AHA/ACC	American Heart Association/American College of Cardiology
ARB	Angiotensin II type I receptor blockers
ARNI	Angiotensin receptor-neprilysin inhibitor
CRT-D	Cardiac resynchronization therapy-defibrillator
CRT-P	Cardiac resynchronization therapy-pacemaker
DCM	Dilated cardiomyopathy
ESC	European Society of Cardiology
FMR	Functional mitral regurgitation
HF	Heart failure
HT	Heart transplantation
ICD	Implantable cardioverter-defibrillator
LBBB	Left bundle branch block
LV	Left ventricular
LVAD	Implantable left ventricular assist device
LVEF	Left ventricular ejection fraction
MCS	Mechanical circulatory support
MRA	Mineralocorticoid receptor antagonists
MRI	Magnetic resonance imaging

A. Altinier (✉) · A. Paldino · M. Gigli · A. Pappalardo
Cardiovascular Department, Azienda Sanitaria Universitaria Integrata, University of Trieste (ASUITS), Trieste, Italy
e-mail: aniello.pappalardo@asuits.sanita.fvg.it

G. Sinagra
Cardiovascular Department, Azienda Sanitaria Universitaria Integrata, Trieste, Italy
e-mail: gianfranco.sinagra@asuits.sanita.fvg.it

NIDCM Nonischemic dilated cardiomyopathy
RV Right ventricular
SCD Sudden cardiac death
VT Ventricular tachycardia

Dilated cardiomyopathy (DCM) is a frequent cause of heart failure (HF) and is characterized by dilation and impaired contraction of one or both ventricles. Patients affected by DCM have impaired systolic function and may or may not develop overt HF and atrial and/or ventricular arrhythmias. Sudden cardiac death (SCD) can occur at any stage of the disease. Important breakthroughs have redefined opportunities to change the natural history of the disease with familial and sport activity screening programs and a broad range of medical therapies, devices, and care strategies, including readmission reduction programs and ambulatory outpatient disease management for those with more advanced disease (Table 13.1, Fig. 13.1).

Table 13.1 Screening programs and pharmacological and non-pharmacological treatments of HF in DCM patients: levels of recommendations from ESC guidelines

	When?	Recommendation
Screening		
Familial screening program	– First-degree relatives, if a specific gene mutation is identified in the proband	Recommended (from age 10 to 12 years)
	– Family history of SCD in a first-degree relative	Can be useful
Sport activity screening	– For all young competitive athletes by history, physical examination, and ECG	Recommended by ESC
	– For all young competitive athletes with history and physical examination	Recommended by AHA/ACC
Pharmacological treatment		
ACEi	– Patients with asymptomatic LV systolic dysfunction, in order to prevent or delay the onset of HF	Recommended (**I B**)
	– Patients with symptomatic LV systolic dysfunction, in order to reduce HF, hospitalization, and death	Recommended (**I A**)
ARB	– Patients with symptomatic LV systolic dysfunction, in order to reduce HF hospitalization and death, unable to tolerate an ACE-I	Recommended (**I B**)
Beta-blocker	– Patients with symptomatic LV systolic dysfunction, in order to reduce HF, hospitalization, and death	Recommended (**I A**)
MRA	– Patients with LV systolic dysfunction still symptomatic with an optimized dosage of ACEi and beta-blocker, in order to reduce HF hospitalization and death	Recommended (**I A**)
Sacubitril/ Valsartan	– Patients with LV systolic dysfunction (EF $\leq$ 35%) still symptomatic (NYHA II–III) with an optimized dosage of ACEi (or ARB), beta-blocker, and MRA in order to reduce HF hospitalization and death	Recommended (**I B**)
Ivabradine	– Patients with LV systolic dysfunction (EF $\leq$ 35%) still symptomatic, in sinus rhythm and a resting heart rate $\geq$70 bpm, with an optimized dosage of ACEi(or ARB), beta-blocker, and MRA in order to reduce HF hospitalization and cardiovascular death	Recommended (**IIa B**)

Table 13.1 (continued)

	When?	Recommendation
Diuretics	– To reduce symptoms and signs of congestion	Recommended (**I B**)
Hydralazine and isosorbide dinitrate	– Black patients with symptomatic LV systolic dysfunction in case of intolerance or contraindication to ACEi or ARB, in order to reduce mortality	Recommended (**IIb B**)
	– Patients with LV systolic dysfunction (EF ≤ 35%) and still symptomatic (NYHA III–IV) with an optimized dosage of ACEi and beta-blocker, in order to reduce HF hospitalization and death	Recommended (**IIa B**)
Non-pharmacological treatment		
ICD	– Patients with LV systolic dysfunction (EF ≤ 35%) and symptomatic (NYHA II–III) despite 3 months of OMT, in order to reduce SCD and all-cause mortality	Recommended (**I B**)
CRT	– Patients with LV systolic dysfunction (EF ≤ 35%), in sinus rhythm and symptomatic despite OMT, in order to reduce morbidity and mortality	
	• QRS duration ≥150 ms and LBBB QRS	Recommended (**I A**)
	• QRS duration 130–149 ms and LBBB QRS	Recommended (**I B**)
	• QRS duration ≥150 and non-LBBB QRS	Recommended (**IIa B**)
	• QRS duration 130–149 ms	Recommended (**IIb B**)
IABP or VA-ECMO	– Refractory acute HF or cardiogenic shock, with a short-term MCS, depending on patient age, comorbidities, and neurological function	Recommended (**IIb C**)
MitraClip	– HF patients with moderate to severe secondary FMR, inoperable or at high surgical risk, in order to improve symptoms and quality of life	Recommended (**IIb C**)
LVAD	– Patients with LV systolic dysfunction (LVEF ≤ 35%), end-stage HF despite OMT/device and eligible for HT, in order to improve symptoms and reduce the HF hospitalization and premature death (bridge to transplant)	Recommended (**IIa C**)
	– Patients with LV systolic dysfunction (LVEF ≤ 35%), end-stage HF despite OMT/device and not eligible for HT, in order to improve symptoms and reduce the HF hospitalization and premature death	Recommended (**IIa B**)
HT	– Patients with LV systolic dysfunction (LVEF ≤ 35%), end-stage HF despite OMT in the absence of contraindications, in order to increase survival, exercise capacity, and quality of life	Recommended

SCD sudden cardiac death, *ESC* European Society of Cardiology, *AHA* American Heart Association, *ACC* American College of Cardiology, *LV* left ventricle, *HF* heart failure, *ACEi* angiotensin-converting enzyme inhibitor, *ARB* angiotensin II type I receptor blockers, *MRA* mineralocorticoid/aldosterone receptor antagonists, *EF* ejection fraction, *ICD* implantable cardioverter-defibrillator, *CRT* cardiac resynchronization therapy, *FMR* functional mitral regurgitation, *IABP* intra-aortic balloon pump, *VA-ECMO* venoarterial extracorporeal membrane oxygenation, *LVAD* implantable left ventricular assist device, *HT* heart transplantation

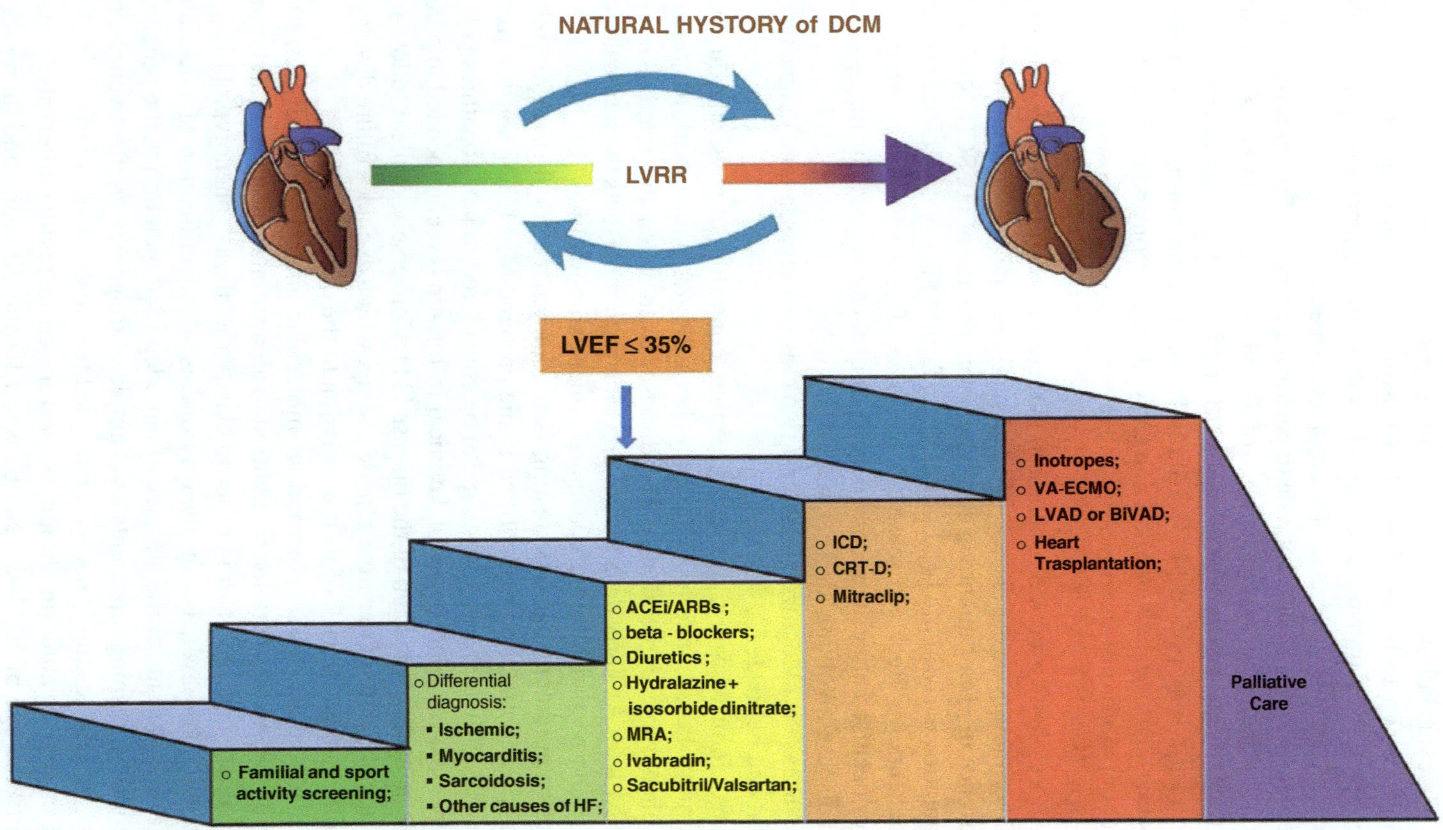

Fig. 13.1 Management and escalation therapy for HF in DCM. *ACEi* angiotensin-converting enzyme inhibitor, *ARB* angiotensin II type I receptor blockers, *MRA* mineralocorticoid/aldosterone receptor antagonists, *ICD* implantable cardioverter defibrillator, *CRT* cardiac resynchronization therapy, *VA-ECMO* veno-arterial extracorporeal membrane oxygenation, *LVAD* implantable left ventricular assist device, *BiVAD* biventricular assist device

13.1 Familial Screening Program

Contrary to what was believed in the past, in the broad spectrum of DCM, 20–50% forms are now known to be familial [1]. Autosomal dominant inheritance is the most frequent pattern of transmission, with less than 50% chance of inheriting the disease for each pregnancy because of incomplete penetrance [2].

These elements represent the rationale to perform a complete family screening in order to identify preclinic manifestations of DCM among relatives, taking into account that DCM has a progressive course [3] and family members can remain asymptomatic for a long period [4–7]. Familial screening program, recommended to proband's first-degree relatives, allows an early identification and treatment of the disease, reducing morbidity and mortality and preventing the high costs of advanced HF management [8].

Family history of at least three generations is recommended in order to recognize the potential heritability of the disease [9]. The pedigree analysis should investigate family occurrence of HF of unknown etiology before the age of 60, SCD, and pacemaker implantation early in life [4]. Furthermore, family history of skeletal myopathies (as Duchenne or Becker disease) or presence of sensorineural hearing loss (congenital or occurred after the second decade of life) can suggest the diagnosis of a syndromic disease involving also the heart.

When the disease is recognized in at least two close relatives, a final diagnosis of familial DCM can be made [3, 4, 10].

In addition to family history, periodic screening, consisting of physical examination and instrumental evaluation (ECG and echocardiogram), can mark the transition to the phenotypic expression of the disease, even when the relative is yet asymptomatic [4, 6]. An early detection of this transition represents the rationale for familial screening proposed by European and American guidelines [11, 12].

According to guidelines, genetic testing is recommended for first-degree relatives when a specific mutation is identified in the proband [4, 11, 13], starting from the age of 10–12, although earlier testing can be considered in laminopathies [11].

In genotype-positive relatives, annual clinical follow-up is recommended in order to recognized an early expression of the disease [11]. Conversely, clinical follow-up is not required in the case of negative genetic testing, which excludes future development of the disease and the risk of its transmission to the offspring [11].

In case of proband's death, postmortem molecular analyses can be useful to detect the disease-causing mutation in addition to an accurate histological and morphological evaluation of the heart in order to clarify the disease phenotype [14].

Genetic testing, however, is not always conclusive: identification of uncertain significant genetic variants or the absence of any identified mutation in the proband on extensive gene screening represents an example of diagnostic ineffectiveness. In these settings, genetic testing is not recommended for close relatives [15].

Repeated cardiac evaluation should be performed at regular intervals: every 1–3 years until the age of 10, 1–2 years between 10 and 20 years, and then every 2–5 years until the age of 50–60, when the penetrance of DCM is usually complete [11].

When a relative is diagnosed as a new case of DCM, even if asymptomatic, the clinical work-up described for the proband starts, including additional tests, such as cardiopulmonary exercise and/or cardiac magnetic resonance imaging (MRI) [11].

13.2 Sport Activity Screening Program

SCD has been associated to competitive sport activity in the adolescents and young adult athletes [16, 17], with an increased risk compared with nonathletic counterparts [18]. Specific cardiomyopathies have been recognized as leading causes of sport-related cardiac arrest such as hypertrophic cardiomyopathy in the USA and arrhythmogenic right ventricular cardiomyopathy in Italy [18, 19].

DCM has been also taken into account as a possible cause of SCD: in international records 1–8% of fatalities of cardiovascular origin have been related to DCM [18–20]. In this context, clinical evaluation of athletes has the important goal of identifying the disease when asymptomatic and protecting them from SCD by sport competition restriction and specific treatment.

American Heart Association/American College of Cardiology (AHA/ACC) and European Society of Cardiology (ESC) recommendations agree that cardiovascular screening for young athletes is justifiable and compelling on ethical, legal, and medical grounds [21, 22], but the two societies propose different screening programs.

The AHA/ACC focuses screening only on physical examination and medical history with consequent cost restriction and reduction of false-positive ECG [22]. On the other hand, ESC and International Olympic Committee recommend also to perform a resting 12-lead ECG [21, 23], in order to detect abnormalities connected to preclinical pathological cardiovascular conditions that cannot be identified by the only clinical approach [21, 23, 24].

The most frequent ECG abnormal findings always requiring further assessment to exclude the presence of a cardiomyopathy are the following:

- T-wave inversion in lateral, infero-lateral, or extended to anterior leads
- ST-segment depression
- Pathologic Q waves
- Complete left bundle branch block (LBBB)
- Multiple premature ventricular beats

When pathological findings emerge, the initial evaluation requires additional tests [18, 21], as recommended by the ESC section of *Sports Cardiology*, based itself on the Italian protocol [21]: echocardiography, stress testing, Holter ECG monitoring, and eventually cardiac MRI in selected cases [24, 25].

In some cases, differential diagnosis between DCM and athlete's heart may be challenging. Indeed, athlete's heart is a clinical phenotype derived from cardiac remodeling induced by sport activity, mostly in endurance sports, and is characterized by enlarging left ventricle with borderline or mildly reduced left ventricular ejection fraction (LVEF) (i.e., between 45 and 55%) [26]. There are many hints helping to distinguish DCM from athlete's heart [25]:

- Positive family history of SCD, cardiac arrest, or cardiac disease
- ECG abnormalities
- Ventricular arrhythmias at 24-h Holter ECG monitoring or stress testing
- LVEF below 45% and regional wall motion abnormalities
- Right ventricular dysfunction associated with LV dysfunction
- Late gadolinium enhancement (LGE) at cardiac MRI

In doubt or borderline cases, demonstrating a significant increase in LVEF during exercise echocardiography or LVEF and diameter normalization at cardiac MRI after an adequate period of detraining may support the diagnosis of athlete's heart [27]. Sport screening benefits go beyond the detection of DCM in the single athlete: when the disease is recognized, a cardiological evaluation can be extended to the first-degree relatives in order to identify other potential affected family members [18].

Athletes recognized to be affected by DCM should not participate in competitive sports because of an increased risk of SCD during exercise [21]. Finally, there are no sufficient evidences supporting that sport activity increases the risk of DCM development or SCD in genotype-positive/phenotype-negative athletes [25].

13.3 Medical Treatment

DCM is a common cause of HF and treatment reflects the management of chronic HF. DCM patients, indeed, can be divided into two different classes on the base of the presence of clinical symptoms:

- Asymptomatic left ventricular systolic dysfunction: in patients with depressed LV systolic function in the absence of symptoms, onset of HF should be delayed or prevented primarily by controlling hypertension [28] and, when the LVEF is ≤40%, by initiating angiotensin-converting enzyme inhibitor (ACEi) therapy [29] prior to beta-blocker therapy, since the evidences supporting ACEi therapy are stronger [30].
- Symptomatic HF with reduced ejection fraction: patients of this category should all be treated. The goals of therapy are to reduce mortality and morbidity; improve symptoms, quality of life, and functional status and decrease hospitalization rate [31].

Pharmacologic and device therapy should be primarily accompanied by the management of contributing factors of HF and by lifestyle modification. For instance, hypertension and ischemic heart disease can impair cardiac function and exacerbate HF clinical symptoms; therefore, they should be considered and treated in DCM patients [12]. The main lifestyle recommendations are sodium and fluid restriction, abstinence from alcohol intake, and adequate body weight loss [31].

For patients with symptomatic HF, a new therapeutic algorithm has been proposed by the current European guidelines [31]. Neurohormonal antagonists, ACEi or angiotensin II type I receptor blockers (ARB) in case of ACEi intolerance, are recommended from the beginning in association with beta-blocker. The addition of mineralocorticoid receptor antagonists (MRA) should be considered in patients still symptomatic with an optimized dosage of ACEi and beta-blocker. ACEi [29, 32, 33], ARB [34, 35], beta-blocker [36–38], and MRA [39, 40] have demonstrated, in several clinical trials, to reduce risk of HF hospitalization and death in patient with HF and reduced EF.

More recently, two new molecules have been included to the recommended pharmacological therapy: an angiotensin receptor-neprilysin inhibitor (ARNI) and the hyperpolarization channel blocker ivabradine [31]. In particular, Sacubitril/Valsartan, tested in PARADIGM trial, is recommended for patients on optimal medical therapy, tolerating ACEi or ARB, but still in II–III NYHA class [31, 41]. Ivabradine is indicated for patients in sinus rhythm that continue to have a resting heart rate over 70 bpm even on beta-blocker therapy based on SHIFT trial [31, 42]. Both these two drugs have shown to improve survival and reduce hospitalization in patients with HF [41, 42].

Diuretic therapy is intended to reduce symptoms and signs of congestion, but no clinical trial could demonstrate any effect on morbidity and mortality [31].

Finally, in case of intolerance or contraindication to ACEi or ARB, combination of hydralazine and isosorbide dinitrate (not approved in Italy) in symptomatic patients with HF and reduced LVEF has demonstrated to reduce mortality [43]. The same association, combined with conventional HF therapy, in NYHA class III–IV black patients, can reduce mortality and HF hospitalizations [44].

Cardioactive pharmacological drugs should be adjusted and up-titrated every 2 weeks to the maximally tolerated doses that should be achieved within 3–6 months from initial diagnosis of HF [45]. During follow-up, frequent reassessment of the clinical status, biohumoral parameters, and ventricular function should be performed in order to achieve therapeutic decision about possible defibrillator or biventricular pacing implantation [31].

13.4 Ventricular and Supraventricular Arrhythmias

Ventricular and supraventricular arrhythmias often coexist with DCM and HF. The treatment of atrial fibrillation (AF) can substantially alter long-term outcomes in patients with heart failure, but the subject of what is the most effective management strategy is debated. Rhythm control with antiarrhythmic drugs is not superior to rate control in patients with coexisting HF and AF [46]. Catheter ablation is a well-established option for symptomatic atrial fibrillation that is resistant to drug therapy in patients with otherwise normal cardiac function, and various studies have shown that ablation is associated with positive outcomes in patients with heart failure [47]. A recent study showed that catheter ablation for AF in patients with HF was associated with a significantly lower rate of a composite end point of death from any cause or hospitalization for worsening heart failure than was medical therapy [48].

Finally, a common feature of DCM regardless of the underlying cause is a propensity to ventricular arrhythmias, being expression of disease's end stage or an intrinsic characteristic of the disease, often connected to particular genotype (i.e., laminopathies). Therapy for ventricular arrhythmias is also needed for recurrent arrhythmias that cause symptoms, most commonly recurrent ICD shocks. Amiodarone is the preferred major antiarrhythmic agent, particularly when ventricular function is severely depressed. In patients with compensated heart failure, sotalol is an option. For patients with recurrent sustained monomorphic ventricular tachycardia (VT), catheter ablation is a therapeutic option to consider, but experience is limited in comparison with that for VTs that occur in patients with coronary artery disease. Success rates depend on VT substrate location, which can be endocardial, intramural, or epicardial. Endocardial VTs can be generally ablated, whereas an epicardial approach is necessary in one-third of cases, but it is associated with higher complication rates. However, sustained monomorphic VT that triggers frequent ICD shocks or electrical storms can be controlled with ablation and adjunctive antiarrhythmic medications in the majority of cases. Experienced centers performing catheter ablation in patients with nonischemic cardiomyopathy have reported that complete absence of inducible VT can be achieved in 38–67% of patients [49].

13.5 Implantable Cardioverter-Defibrillator

Prophylactic implantation of an ICD is a class I recommendation for patients with nonischemic dilated cardiomyopathy (NIDCM), symptomatic HF with NYHA class II–III, and an LVEF $\leq$ 35% [31]. However, the evidence for a benefit is stronger for patients with ischemic heart disease than it is for patients with other HF etiologies. Among patients with NIDCM, these indications are based on two randomized trials, the DEFINITE and SCD-HeFT trial, performed in the 2000s, which showed a trend toward a reduction of mortality in the ICD arm [50–52]. Accordingly, the current recommendation is based on analysis of subgroup of NIDCM patients of minor trials or on meta-analysis of smaller studies with NIDCM patients [51].

The recent DANISH trial [53] casts a shadow on this strong recommendation: 1156 patients with severe nonischemic LV systolic impairment were randomly assigned to receive an ICD on top of medical therapy or medical therapy alone and followed for a median of 5.6 years. In both ICD and control arms, 58% of the patients received cardiac resynchronization therapy (CRT). Although ICD was associated with a risk of SCD that was half that associated with conventional therapy, mortality from any cause was similar in the ICD and control groups (HR 0.87; 95% CI 0.68–1.12), as well as in patients with CRT-defibrillator (CRT-D) and CRT-pacemaker (CRT-P) ($p = 0.59$), leaving unclear whether patients eligible for CRT should routinely receive an ICD. These results, probably due to lower rates of events in NIDCM than ischemic patients and the comprehensive medical therapy plus CRT of study population, urge the search for other predictors of sudden death over LVEF, in order to identify the patient who can best benefit from ICD, potentially reducing device-related adverse events in those who will not experience appropriate ICD interventions. Other noninvasive markers of arrhythmic risk may help to improve the appropriateness of ICD implantation: fibrosis identification by late gadolinium enhancement in cardiac MRI seems the most promising risk predictor [54].

13.6 Cardiac Resynchronization Therapy

Approximately 30% of patients with HF and LV systolic function impairment have a wide QRS complex on the surface electrocardiogram [55], and cumulative mortality increases proportionally with QRS duration [56]. Left bundle branch block (LBBB), associated itself with increased mortality, determines ventricular dyssynchrony as the final result of transmural functional line of block located between the LV septum and the lateral wall with a prolonged activation time [57]. Use of biventricular pacing had been proposed in pharmacological refractory HF patients with intraventricular conduction delay to optimize cardiac performance, through epicardial and then transvenous electrodes. Since then, many trials have demonstrated that CRT, in appropriately selected patients, reduces mortality and morbidity [58] and improves systolic function, symptoms, and quality of life [59, 60].

The effect of CRT, compared to optimized medical therapy, was evaluated by two trials. The COMPANION study demonstrated for the first time a better outcome in patients implanted with CRT plus a defibrillator with advanced HF and a QRS interval > 120 ms than those under pharmacological therapy alone [61]: in the subgroup analyses, hazard ratios for death from any cause of CRT-D as compared with pharmacologic therapy were 0.50 (95% CI, 0.29–0.88) in NIDCM. In the CARE-HF study, CRT reduced all-cause mortality, and the survival benefit with CRT-D over an implantable ICD was consistent in a subgroup analysis of patients with ischemic and nonischemic DCM [62].

Patients enrolled in CRT trials had severe LV systolic dysfunction: most patients had a LVEF < 35%, but other, as MADIT-CRT [59] or RAFT [63], considered LVEF < 30%. Only few patients with an LVEF of 35–40% have been randomized.

As a result, CRT is indicated, according to ESC guidelines [31], as class I recommendation for patients in sinus rhythm, with LBBB, a QRS longer than 130 ms, and LVEF of 35% or less. Evidences are weaker for non-LBBB intraventricular conduction delay and QRS < 150 ms. CRT is contraindicated when QRS is not prolonged: a recent study demonstrated that in patients with systolic HF and a QRS duration < 130 ms, CRT may increase mortality and has no effect on the rate of death or hospitalization for HF [64].

Reverse remodeling is one of the most important mechanisms of action of CRT, but not all patients respond successfully: patients with nonischemic etiology have greater improvement in LV function and decrease in NYHA class after CRT [65]. Data from MADIT-CRT were used to identify factors associated with positive response: female sex, nonischemic etiology, QRS ≥ 150 ms, LBBB, prior HF hospitalization, baseline LVEDV < 125 mL/m^2, and LAVI (left atrial volume index) < 40 mL/m^2 were associated with favorable reverse modeling after CRT implantation [66].

Choice between CRT-P and CRT-D may be hard in selected patients, since most of them with LVEF ≤ 35% have an indication for a concomitant ICD. There are no prospective data proving a benefit of CRT-D over CRT-P, and the only randomized trial to compare CRT-P and CRT-D failed to demonstrate a difference in morbidity or mortality between these strategies [61]. Observational and retrospective studies show that older patients (age ≥ 75 years), particularly if without dilated LV and with nonischemic etiology, and pacemaker-dependent patients are less likely to benefit from CRT-D compared with CRT-P [67, 68].

13.7 Advanced Heart Failure, Mechanical Circulatory Support, Functional Mitral Regurgitation Correction, Heart Transplantation, and Palliative Care

Use of optimal medical therapy, cardiac resynchronization, and implantable defibrillators has changed HF prognosis dramatically. However, 0.5–5% of patients respond poorly to recommended therapy and can develop severe chronic advanced HF with a wide scenario going from refractory deterioration up to cardiogenic shock [69].

Mechanical circulatory support (MCS) devices can be used in critically ill HF patients who can't be stabilized by medical therapy alone. Their goals are to unload the failing ventricle and maintain an adequate end-organ perfusion. Acute and chronic settings require different types of MCS, with short- or mid-/long-term action.

Short-term MCS (few days to weeks) are the systems of choice in patients with acute HF or cardiogenic shock: they include intra-aortic balloon pump and venoarterial extracorporeal membrane oxygenation. They permit to stabilize hemodynamics and gain time for recovery or reevaluation for the possibility of either a more durable MCS or heart transplant.

In a more chronic setting, functional mitral regurgitation (FMR) is a common finding in patients with DCM and left ventricular impairment and is associated with a poor prognosis [70]. In recent years percutaneous correction of mitral regurgitation with the MitraClip system has been established as an alternative treatment option for surgically high-risk patients with degenerative and FMR [71]. Worldwide experience reports high procedural success rates and favorable clinical outcomes in patients with systolic HF and FMR [71, 72]. Patient selection is a crucial issue to obtain the best benefit for patients. A recent report showed that anteroposterior diameter of the mitral annulus and LV end-diastolic volume were significantly associated with device failure during follow-up, and the assessment of these two parameters might be particularly useful for the selection of the optimal candidates to percutaneous treatment of FMR [73].

Heart transplantation (HT) is a well-recognized treatment that significantly increases quality of life and survival for eligible patients with advanced HF, severe symptoms, poor prognosis, and no remaining alternative choices [74]. Unfortunately suitable donor availability is extremely limited. In these cases, implantable left ventricular assist device (LVAD) technology has improved considerably in the last years. This MCS, historically used only for short periods as bridge-to-transplantation, nowadays is being used increasingly also as a permanent treatment or "destination therapy" [75]. In this scenario, right ventricular (RV) assessment is crucial considering RV failure to occur in up to 50% of cases following LVAD implantation and resulting in high perioperative mortality and morbidity rates [76–78]. An important contribution to evaluation for candidacy to LVAD was the introduction of the INTERMACS classification, which categorizes patients for the purpose of risk assessment prior to LVAD implant or HT [79], ranging from 1 (cardiogenic shock) to 7 (advanced NYHA III), and describes patient's clinical status in terms of hemodynamic stability, inotrope dependence, and functional capacity. Since outcomes in INTERMACS 3 (stable on inotropes) are better than in class I–II, this class has been advocated as the optimal group for implantation. However, the choice remains tough for clinicians, since patients can experience adverse events and complications in up to 60% of cases by 6 months postimplantation, including bleeding, thromboembolic events, infections, and right ventricle failure [80].

Advanced ages, multiple comorbidities, and poorly controlled symptoms characterize the HF terminal stage. In this setting, symptoms management and emotional support of the patients and their family are the principal components of palliative care in advanced HF, in order to improve quality of life [31]. Currently, no consensus has been reached in international guidelines about the right time to start palliative care because of the absence of end-of-life objective criteria. However, the decisions should be always taken by physicians according to the patient and the family.

References

1. Hershberger RE, Cowan J, Morales A, Siegfried JD. Progress with genetic cardiomyopathies: screening, counseling, and testing in dilated, hypertrophic, and arrhythmogenic right ventricular dysplasia/cardiomyopathy. Circ Heart Fail. 2009;2(3):253–61. https://doi.org/10.1161/CIRCHEARTFAILURE.108.817346.
2. Mestroni L, Brun F, Spezzacatene A, Sinagra G, Taylor MR. Genetic causes of dilated cardiomyopathy. Prog Pediatr Cardiol. 2014;37(1–2):13–8.
3. Sisakian H. Cardiomyopathies: evolution of pathogenesis concepts and potential for new therapies. World J Cardiol. 2014;6(6):478. https://doi.org/10.4330/wjc.v6.i6.478.
4. Burkett EL, Hershberger RE. Clinical and genetic issues in familial dilated cardiomyopathy. J Am Coll Cardiol. 2005;45(7):969–81.
5. Mahon NG, Murphy RT, MacRae CA, Caforio ALP, Elliott PM, McKenna WJ. Echocardiographic evaluation in asymptomatic relatives of patients with dilated cardiomyopathy reveals preclinical disease. Ann Intern Med. 2005;143(2):108–15.
6. Crispell KA, Hanson EL, Coates K, Toy W, Hershberger RE. Periodic rescreening is indicated for family members at risk of developing familial dilated cardiomyopathy. J Am Coll Cardiol. 2002;39(9):1503–7.
7. Hershberger RE, Lindenfeld J, Mestroni L, Seidman CE, Taylor MRG, Towbin JA, et al. Genetic evaluation of cardiomyopathy—a Heart Failure Society of America practice guideline. J Card Fail. 2009;15(2):83–97. https://doi.org/10.1016/j.cardfail.2009.01.006.
8. Hershberger RE, Morales A. Dilated cardiomyopathy overview. GeneReviews®. Seattle: University of Washington; 1993.

9. Ackerman MJ, Priori SG, Willems S, Berul C, Brugada R, Calkins H, et al. HRS/EHRA expert consensus statement on the state of genetic testing for the channelopathies and cardiomyopathies: this document was developed as a partnership between the Heart Rhythm Society (HRS) and the European Heart Rhythm Association (EHRA). Heart Rhythm. 2011;8(8):1308–39. https://doi.org/10.1016/j.hrthm.2011.05.020.
10. Hershberger RE, Siegfried JD. Update 2011: clinical and genetic issues in familial dilated cardiomyopathy. J Am Coll Cardiol. 2011;57(16):1641–9. https://doi.org/10.1016/j.jacc.2011.01.015.
11. Charron P, Arad M, Arbustini E, Basso C, Bilinska Z, Elliott P, et al. Genetic counselling and testing in cardiomyopathies: a position statement of the European Society of Cardiology Working Group on Myocardial and Pericardial Diseases. Eur Heart J. 2010;31(22):2715–28. https://doi.org/10.1093/eurheartj/ehq271.
12. Yancy CW, Jessup M, Bozkurt B, Butler J, Casey DE, Drazner MH, et al. 2013 ACCF/AHA guideline for the management of heart failure: a report of the American College of Cardiology Foundation/American Heart Association Task Force on practice guidelines. J Am Coll Cardiol. 2013;62(16):e147–239. https://doi.org/10.1016/j.jacc.2013.05.019.
13. van Spaendonck-Zwarts KY, van den Berg MP, van Tintelen JP. DNA analysis in inherited cardiomyopathies: current status and clinical relevance. Pacing Clin Electrophysiol. 2008;31(Suppl 1):S46–9. https://doi.org/10.1111/j.1540-8159.2008.00956.x.
14. Basso C, Burke M, Fornes P, Gallagher PJ, de Gouveia RH, Sheppard M, et al. Guidelines for autopsy investigation of sudden cardiac death. Virchows Arch. 2008;452(1):11–8.
15. Wolf MJ, Noeth D, Rammohan C, Shah SH. Complexities of genetic testing in familial dilated cardiomyopathy. Circ Cardiovasc Genet. 2016;9(1):95–9. https://doi.org/10.1161/CIRCGENETICS.115.001157.
16. Corrado D, Thiene G, Nava A, Rossi L, Pennelli N. Sudden death in young competitive athletes: clinicopathologic correlations in 22 cases. Am J Med. 1990;89(5):588–96.
17. Maron BJ, Shirani J, Poliac LC, Mathenge R, Roberts WC, Mueller FO. Sudden death in young competitive athletes. JAMA. 1996;276(3):199.
18. Corrado D, Basso C, Rizzoli G, Schiavon M, Thiene G. Does sports activity enhance the risk of sudden death in adolescents and young adults? J Am Coll Cardiol. 2003;42(11):1959–63.
19. Maron BJ, Doerer JJ, Haas TS, Tierney DM, Mueller FO. Sudden deaths in young competitive athletes: analysis of 1866 deaths in the United States, 1980–2006. Circulation. 2009;119(8):1085–92. https://doi.org/10.1161/CIRCULATIONAHA.108.804617.
20. Harmon KG, Drezner JA, Maleszewski JJ, Lopez-Anderson M, Owens D, Prutkin JM, et al. Pathogeneses of sudden cardiac death in National Collegiate Athletic Association Athletes. Circ Arrhythm Electrophysiol. 2014;7(2):198–204. https://doi.org/10.1161/CIRCEP.113.001376.
21. Corrado D, Pelliccia A, Bjørnstad HH, Vanhees L, Biffi A, Borjesson M, et al. Cardiovascular pre-participation screening of young competitive athletes for prevention of sudden death: proposal for a common European protocol. Consensus statement of the study Group of Sport Cardiology of the Working Group of Cardiac Rehabilitation and Exercise Physiology and the Working Group of Myocardial and Pericardial Diseases of the European Society of Cardiology. Eur Heart J. 2005;26(5):516–24.
22. Maron BJ, Thompson PD, Ackerman MJ, Balady G, Berger S, Cohen D, et al. Recommendations and considerations related to preparticipation screening for cardiovascular abnormalities in competitive athletes: 2007 update: a scientific statement from the American Heart Association Council on Nutrition, Physical Activity, and Metabolism: endorsed by the American College of Cardiology Foundation. Circulation. 2007;115(12):1643–455.
23. Pelliccia A, Fagard R, Bjørnstad HH, Anastassakis A, Arbustini E, Assanelli D, et al. Recommendations for competitive sports participation in athletes with cardiovascular disease: a consensus document from the Study Group of Sports Cardiology of the Working Group of Cardiac Rehabilitation and Exercise Physiology and the Working Group of Myocardial and Pericardial Diseases of the European Society of Cardiology. Eur Heart J. 2005;26(14):1422–45.

24. Corrado D, Schmied C, Basso C, Borjesson M, Schiavon M, Pelliccia A, et al. Risk of sports: do we need a pre-participation screening for competitive and leisure athletes? Eur Heart J. 2011;32(8):934–44. https://doi.org/10.1093/eurheartj/ehq482.
25. Zorzi A, Pelliccia A, Corrado D. Inherited cardiomyopathies and sports participation. Neth Heart J. 2018;26(3):154–65. https://doi.org/10.1007/s12471-018-1079-3.
26. Baggish AL, Wood MJ. Athlete's heart and cardiovascular care of the athlete: scientific and clinical update. Circulation. 2011;123(23):2723–35. https://doi.org/10.1161/CIRCULATIONAHA.110.981571.
27. Galderisi M, Cardim N, D'Andrea A, Bruder O, Cosyns B, Davin L, et al. The multi-modality cardiac imaging approach to the athlete's heart: an expert consensus of the European Association of Cardiovascular Imaging. Eur Hear J Cardiovasc Imaging. 2015;16(4):353–353r.
28. Wright JT Jr, Williamson JD, Whelton PK, Snyder JK, Sink KM, Rocco MV, et al. A randomized trial of intensive versus standard blood-pressure control. N Engl J Med. 2017; 377(25):2506.
29. Yusuf S, Pitt B, Davis CE, Hood WB, Cohn JN. Effect of enalapril on survival in patients with reduced left ventricular ejection fractions and congestive heart failure. N Engl J Med. 1991;325(5):293–302.
30. Exner DV, Dries DL, Waclawiw MA, Shelton B, Domanski MJ. Beta-adrenergic blocking agent use and mortality in patients with asymptomatic and symptomatic left ventricular systolic dysfunction: a post hoc analysis of the studies of left ventricular dysfunction. J Am Coll Cardiol. 1999;33(4):916–23.
31. Ponikowski P, Voors AA, Anker SD, Bueno H, Cleland JGF, Coats AJS, et al. 2016 ESC guidelines for the diagnosis and treatment of acute and chronic heart failure: the task force for the diagnosis and treatment of acute and chronic heart failure of the European Society of Cardiology (ESC) developed with the special contribution of the Heart Failure Association (HFA) of the ESC. Eur Heart J. 2016;37(27):2129–200. https://doi.org/10.1093/eurheartj/ehw128.
32. CONSENSUS Trial Study Group. Effects of enalapril on mortality in severe congestive heart failure. N Engl J Med. 1987;316(23):1429–35.
33. Wollert KC, Studer R, von Bülow B, Drexler H, Horowitz JD, Massie BM, et al. Survival after myocardial infarction in the rat. Role of tissue angiotensin-converting enzyme inhibition. Circulation. 1994;90(5):2457–67.
34. Young JB, Dunlap ME, Pfeffer MA, Probstfield JL, Cohen-Solal A, Dietz R, et al. Mortality and morbidity reduction with candesartan in patients with chronic heart failure and left ventricular systolic dysfunction: results of the CHARM low-left ventricular ejection fraction trials. Circulation. 2004;110(17):2618–26.
35. Cohn JN, Tognoni G. A randomized trial of the angiotensin-receptor blocker valsartan in chronic heart failure. N Engl J Med. 2001;345(23):1667–75.
36. CIBIS-II Investigators and Committees. The cardiac insufficiency bisoprolol study II (CIBIS-II): a randomised trial. Lancet. 1999;353(9146):9–13.
37. Packer M, Fowler MB, Roecker EB, Coats AJS, Katus HA, Krum H, et al. Effect of carvedilol on the morbidity of patients with severe chronic heart failure: results of the carvedilol prospective randomized cumulative survival (COPERNICUS) study. Circulation. 2002;106(17):2194–9.
38. Hjalmarson A, Goldstein S, Fagerberg B, Wedel H, Waagstein F, Kjekshus J, et al. Effects of controlled-release metoprolol on total mortality, hospitalizations, and well-being in patients with heart failure: the metoprolol CR/XL randomized intervention trial in congestive heart failure (MERIT-HF). MERIT-HF Study Group. JAMA. 2000;283(10):1295–302.
39. Pitt B, Zannad F, Remme WJ, Cody R, Castaigne A, Perez A, et al. The effect of spironolactone on morbidity and mortality in patients with severe heart failure. N Engl J Med. 1999;341(10):709–17.
40. Zannad F, McMurray JJV, Krum H, van Veldhuisen DJ, Swedberg K, Shi H, et al. Eplerenone in patients with systolic heart failure and mild symptoms. N Engl J Med. 2011;364(1):11–21. https://doi.org/10.1056/NEJMoa1009492.

41. McMurray JJV, Packer M, Desai AS, Gong J, Lefkowitz MP, Rizkala AR, et al. Angiotensin–neprilysin inhibition versus enalapril in heart failure. N Engl J Med. 2014;371(11):993–1004. https://doi.org/10.1056/NEJMoa1409077.
42. Swedberg K, Komajda M, Böhm M, Borer JS, Ford I, Dubost-Brama A, et al. Ivabradine and outcomes in chronic heart failure (SHIFT): a randomised placebo-controlled study. Lancet. 2010;376(9744):875–85. https://doi.org/10.1016/S0140-6736(10)61198-1.
43. Cohn JN, Archibald DG, Ziesche S, Franciosa JA, Harston WE, Tristani FE, et al. Effect of vasodilator therapy on mortality in chronic congestive heart failure. N Engl J Med. 1986;314(24):1547–52.
44. Taylor AL, Ziesche S, Yancy C, Carson P, D'Agostino R, Ferdinand K, et al. Combination of isosorbide dinitrate and hydralazine in blacks with heart failure. N Engl J Med. 2004;351(20):2049–57.
45. Yancy CW, Januzzi JL, Allen LA, Butler J, Davis LL, Fonarow GC, et al. 2017 ACC expert consensus decision pathway for optimization of heart failure treatment: answers to 10 pivotal issues about heart failure with reduced ejection fraction. J Am Coll Cardiol. 2018;71(2):201–30. https://doi.org/10.1016/j.jacc.2017.11.025.
46. Roy D, Talajic M, Nattel S, Wyse DG, Dorian P, Lee KL, et al. Rhythm control versus rate control for atrial fibrillation and heart failure. N Engl J Med. 2008;358(25):2667–77. https://doi.org/10.1056/NEJMoa0708789.
47. Khan MN, Jaïs P, Cummings J, Di Biase L, Sanders P, Martin DO, et al. Pulmonary-vein isolation for atrial fibrillation in patients with heart failure. N Engl J Med. 2008;359(17):1778–85. https://doi.org/10.1056/NEJMoa0708234.
48. Marrouche NF, Brachmann J, Andresen D, Siebels J, Boersma L, Jordaens L, et al. Catheter ablation for atrial fibrillation with heart failure. N Engl J Med. 2018;378(5):417–27. https://doi.org/10.1056/NEJMoa1707855.
49. Dinov B, Fiedler L, Schönbauer R, Bollmann A, Rolf S, Piorkowski C, et al. Outcomes in catheter ablation of ventricular tachycardia in dilated nonischemic cardiomyopathy compared with ischemic cardiomyopathy: results from the prospective heart Centre of Leipzig VT (HELP-VT) study. Circulation. 2014;129(7):728–36. https://doi.org/10.1161/CIRCULATIONAHA.113.003063.
50. Priori SG, Blomström-Lundqvist C, Mazzanti A, Blom N, Borggrefe M, Camm J, et al. 2015 ESC guidelines for the management of patients with ventricular arrhythmias and the prevention of sudden cardiac death: the task force for the management of patients with ventricular arrhythmias and the prevention of sudden cardiac death of the European Society of Cardiology (ESC). Eur Heart J. 2015;36(41):2793–867. https://doi.org/10.1093/eurheartj/ehv316.
51. Kadish A, Dyer A, Daubert JP, Quigg R, Estes NAM, Anderson KP, et al. Prophylactic defibrillator implantation in patients with nonischemic dilated cardiomyopathy. N Engl J Med. 2004;350:2151–8.
52. Bardy GH, Lee KL, Mark DB, Poole JE, Packer DL, Boineau R, et al. Amiodarone or an implantable cardioverter–defibrillator for congestive heart failure. N Engl J Med. 2005;352(21):225–37.
53. Kober L, Thune JJ, Nielsen JC, Haarbo J, Videbaek L, Korup E, et al. Defibrillator implantation in patients with nonischemic systolic heart failure. N Engl J Med. 2016;375(13):1221–30. https://doi.org/10.1056/NEJMoa1608029.
54. Di Marco A, Anguera I, Schmitt M, Klem I, Neilan T, White JA, et al. Late gadolinium enhancement and the risk for ventricular arrhythmias or sudden death in dilated cardiomyopathy: systematic review and meta-analysis. JACC Heart Fail. 2017;5(1):28–38. https://doi.org/10.1016/j.jchf.2016.09.017.
55. Khan NK, Goode KM, Cleland JGF, Rigby AS, Freemantle N, Eastaugh J, et al. Prevalence of ECG abnormalities in an international survey of patients with suspected or confirmed heart failure at death or discharge. Eur J Heart Fail. 2007;9(5):491–501.
56. Iuliano S, Fisher SG, Karasik PE, Fletcher RD, Singh SN. Department of Veterans Affairs Survival Trial of antiarrhythmic therapy in congestive heart failure. QRS duration and mortality in patients with congestive heart failure. Am Heart J. 2002;143(6):1085–91.

57. Auricchio A, Fantoni C, Regoli F, Carbucicchio C, Goette A, Geller C, et al. Characterization of left ventricular activation in patients with heart failure and left bundle-branch block. Circulation. 2004;109(9):1133–9.
58. Cleland JG, Abraham WT, Linde C, Gold MR, Young JB, Claude Daubert J, et al. An individual patient meta-analysis of five randomized trials assessing the effects of cardiac resynchronization therapy on morbidity and mortality in patients with symptomatic heart failure. Eur Heart J. 2013;34(46):3547–56. https://doi.org/10.1093/eurheartj/eht290.
59. Moss AJ, Hall WJ, Cannom DS, Klein H, Brown MW, Daubert JP, et al. Cardiac-resynchronization therapy for the prevention of heart-failure events. N Engl J Med. 2009;361(14):1329–38. https://doi.org/10.1056/NEJMoa0906431.
60. Cleland JGF, Calvert MJ, Verboven Y, Freemantle N. Effects of cardiac resynchronization therapy on long-term quality of life: an analysis from the CArdiac Resynchronisation-Heart Failure (CARE-HF) study. Am Heart J. 2009;157(3):457–66. https://doi.org/10.1016/j.ahj.2008.11.006.
61. Bristow MR, Saxon LA, Boehmer J, Krueger S, Kass DA, De Marco T, et al. Cardiac-resynchronization therapy with or without an implantable defibrillator in advanced chronic heart failure. N Engl J Med. 2004;350(21):2140–50.
62. Cleland JGF, Daubert J-C, Erdmann E, Freemantle N, Gras D, Kappenberger L, et al. The effect of cardiac resynchronization on morbidity and mortality in heart failure. N Engl J Med. 2005;352(15):1539–49.
63. Tang ASL, Wells GA, Talajic M, Arnold MO, Sheldon R, Connolly S, et al. Cardiac-resynchronization therapy for mild-to-moderate heart failure. N Engl J Med. 2010;363(25):2385–95. https://doi.org/10.1056/NEJMoa1009540.
64. Ruschitzka F, Abraham WT, Singh JP, Bax JJ, Borer JS, Brugada J, et al. Cardiac-resynchronization therapy in heart failure with a narrow QRS complex. N Engl J Med. 2013;369(15):1395–405. https://doi.org/10.1056/NEJMoa1306687.
65. Gasparini M, Mantica M, Galimberti P, Genovese L, Pini D, Faletra F, et al. Is the outcome of cardiac resynchronization therapy related to the underlying etiology? Pacing Clin Electrophysiol. 2003;26(1 Pt 2):175–80.
66. Goldenberg I, Moss AJ, Hall WJ, Foster E, Goldberger JJ, Santucci P, et al. Predictors of response to cardiac resynchronization therapy in the multicenter automatic defibrillator implantation trial with cardiac resynchronization therapy (MADIT-CRT). Circulation. 2011;124(14):1527–36. https://doi.org/10.1161/CIRCULATIONAHA.110.014324.
67. Morani G, Gasparini M, Zanon F, Casali E, Spotti A, Reggiani A, et al. Cardiac resynchronization therapy-defibrillator improves long-term survival compared with cardiac resynchronization therapy-pacemaker in patients with a class IA indication for cardiac resynchronization therapy: data from the Contak Italian Registry. Europace. 2013;15(9):1273–9. https://doi.org/10.1093/europace/eut032.
68. Looi K-L, Gajendragadkar PR, Khan FZ, Elsik M, Begley DA, Fynn SP, et al. Cardiac resynchronisation therapy: pacemaker versus internal cardioverter-defibrillator in patients with impaired left ventricular function. Heart. 2014;100(10):794–9. https://doi.org/10.1136/heartjnl-2014-305537.
69. Lloyd-Jones D, Adams RJ, Brown TM, Carnethon M, Dai S, De Simone G, et al. Executive summary: heart disease and stroke statistics—2010 update: a report from the American Heart Association. Circulation. 2010;121(7):948–54. https://doi.org/10.1161/CIRCULATIONAHA.109.192666.
70. Stolfo D, Merlo M, Pinamonti B, Poli S, Gigli M, Barbati G, et al. Early improvement of functional mitral regurgitation in patients with idiopathic dilated cardiomyopathy. Am J Cardiol. 2015;115(8):1137–43. https://doi.org/10.1016/j.amjcard.2015.01.549.
71. Franzen O, van der Heyden J, Baldus S, Schlüter M, Schillinger W, Butter C, et al. MitraClip® therapy in patients with end-stage systolic heart failure. Eur J Heart Fail. 2011;13(5):569–76. https://doi.org/10.1093/eurjhf/hfr029.
72. Auricchio A, Schillinger W, Meyer S, Maisano F, Hoffmann R, Ussia GP, et al. Correction of mitral regurgitation in nonresponders to cardiac resynchronization therapy by MitraClip

improves symptoms and promotes reverse remodeling. J Am Coll Cardiol. 2011;58(21):2183–9. https://doi.org/10.1016/j.jacc.2011.06.061.

73. Berardini A, Biagini E, Saia F, Stolfo D, Previtali M, Grigioni F, et al. Percutaneous mitral valve repair: the last chance for symptoms improvement in advanced refractory chronic heart failure? Int J Cardiol. 2017;228:191–7. https://doi.org/10.1016/j.ijcard.2016.11.241.
74. Mehra MR, Canter CE, Hannan MM, Semigran MJ, Uber PA, Baran DA, et al. The 2016 International Society for Heart Lung Transplantation listing criteria for heart transplantation: a 10-year update. J Heart Lung Transplant. 2016;35(1):1–23. https://doi.org/10.1016/j.healun.2015.10.023.
75. Rose EA, Gelijns AC, Moskowitz AJ, Heitjan DF, Stevenson LW, Dembitsky W, et al. Long-term use of a left ventricular assist device for end-stage heart failure. N Engl J Med. 2001;345(20):1435–43.
76. Lietz K, Long JW, Kfoury AG, Slaughter MS, Silver MA, Milano CA, et al. Outcomes of left ventricular assist device implantation as destination therapy in the post-REMATCH era: implications for patient selection. Circulation. 2007;116(5):497–505.
77. Matthews JC, Koelling TM, Pagani FD, Aaronson KD. The right ventricular failure risk score. J Am Coll Cardiol. 2008;51(22):2163–72. https://doi.org/10.1016/j.jacc.2008.03.009.
78. Ochiai Y, McCarthy PM, Smedira NG, Banbury MK, Navia JL, Feng J, et al. Predictors of severe right ventricular failure after implantable left ventricular assist device insertion: analysis of 245 patients. Circulation. 2002;106(12 Suppl 1):I198–202.
79. Stevenson LW, Pagani FD, Young JB, Jessup M, Miller L, Kormos RL, et al. INTERMACS profiles of advanced heart failure: the current picture. J Heart Lung Transplant. 2009;28(6):535–41. https://doi.org/10.1016/j.healun.2009.02.015.
80. Kilic A, Acker MA, Atluri P. Dealing with surgical left ventricular assist device complications. J Thorac Dis. 2015;7(12):2158–64. https://doi.org/10.3978/j.issn.2072-1439.2015.10.64.

14

Unresolved Issues and Future Perspectives

Marco Merlo, Giulia De Angelis, Antonio Cannatà, Laura Massa, and Gianfranco Sinagra

Abbreviations and Acronyms

ARVC	Arrhythmogenic right ventricular cardiomyopathy
CMR	Cardiac magnetic resonance
DCM	Dilated cardiomyopathy
DMD	Dystrophin
ECG	Electrocardiogram
FLNC	Filamin C
HCM	Hypertrophic cardiomyopathy
ICD	Implantable cardioverter-defibrillator
LAEF	Left atrial emptying fraction
LGE	Late gadolinium enhancement
LMNA	Lamin A/C
LVEF	Left ventricular ejection fraction
NYHA	New York Heart Association
OMT	Optimal medical therapy
PLN	Phospholamban
RBM20	RNA-binding motif protein 20
RCM	Restrictive cardiomyopathy
RNA	Ribonucleic acid
SCD	Sudden cardiac death
TNNT2	Troponin T2
TTN	Titin

M. Merlo (✉) · G. Sinagra
Cardiovascular Department, Azienda Sanitaria Universitaria Integrata, Trieste, Italy
e-mail: gianfranco.sinagra@asuits.sanita.fvg.it

G. De Angelis · A. Cannatà · L. Massa
Cardiovascular Department, Azienda Sanitaria Universitaria Integrata, University of Trieste (ASUITS), Trieste, Italy
e-mail: laura.massa@asuits.sanita.fvg.it

14.1 Toward a Personalized Medicine: A Genetic Approach

One of the major challenges in nonischemic Dilated Cardiomyopathy (DCM) is the complex and heterogeneous etiology of the disease [1].

Indeed, DCM is the final common pathway of different pathogenic processes, and distinguishing between this complex etiological diversity is emerging as a useful tool to a better prognostic stratification and a targeted therapy.

It has already been shown that post-myocarditis DCM could have a better prognosis compared to the idiopathic form [2]. Moreover, it is well known that secondary forms show reversibility after removing the trigger factors [3–5]. More undefined is the prognostic relevance of certain gene mutations in the setting of genetically determined DCM.

Over the years, there has been increasing evidence that DCM is a familial or genetic disease in a consistent proportion of cases. In this setting, the mere morpho-functional classification doesn't allow proper risk stratification, and the important information on the causal gene gets lost as well as the cascade familial genetic screening.

The relatively recent proposal of a new classification that integrates phenotype description and genetic information at the same level moves in this direction [6]. At the same time when genetic testing is becoming part of a routine, its role in decision-making is still very limited.

The cascade genetic familial screening remains the most direct consequence of a positive genetic test, in order to obtain an early diagnosis in relatives, as this facilitates prompt prophylactic therapy in early or preclinical disease with a subsequent improved clinical outcome [7].

Relatives without the mutation can be discharged, although the complex interaction between environmental factors and predisposing gene variants and the possible coexistence of multiple mutations in developing the dilated phenotype make it impossible to exclude at all a pathogenic evolution, even in the absence of the causal pathogenic mutation. On the contrary, mutation carriers deserve more frequent clinical surveillance. Given the incomplete penetrance of such mutations, the early identification of pathogenic predictors represents an intriguing issue to be deeper investigated.

In the past years, left ventricular enlargement in the absence of systolic dysfunction emerged as a possible predictor of progression to overt DCM in asymptomatic relatives [8].

More recently, modern imaging techniques, such as speckle tracking echocardiography, are getting ahead in the hazy area of preclinical diagnosis [9]. Interesting data on their capacity to identify subtle abnormalities in contractile function need to be improved with larger numbers and should be extended to cardiac magnetic resonance (CMR) feature tracking analysis.

A flash-forward to the future of personalized medicine could be the understanding of a precise genotype-phenotype correlation. Actually, many efforts of the clinical research are moving in this direction. The implications in terms of early diagnosis, prognostic stratification, and targeted therapy would be revolutionary.

Lamin A/C (*LMNA*) mutations represent the example on how the identification of a specific mutation can change the routine management, by gaining a class IIa indication for ICD implantation in the presence of certain additional risk factors, regardless of left ventricular dysfunction severity [10].

The same gene is targeted by a new molecule, ARRY-797, which showed promising results in a phase II clinical trial. The small molecule is an inhibitor of the p38-MAPK pathway, which appears to be upregulated in *LMNA*-deficient mouse.

Other attempts to identify a genotype-phenotype correlation have been made riding the wave of *LMNA*, leading to interesting results.

For example, rare sarcomeric gene variants could harbor a poor long-term prognosis [11], while cytoskeleton Z-disk mutations demonstrate a lower rate of left ventricular reverse remodeling after optimized medical therapy [12].

Filling the gap of knowledge in this area requires many other efforts. The interpretation of the results of genetic testing is often hard, given the high prevalence of private mutations. To generate a response, it's necessary to assess the possible pathogenicity, based on structure-function models and evidence of interspecies conservation [13].

The pathogenic role of several mutations is still not well characterized. For example, some *titin* (*TTN*) missense variants could have a potential pathogenic role, suggested by their nonrandom distribution in affected members [14].

Moreover, little is known about the role of modifier genes and environmental interaction on the development of an overt phenotype. A recent study highlighted a shared genetic predisposition in women with peripartum cardiomyopathy compared with patients with idiopathic dilated cardiomyopathy, suggesting that different insults could unmask the same dilative phenotype in patients with similar genetic background [15]. It is also probable that a genetic predisposition favors the development of a dilative phenotype in the presence of different trigger factors, such as inflammation, toxic insults from alcohol [16] or drugs, and tachycardia. Furthermore, the association of two or more potentially pathogenic factors has been associated with worse prognosis [17].

The complexity of mutational status in DCM is made more difficult by the absence of co-segregation of modifier genes. Variance component analysis may help to identify the relative impact of genetic and environmental factors. This technique allows a comparison of phenotypic variability within and between families carrying the same primary mutation [18].

Adding complexity to this context, the majority of genes responsible for DCM are not specific, but show a significant overlap with hypertrophic (HCM), restrictive (RCM), arrhythmogenic right ventricular cardiomyopathy (ARVC), and channelopathies [19]. Moreover, the distinctive phenotype of DCM (left ventricular dilation and dysfunction) can frequently overlap with other distinctive traits of different cardiomyopathies (Fig. 14.1). It is intriguing how the same mutation in the gene coding for troponin T (TNNT2) has shown variable phenotypic expression ranging from DCM to HCM and RCM within the same family [20]. Many genes are associated with arrhythmic tendency and are reviewed in the next paragraph.

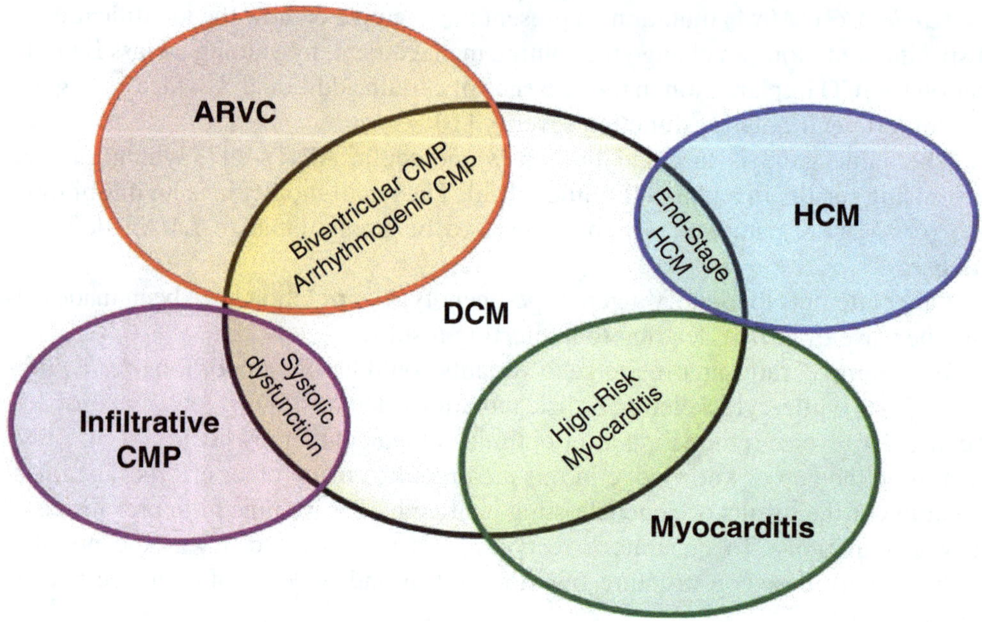

Fig. 14.1 Overlap phenotypes between DCM and other cardiomyopathies. *ARVC* arrhythmogenic right ventricular cardiomyopathy, *CMP* cardiomyopathy, *DCM* dilated cardiomyopathy, *HCM* hypertrophic cardiomyopathy

Summing up, genetics currently represents one of the most important fields of increasing knowledge in order to further improve the outcomes of DCM. Early diagnosis, the complexity of genotype-phenotype interaction, the pathogenic role of certain mutations, and the interplay with environmental factors all represent unresolved issues to be better understood for improving care.

14.2 The Challenge of Arrhythmic Stratification

To date, another important open issue is the arrhythmic stratification, in order to carefully identify patients who are most likely to die from arrhythmia and could benefit from an implantable cardioverter-defibrillator (ICD), mostly in the first phases after diagnosis.

Mortality in DCM results typically from pump failure or sudden cardiac death (SCD). The latter occurs out of hospital in the majority of patients and could be prevented by an appropriate ICD intervention [21].

ICD implantation for primary prevention is recommended in patients with DCM, New York Heart Association (NYHA) classes II–III, and a left ventricular ejection fraction (LVEF) ≤ 35% despite optimized medical therapy [22].

The capacity of this device to interrupt malignant arrhythmias, thus preventing death, is unquestionable. However, its role in preventing overall mortality in nonischemic DCM is still debated, given the negative results of many trials in the past years [23–25] and only one demonstrating benefit in both ischemic and nonischemic populations [26].

The recent publication of the DANISH trial has once again raised this issue [27]. While overall mortality was similar in both study groups, younger patients had a clear benefit from ICD implantation, resulting in reduction of overall mortality, other than SCD. The lower prevalence of comorbidities and competing causes of death in this population could explain this outcome.

This result would encourage the development of a new decisional algorithm for ICD implantation, in order to guarantee greater quality-adjusted life years and prevent futile inappropriate shocks and complications, such as device infections (respectively, 4.9% and 5.9% over 5.6 years in DANISH trial). It is well demonstrated in fact the negative prognostic impact of inappropriate ICD implantation [28].

The novel approach should at first make a negative selection, excluding patients with high mortality risk from competing causes. Several models have been developed to predict non-sudden mortality, based on clinical parameters [29] and serum biomarkers [30], claiming for a multiparametric algorithm that possibly combines clinical data, biomarker quantification, CMR evaluation, and genetic testing to predict the risk of death from pump failure rather than from malignant arrhythmia.

Once this negative selection has been made, patients at higher risk for SCD should be identified. By now, the only validated parameter is LVEF, being its relationship with the extent of myocardial lesion, and thus the arrhythmogenic risk, the physiopathological rationale.

Nonetheless, as discussed above, the selection of patients with nonischemic DCM based on this parameter has shown poor specificity and low incidence of appropriate therapies.

Useful information comes from a basic clinical approach. Easily collectable data, such as unexplained syncope, Holter ECG monitoring showing rapid nonsustained ventricular tachycardia, and frequent premature ventricular contraction and couplets, have been related to a higher incidence of SCD and malignant arrhythmias, even in the absence of overt heart failure. When combined with a family history of major arrhythmias or SCD, the risk was increased [31].

Integrating clinical data with the aforementioned genetic testing could increase the capacity to identify at-risk patients. Beyond the widely known *LMNA* mutations, other mutations have been related to arrhythmic phenotypes. Future-focused research should be developed, but some preliminary results are already available.

Truncating *filamin C* (*FLNC*) mutations have been associated with an overlapping phenotype of dilated and left-dominant arrhythmogenic cardiomyopathies, complicated by frequent premature SCD [32]. The same arrhythmic tendency has been shown in carriers of *TNNT2* [33], *phospholamban* (*PLN*) [34], *RNA-binding motif protein 20* (*RBM20*) [35], *TTN* [36], and desmosomal mutations. Together, these data suggest that, in the future, genotypes other than *LMNA* could benefit from an early ICD implantation independently from LVEF reduction.

Conversely, *dystrophin* (*DMD*) mutations have been related to a DCM phenotype more susceptible to heart failure than arrhythmic events. This mutation could identify patients whose treatment could be directed toward advanced heart failure therapies rather than protection from SCD.

A helpful prognostic tool could come from imaging techniques. Global longitudinal strain (GLS), assessed by means of echocardiography, could be a useful tool to evaluate arrhythmic risk in DCM patients, by identifying those with mechanical dispersion, which show higher arrhythmic propensity [37]. More recently, CMR strain imaging was shown to predict outcome in a nonischemic DCM population independently from validated parameters such as NYHA class and LVEF, but more studies are needed to clarify its role also in the setting of SCD.

Actually, CMR represents the most promising tool in assessing arrhythmic risk. The presence of late gadolinium enhancement (LGE), a marker of fibrosis, has been shown in approximately 30% of DCM patients [38]. Its presence and, less certainly, its extent have been related to a higher risk of SCD and aborted SCD, identifying a subgroup of patients at high risk of arrhythmic events independently from LVEF [39].

LGE is now widely assessed during follow-up of DCM patients, although its use as a marker of arrhythmogenicity has not yet been mentioned in clinical guidelines. But its robust correlation with SCD makes it the most suitable tool to be incorporated into combined models of prediction.

Less clear is the possible association between interstitial fibrosis, assessed by T1-mapping, and SCD. An association between T1 values and overall mortality has been shown, as well as with major arrhythmic endpoints [40].

Right ventricular systolic dysfunction at diagnosis and during follow-up appears as a powerful and independent predictor of mortality outcome in large series, although its role in favoring SCD itself is still not clarified [41, 42].

Finally, recent reports identified left atrial emptying fraction (LAEF), assessed by CMR, as an independent predictor of appropriate device therapy in patients with ischemic and dilated cardiomyopathy, who had an ICD in primary prevention [43].

Parameters of electrical instability, such as T-wave alternans or fragmented QRS at ECG, could improve models of prediction, but yet no single index of electrical instability was more accurate than LVEF in predicting arrhythmic events, although some showed high negative predictive value [44].

The same importance as the selection of patients is the correct timing of ICD implantation.

Only one third of patients with DCM, satisfying criteria for ICD implantation, maintain their eligibility after 3–9 months of OMT (optimal medical therapy) [45], making it mandatory a waiting period of at least 3 months of OMT. This period is very important, because inappropriate ICD implantation has not only an economic impact on public healthcare system but is also associated with higher in-hospital death and post-procedural complication rate [28].

Importantly, a non-negligible proportion of patients could die in the first 6 months, during therapy titration. These patients should be carefully identified, because they could benefit from an early ICD implantation or from a wearable cardioverter-defibrillator. Higher left ventricular end-systolic indexed volumes, longer QRS, and intolerance to beta-blockers have been shown to characterize this high-risk population [46], but further studies are needed to integrate these parameters into a validated, universally accepted multiparametric model. The role of wearable cardioverter-defibrillators in this setting is still debated, and registry studies failed to demonstrate a clear benefit of this bridge solution in nonischemic DCM [47]. Properly selected higher-risk patients should be evaluated into a randomized controlled trial, in order to obtain more robust data.

Periodic reassessment of arrhythmic risk should also be performed, as DCM is a dynamic condition, with the possibility of exacerbation also after many years of stability. Moreover, the predictors of arrhythmogenicity may change at subsequent evaluations. Surprisingly, impaired LVEF was associated with worse arrhythmic outcome only in the long term, while best early predictors were, respectively, QRS duration, mitral regurgitation, and disease duration at baseline and NYHA functional class III or IV, syncope, disease duration, and left ventricular end-diastolic volume at 12-month evaluation [48].

In conclusion, the current guidelines show poor capacity to identify nonischemic DCM patients likely to benefit from primary prevention ICD implantation.

The way forward needs the identification of parameters, which should be incorporated together into a multiparametric and dynamic model, which permit an early identification of higher-risk patients and a periodic risk reassessment.

To pursue this objective, different approaches should be combined, ranging from clinical data, genetics, standard and modern imaging techniques, to electrophysiological data.

14.3 Toward Innovation in Therapy

Mortality rates in patients with DCM have significantly decreased over years. The basis of this success lies in the sequential introduction of drugs and the appropriate use of device therapy, which contributed to the decline of both cardiovascular and SCD risk [49].

The major leap came with the use of angiotensin-converting enzyme inhibitors, promptly followed by beta-blockers and mineralocorticoid-receptor antagonists. Despite the efficacy of these therapies, the spectrum of drugs used in heart failure due to DCM still remains very limited.

The recent introduction of the angiotensin receptor-neprilysin inhibitor sacubitril/valsartan raises the possibility for a further improvement of prognosis in DCM [50].

Nevertheless, all the currently approved drugs act on the common physiopathological mechanisms of heart failure. A big improvement would come from the development of therapies more specifically focused on DCM itself and its underlying mechanisms.

In this setting, the stimulation of the endogenous regenerative capacity of the myocardium and its replacement by new cells or tissue are promising paths to be further investigated.

The myocardium has poor intrinsic regenerative capacity, although resident cardiac progenitor cells have been shown to persist in adult mammalian hearts.

Given the role of paracrine signaling pathways in myocardial repair, a promising approach comes from the development of exosomes, whose effect has been investigated in several preclinical studies, targeted by now to the regeneration after myocardial infarction [51].

A similar mechanism of action is shared by autologous and allogenic mesenchymal stem cells derived from bone marrow and myocardial biopsies.

The capacity of these cells to promote angiogenesis, mitigate inflammation and apoptotic cell death, and reduce myocardial fibrosis represents a good opportunity for their use in DCM.

In this sense, the demonstration of feasibility and safety of their transendocardial injection in 37 patients with nonischemic DCM is encouraging and should promote future research [52]. A caveat remains the risk of sensitization against donor cell-specific HLA that could hamper a future heart transplantation.

Likewise, in animal studies, gene therapy showed potential beneficial effects in the setting of nonischemic heart failure [53].

Last but not least, the small RNA-based therapeutics, hanging on the evidence of a pivotal role of microRNAs in the postnatal cardiomyocyte proliferation in animal models, represents a potential targeted therapy for myocardial regeneration [54].

Hence there are still many open issues to be deeper investigated by translational research in the way of understanding the mechanisms and developing targeted therapies in the field of DCM.

In conclusion, the very next future of DCM management should go through the better understanding of the etiology of the disease, the correct risk stratification, and the development of new therapies (Table 14.1). The rapidly increasing knowledge should be combined into an interconnected network with the purpose of a multiparametric evaluation of the disease.

Table 14.1 Unresolved issues and future perspectives in arrhythmic stratification of idiopathic dilated cardiomyopathy

Unresolved issues and future perspectives in arrhythmic risk stratification		
Critical issue	What is known	Future directions
Proper risk stratification	Primary prevention ICD: Is recommended in NYHA class II–III DCM patients with LVEF ≤ 35% despite OMT, with survival expectancy >1 year Should be considered in DCM patients with LMNA mutation and clinical risk factors (NSVT during ambulatory ECG monitoring, LVEF < 45% at first evaluation, male sex, non-missense mutations)	Creation of a multiparametric score, which encompasses: Clinical data (syncope; NSVT; family history) Search for proarrhythmic mutations (LMNA; FLNC, etc.) Functional imaging parameters (GLS; LAEF) Structural imaging parameters (LGE; T1 mapping) Parameters of electrical instability (T-wave alternans, fragmented QRS)
Proper timing of implantation	ICD should be implanted in primary prevention only after at least 3 months of OMT	Identification of higher-risk patients who could benefit from early ICD implantation (higher LVESVi; larger QRS; intolerance to beta-blockers) Defining a role for wearable cardioverter-defibrillators
Periodic reassessment of arrhythmic risk	Currently, no time-dependent parameters are known	Creation of a dynamic score, with different predictors at subsequent evaluations

DCM dilated cardiomyopathy, *FLNC* filamin, *GLS* global longitudinal strain, *ICD* implantable cardioverter-defibrillator, *LAEF* left atrial emptying fraction, *LGE* late gadolinium enhancement, *LMNA* lamin, *LVEF* left ventricular ejection fraction, *LVESVi* left ventricular end-systolic volume indexed, *NYHA* New York Heart Association, *NSVT* nonsustained ventricular tachycardia, *OMT* optimized medical therapy

References

1. Elliott P, Andersson B, Arbustini E, Bilinska Z, Cecchi F, Charron P, et al. Classification of the cardiomyopathies: a position statement from the European Society of Cardiology Working Group on Myocardial and Pericardial Diseases. Eur Heart J. 2008;29:270–6.
2. Merlo M, Anzini M, Bussani R, Artico J, Barbati G, Stolfo D, et al. Characterization and long-term prognosis of postmyocarditic dilated cardiomyopathy compared with idiopathic dilated cardiomyopathy. Am J Cardiol. 2016;118:895–900.
3. Brembilla-Perrot B, Ferreira JP, Manenti V, Sellal JM, Olivier A, Villemin T, et al. Predictors and prognostic significance of tachycardiomyopathy: insights from a cohort of 1269 patients undergoing atrial flutter ablation. Eur J Heart Fail. 2016;18:394–401.
4. Cooper LT, Mather PJ, Alexis JD, Pauly DF, Torre-Amione G, Wittstein IS, et al. Myocardial recovery in peripartum cardiomyopathy: prospective comparison with recent onset cardiomyopathy in men and nonperipartum women. J Card Fail. 2012;18:28–33.
5. Guzzo-Merello G, Segovia J, Dominguez F, Cobo-Marcos M, Gomez-Bueno M, Avellana P, et al. Natural history and prognostic factors in alcoholic cardiomyopathy. JACC Heart Fail. 2015;3:78–86.
6. Arbustini E, Narula N, Tavazzi L, Serio A, Grasso M, Favalli V, et al. The MOGE(S) classification of cardiomyopathy for clinicians. J Am Coll Cardiol. 2014;64:304–18.
7. Moretti M, Merlo M, Barbati G, Di Lenarda A, Brun F, Pinamonti B, et al. Prognostic impact of familial screening in dilated cardiomyopathy. Eur J Heart Fail. 2010;12:922–7.
8. Fatkin D, Yeoh T, Hayward CS, Benson V, Sheu A, Richmond Z, et al. Evaluation of left ventricular enlargement as a marker of early disease in familial dilated cardiomyopathy. Circ Cardiovasc Genet. 2011;4:342–8.
9. Lakdawala NK, Thune JJ, Colan SD, Cirino AL, Farrohi F, Rivero J, et al. Subtle abnormalities in contractile function are an early manifestation of sarcomere mutations in dilated cardiomyopathy. Circ Cardiovasc Genet. 2012;5:503–10.
10. Priori SG, Blomström-Lundqvist C, Mazzanti A. 2015 ESC guidelines for the management of patients with ventricular arrhythmias and the prevention of sudden cardiac death. Eur Heart J. 2015;8:746–837.
11. Merlo M, Sinagra G, Carniel E, Slavov D, Zhu X, Barbati G, et al. Poor prognosis of rare sarcomeric gene variants in patients with dilated cardiomyopathy. Clin Transl Sci. 2013;6:424–8.
12. Dal Ferro M, Stolfo D, Altinier A, Gigli M, Perrieri M, Ramani F, et al. Association between mutation status and left ventricular reverse remodelling in dilated cardiomyopathy. Heart. 2017;103:1704–10.
13. Jacoby D, McKenna WJ. Genetics of inherited cardiomyopathy. Eur Heart J. 2012;33:296–304.
14. Begay RL, Graw S, Sinagra G, Merlo M, Slavov D, Gowan K, et al. Role of titin missense variants in dilated cardiomyopathy. J Am Heart Assoc. 2015;4(11).
15. Ware JS, Li J, Mazaika E, Yasso CM, DeSouza T, Cappola TP, et al. Shared genetic predisposition in peripartum and dilated cardiomyopathies. N Engl J Med. 2016;374:233–41.
16. Ware JS, Amor-Salamanca A, Tayal U, Govind R, Serrano I, Pascual-figal DA, et al. Genetic etiology for alcohol-induced cardiac toxicity. J Am Coll Cardiol. 2018;71:2293–302.
17. Hazebroek MR, Moors S, Dennert R, van den Wijngaard A, Krapels I, Hoos M, et al. Prognostic relevance of gene-environment interactions in patients with dilated cardiomyopathy: applying the MOGE(S) classification. J Am Coll Cardiol. 2015;66:1313–23.
18. Sen-Chowdhry S, Syrris P, Pantazis A, Quarta G, McKenna WJ, Chambers JC. Mutational heterogeneity, modifier genes, and environmental influences contribute to phenotypic diversity of arrhythmogenic cardiomyopathy. Circ Cardiovasc Genet. 2010;3:323–30.
19. Hershberger RE, Hedges DJ, Morales A. Dilated cardiomyopathy: the complexity of a diverse genetic architecture. Nat Rev Cardiol. 2013;10:531–47.
20. Menon SC, Michels VV, Pellikka PA, Ballew JD, Karst ML, Herron KJ, et al. Cardiac troponin T mutation in familial cardiomyopathy with variable remodeling and restrictive physiology. Clin Genet. 2008;74:445–54.
21. Halliday BP, Cleland JGF, Goldberger JJ, Prasad SK. Personalizing risk stratification for sudden death in dilated cardiomyopathy. Circulation. 2017;136:215–31.

22. Ponikowski P, Voors AA, Anker SD, Bueno H, Cleland JGF, Coats AJS, et al. 2016 ESC guidelines for the diagnosis and treatment of acute and chronic heart failure. Eur Heart J. 2016;37:2129–2200m.
23. Bansch D. Primary prevention of sudden cardiac death in idiopathic dilated cardiomyopathy: the cardiomyopathy trial (CAT). Circulation. 2002;105:1453–8.
24. Strickberger SA, Hummel JD, Bartlett TG, Frumin HI, Schuger CD, Beau SL, et al. Amiodarone versus implantable cardioverter-defibrillator: randomized trial in patients with nonischemic dilated cardiomyopathy and asymptomatic nonsustained ventricular tachycardia—AMIOVIRT. J Am Coll Cardiol. 2003;41:1707–12.
25. Kadish A, Dyer A, Daubert JP, Quigg R, Estes NAM, Anderson KP, et al. Prophylactic defibrillator implantation in patients with nonischemic dilated cardiomyopathy for the defibrillators in non-ischemic cardiomyopathy treatment evaluation (DEFINITE) investigators. N Engl J Med. 2004;350:2151–8.
26. Bardy GH, Lee KL, Mark DB, Poole JE, Packer DL, Boineau R, et al. Amiodarone or an implantable cardioverter–defibrillator for congestive heart failure. N Engl J Med. 2005;352:225–37.
27. Køber L, Thune JJ, Nielsen JC, Haarbo J, Videbæk L, Korup E, et al. Defibrillator implantation in patients with nonischemic systolic heart failure. N Engl J Med. 2016;375:1221–30.
28. Al-Khatib SM, Hellkamp A, Curtis J, Mark D, Peterson E, Sanders GD, et al. Non-evidence-based ICD implantations in the United States. JAMA. 2011;305:43–9.
29. Mozaffarian D, Anker SD, Anand I, Linker DT, Sullivan MD, Cleland JGF, et al. Prediction of mode of death in heart failure: the Seattle heart failure model. Circulation. 2007;116:392–8.
30. Zhang Y, Guallar E, Blasco-Colmenares E, Dalal D, Butcher B, Norgard S, et al. Clinical and serum-based markers are associated with death within 1 year of de novo implant in primary prevention ICD recipients. Heart Rhythm. 2015;12:360–6.
31. Spezzacatene A, Sinagra G, Merlo M, Barbati G, Graw SL, Brun F, et al. Arrhythmogenic phenotype in dilated cardiomyopathy: natural history and predictors of life-threatening arrhythmias. J Am Heart Assoc. 2015;4:e002149.
32. Begay RL, Graw SL, Sinagra G, Asimaki A, Rowland TJ, Slavov DB, et al. Filamin C truncation mutations are associated with arrhythmogenic dilated cardiomyopathy and changes in the cell–cell adhesion structures. JACC Clin Electrophysiol. 2018;4:504–14.
33. Fiset C, Giles WR. Cardiac troponin T mutations promote life-threatening arrhythmias. J Clin Invest. 2008;118:3845–7.
34. Van Rijsingen IAW, Van Der Zwaag PA, Groeneweg JA, Nannenberg EA, Jongbloed JDH, Zwinderman AH, et al. Outcome in phospholamban R14del carriers results of a large multicentre cohort study. Circ Cardiovasc Genet. 2014;7:455–65.
35. Refaat MM, Lubitz SA, Makino S, Islam Z, Frangiskakis JM, Mehdi H, et al. Genetic variation in the alternative splicing regulator RBM20 is associated with dilated cardiomyopathy. Heart Rhythm. 2012;9:390–6.
36. Verdonschot JAJ, Hazebroek MR, Derks KWJ, Barandiarán Aizpurua A, Merken JJ, Wang P, et al. Titin cardiomyopathy leads to altered mitochondrial energetics, increased fibrosis and long-term life-threatening arrhythmias. Eur Heart J. 2018;39:864–73.
37. Haugaa KH, Goebel B, Dahlslett T, Meyer K, Jung C, Lauten A, et al. Risk assessment of ventricular arrhythmias in patients with nonischemic dilated cardiomyopathy by strain echocardiography. J Am Soc Echocardiogr. 2012;25:667–73.
38. Gulati A, Jabbour A, Ismail TF, Guha K, Khwaja J, Raza S, et al. Association of fibrosis with mortality and sudden cardiac death in patients with nonischemic dilated cardiomyopathy. JAMA. 2013;309:896–908.
39. Di Marco A, Anguera I, Schmitt M, Klem I, Neilan T, White JA, et al. Late gadolinium enhancement and the risk for ventricular arrhythmias or sudden death in dilated cardiomyopathy: systematic review and meta-analysis. JACC Heart Fail. 2017;5:28–38.
40. Chen Z, Sohal M, Voigt T, Sammut E, Tobon-Gomez C, Child N, et al. Myocardial tissue characterization by cardiac magnetic resonance imaging using T1 mapping predicts ventricular arrhythmia in ischemic and non-ischemic cardiomyopathy patients with implantable cardioverter-defibrillators. Heart Rhythm. 2015;12:792–801.

41. Gulati A, Ismail TF, Jabbour A, Alpendurada F, Guha K, Ismail NA, et al. The prevalence and prognostic significance of right ventricular systolic dysfunction in nonischemic dilated cardiomyopathy. Circulation. 2013;128:1623–33.
42. Merlo M, Gobbo M, Stolfo D, Losurdo P, Ramani F, Barbati G, et al. The prognostic impact of the evolution of RV function in idiopathic DCM. JACC Cardiovasc Imaging. 2016;9:1034–42.
43. Rijnierse MT, Kamali Sadeghian M, Schuurmans Stekhoven S, Biesbroek PS, van der Lingen ALC, van de Ven PM, et al. Usefulness of left atrial emptying fraction to predict ventricular arrhythmias in patients with implantable cardioverter defibrillators. Am J Cardiol. 2017;120:243–50.
44. Goldberger JJ, Subačius H, Patel T, Cunnane R, Kadish AH. Sudden cardiac death risk stratification in patients with nonischemic dilated cardiomyopathy. J Am Coll Cardiol. 2014;63:1879–89.
45. Zecchin M, Merlo M, Pivetta A, Barbati G, Lutman C, Gregori D, et al. How can optimization of medical treatment avoid unnecessary implantable cardioverter-defibrillator implantations in patients with idiopathic dilated cardiomyopathy presenting with "SCD-HeFT criteria?". Am J Cardiol. 2012;109:729–35.
46. Losurdo P, Stolfo D, Merlo M, Barbati G, Gobbo M, Gigli M, et al. Early arrhythmic events in idiopathic dilated cardiomyopathy. JACC Clin Electrophysiol. 2016;2:535–43.
47. Kutyifa V, Moss AJ, Klein H, Biton Y, McNitt S, MacKecknie B, et al. Use of the wearable cardioverter defibrillator in high-risk cardiac patients data from the prospective registry of patients using the wearable cardioverter defibrillator (WEARIT-II registry). Circulation. 2015;132:1613–9.
48. Stolfo D, Ceschia N, Zecchin M, De Luca A, Gobbo M, Barbati G, et al. Arrhythmic risk stratification in patients with idiopathic dilated cardiomyopathy. Am J Cardiol. 2018;121:1601–9.
49. Merlo M, Pivetta A, Pinamonti B, Stolfo D, Zecchin M, Barbati G, et al. Long-term prognostic impact of therapeutic strategies in patients with idiopathic dilated cardiomyopathy: changing mortality over the last 30 years. Eur J Heart Fail. 2014;16:317–24.
50. McMurray JJV, Packer M, Desai AS, Gong J, Lefkowitz MP, Rizkala AR, et al. Angiotensin–neprilysin inhibition versus enalapril in heart failure. N Engl J Med. 2014;371:993–1004.
51. Maring JA, Beez CM, Falk V, Seifert M, Stamm C. Myocardial regeneration via progenitor cell-derived exosomes. Stem Cells Int. 2017;2017:7849851.
52. Hare JM, DiFede DL, Castellanos AM, Florea V, Landin AM, El-Khorazaty J, et al. Randomized comparison of allogeneic vs. autologous mesenchymal stem cells for non-ischemic dilated cardiomyopathy: POSEIDON-DCM trial. J Am Coll Cardiol. 2017;69:526–37.
53. Woitek F, Zentilin L, Hoffman NE, Powers JC, Ottiger I, Parikh S, et al. Intracoronary cytoprotective gene therapy: a study of VEGF-B167 in a pre-clinical animal model of dilated cardiomyopathy. J Am Coll Cardiol. 2015;66:139–53.
54. Giacca M, Zacchigna S. Harnessing the microRNA pathway for cardiac regeneration. J Mol Cell Cardiol. 2015;89(Pt A):68–74.

15

Dilated Cardiomyopathy at the Crossroad: Multidisciplinary Approach

Gianfranco Sinagra, Enrico Fabris, Simona Romani, Francesco Negri, Davide Stolfo, Francesca Brun, and Marco Merlo

Abbreviations and Acronyms

ACEi	Angiotensin converting enzyme inhibitors
BMD	Becker muscular dystrophy
BNP	Brain natriuretic peptide
CK	Creatine kinase
CMR	Cardiac magnetic resonance
CS	Cardiac sarcoidosis
DCM	Dilated cardiomyopathy
DMD	Duchenne muscular dystrophy
ECG	Electrocardiogram
ECG-SA	Signal-averaged electrocardiography
EDMD	Emery-Dreifuss muscular dystrophy
HF	Heart failure
LGMD	Limb-girdle muscular dystrophy
LV	Left ventricular
LVEF	Left ventricular ejection fraction
NYHA	New York Heart Association
SLE	Systemic lupus erythematosus
TTNtv	Truncation variants in the gene encoding titin
VT	Ventricular tachycardia

G. Sinagra · M. Merlo
Cardiovascular Department, Azienda Sanitaria Universitaria Integrata, Trieste, Italy
e-mail: gianfranco.sinagra@asuits.sanita.fvg.it; marco.merlo@asuits.sanita.fvg.it

E. Fabris (✉) · S. Romani · F. Negri · D. Stolfo · F. Brun
Cardiovascular Department, Azienda Sanitaria Universitaria Integrata, University of Trieste (ASUITS), Trieste, Italy
e-mail: davide.stolfo@asuits.sanita.fvg.it; francesca.brun@asuits.sanita.fvg.it

Table 15.1 Clinical "red flags" and potential related DCM subgroup

	Abnormalities	Potential specific DCM subgroup or systemic disease	Laboratory tests suggested
Medical history/ physical examination	Mental retardation	Dystrophinopathies, Mitochondrial diseases, Myotonic dystrophy	Creatine kinase
	Visual impairment	Myotonic dystrophy	Creatine kinase
	Muscle weakness	Desminopathy, Dystrophinopathies, Sarcoglycanopathies, Laminopathies, Myotonic dystrophy	Creatine kinase
	Myotonia	Myotonic dystrophy	Creatine kinase
	Pigmentation of the skin	Hemochromatosis	Serum iron, ferritin, transferrin saturation
	Uveitis; nodular erythema; arthralgias	Sarcoidosis	Serum angiotensin-converting enzyme
	Malar rash, discoid rash, oral ulcers, arthritis, serositis; fibrosis and thickening of the skin	Connective tissue disorder (Systemic lupus erythematosus, scleroderma)	Autoantibody screen, erythrocyte sedimentation rate, proteinuria research
	Chemotherapy exposure (anthracyclines, trastuzumab, etc.)	DCM related to chemotherapeutic agents	Troponin
	History of amphetamines, cocaine intake	DCM related to toxic agents	Urine toxicology screen for cocaine/ amphetamine abuse
	Alcohol abuse	Alcoholic DCM	Liver function Mean corpuscular volume
	Pregnancy	Peripartum-DCM	
Electrocardiography	Atrioventricular block	Myocarditis (Lyme disease, Chagas disease) Sarcoidosis Laminopathy Desminopathy Myotonic dystrophy Emery-Dreifuss 1	Specific serum autoantibodies for suspected infection: Lyme disease, Chagas disease, etc. Serum angiotensin-converting enzyme (sarcoidosis) Creatine kinase
	"Posterolateral infarction" pattern	Dystrophin-related cardiomyopathy, Limb-girdle muscular dystrophy, Sarcoidosis	Creatine kinase, Serum angiotensin-converting enzyme (sarcoidosis)
Echocardiography	Posterolateral akinesia/ dyskinesia	Dystrophin-related cardiomyopathy	Creatine kinase
	Mild dilatation/segment kinetic alterations with non-coronary distribution	Myocarditis, Sarcoidosis	Troponin (myocarditis) Serum angiotensin-converting enzyme (sarcoidosis)

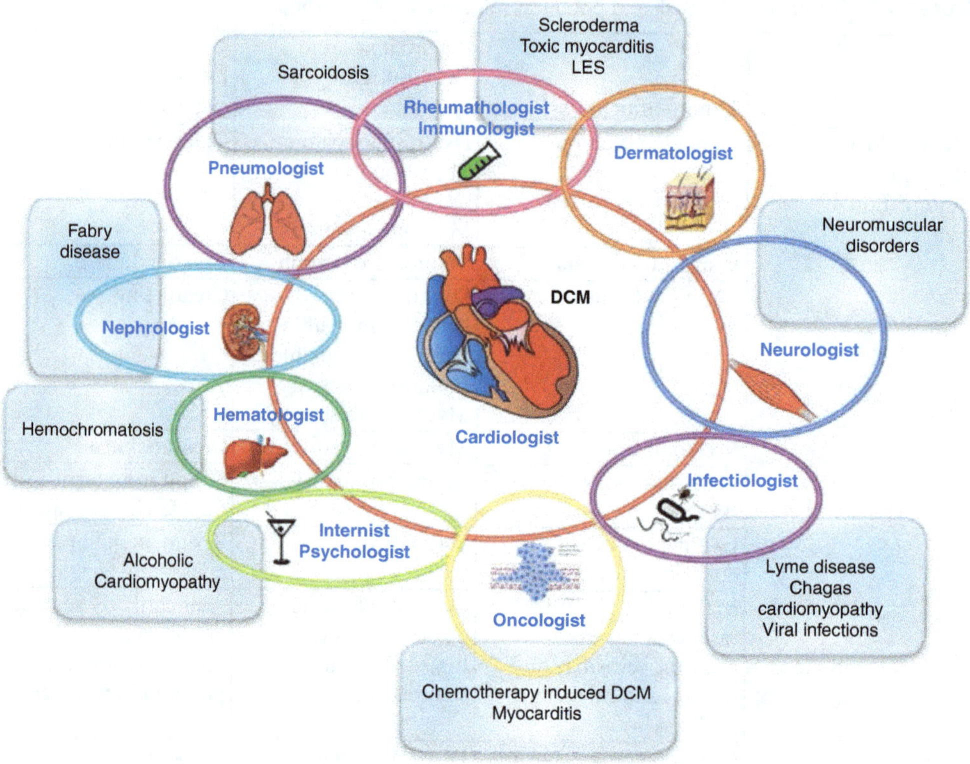

Fig. 15.1 Complex interactions between multiple specialties in the clinical management of DCM

Dilated cardiomyopathy (DCM) constitutes a broad cardiac phenotype that can arise from a multitude of myocardial insults. Rigorous etiological evaluation may allow to identify specific treatments, targeted to the underlying cause [1]. This approach requires clinical acumen (Table 15.1) and a multidisciplinary approach, with close collaboration with other specialists, as represented in Fig. 15.1.

Indeed, evaluation of patients with DCM requires a thorough understanding of potential complex pathophysiology that may be different in each patient [2]. In certain cases, with the elimination of the cause and the appropriate treatment, reversal of myocardial damage and recovery of cardiac dysfunction can occur, and therefore treatment should be individualized and should target the underlying cause, when added to the standard systolic heart failure (HF) therapies.

15.1 Sarcoidosis: Co-working with Pneumologists

Sarcoidosis is a systemic disease, characterized by noncaseating granuloma formation in multiple organ systems. The lung is the most frequently involved organ, and symptomatic patients have usually dry cough and dyspnea. Red flag of the disease is a bilateral lymphadenopathy at chest X-ray that is abnormal in about 90% of patients with pulmonary sarcoidosis [3]. In acute forms the multi-organ involvement suggests the diagnosis (uveitis, nodular erythema, arthralgia, etc.). Clinically manifest cardiac involvement occurs in about 5% of patients with sarcoidosis [4]. The diagnosis of cardiac sarcoidosis (CS) requires appropriate clinical suspicion and the integration of clinical and pathologic data together with the results of advanced cardiac imaging techniques.

See Chap. 4 for diagnosis of sarcoidosis.

15.1.1 Treatment

The management of CS often requires multidisciplinary care teams. Indeed, electrophysiologists, heart failure specialists, imaging experts, pneumologists, and rheumatologists (especially when other organ involvement is present and when "biologic therapy" is required) have to work together to provide optimal patient management. Systemic corticosteroids remain the first-line treatment for sarcoidosis followed, if ineffective, by methotrexate. In patients with ventricular tachycardia (VT), refractory to immunosuppressive therapy, a first-line treatment is with antiarrhythmic drugs; then, if VT still persists, a catheter ablation is indicated (class IIa) [5]. Implantable cardioverter-defibrillator is indicated, over the conventional indication, if a patient with CS (independently of ventricular function) has an indication for permanent pacemaker implantation and presents unexplained syncope or near-syncope and/or inducible sustained ventricular arrhythmias (class IIa) [5]. Many aspects of CS management, however, are not still fully understood, and further studies are needed for a better comprehension of the pathology, adequate risk stratification, treatment, and targeted follow-up.

15.2 Autoimmune Cardiomyopathy: Co-working with Rheumatologists

15.2.1 Systemic Lupus Erythematosus

Autoimmune diseases may be rare causes of cardiomyopathy and heart failure, mediated by several potential mechanisms, including immune-mediated myocarditis, progressive fibrosis, and apoptosis with resultant dilated phenotype.

The association between autoimmune disorders and DCM includes various autoimmune diseases, as the systemic lupus erythematosus (SLE) but also dermatomyositis, scleroderma, rheumatoid arthritis, and polyarteritis nodosa [2].

DCM is not a prominent manifestation of SLE; however myocardial involvement is not uncommon in the disease. At echocardiographic studies about 6% of SLE patients showed global hypokinesia [6], and evidence of myocarditis can be found at postmortem examination in approximately 40% of cases [7]. According to guidelines [8], the diagnosis of SLE can be made by a combination of clinical features and laboratory tests. Immunological tests should be investigated by cardiologists especially in a young woman with unexplained left ventricular dysfunction associated with clinical symptoms suggestive of autoimmune disorder (fatigue, fever, associated with skin, musculoskeletal, and mild hematologic disorders). Among immunological tests, antinuclear antibodies are present in 95% of SLE patients. This test however has a high sensitivity but a low specificity [9].

Cardiovascular manifestations of SLE are heterogeneous and, in addition to pericarditis and less often myocarditis, may include also coronary artery disease, conduction system disease, valvular disease, and pulmonary hypertension in various associations [9]. Particularly, 12-lead ECG abnormalities include non-specific ST-T changes, left ventricular (LV) hypertrophy, and supraventricular/ventricular arrhythmias [10]. Signal-averaged electrocardiography (ECG-SA) is currently used for recording ventricular late potentials which are the expression of slowed and disorganized conduction through zones of myocardial scarring. Left ventricular diastolic dysfunction has been documented both in active and quiescent SLE patients. Active chronic myocarditis can be detected using cardiac magnetic resonance (CMR).

15.2.2 Treatment

Main drugs for disease treatment are corticosteroids and hydroxychloroquine in mild disease; in moderate and severe disease, other immunosuppressive drugs (e.g., methotrexate, cyclosporine, azathioprine, etc.) have to be added [8].

15.3 Infectious Disease and Cardiomyopathy: Co-working with Infectious Disease Specialist

15.3.1 Chagas Cardiomyopathy

Chagas disease is caused by the protozoan parasite *Trypanosoma cruzi*, which is transmitted by large, blood-sucking reduviid bugs of the subfamily Triatominae. This illness was originally confined to poor, rural areas of South and Central America; however in recent years, the disease is also spreading in the USA, Canada, and Europe due to the influx of immigrants from endemic countries [11]. The chronic cardiac involvement manifests as Chagas cardiomyopathy, characterized by a chronic myocarditis that involves all cardiac chambers and damage to the conduction system [12].

The myocardium damage is generally a progressive process that can be classified into stages: those with a normal ECG are considered to have the indeterminate phase of the disease (stage A). The appearance of ECG abnormalities implies disease progression (stage B) and precedes the appearance of symptoms of heart failure (stages C and D) [13]. The most common initial signs are left anterior fascicular block, right bundle branch block, and segmental left ventricular wall motion abnormalities (the segments frequently involved are the infero-lateral wall and the apex). Late manifestations include sinus node dysfunction leading to severe bradycardia, high-degree atrioventricular blocks, non-sustained or sustained ventricular tachycardia, progressive dilated cardiomyopathy with congestive heart failure, apical aneurysms (usually of the left ventricle), and emboli [11].

The diagnosis of chronic infection relies on serological testing, through detection of IgG antibodies against *T. cruzi*. Cardiac involvement should be evaluated through ECG and echocardiography. A direct relationship exists between the number of alterations identified in a single ECG and the severity of myocardial damage. Holter monitoring, exercise stress testing, and cardiac MRI (CMR) should be considered in symptomatic patients [11]. New York Heart Association (NYHA) functional class, left ventricular systolic function, cardiomegaly, and non-sustained ventricular tachycardia have been consistently identified as important prognostic markers [14].

15.3.2 Treatment

The treatment of Chagas cardiomyopathy involves both parasite-specific therapy and adjunctive therapy for the management of heart failure. Treatment with antitrypanosomal drugs, benznidazole or nifurtimox, is generally offered to patients with chronic disease in the indeterminate phase and patients with mild to moderate disease. Sudden death is the main cause of death, followed by refractory heart failure and thromboembolism [11]. Although both amiodarone and implantable cardioverter-defibrillator have been used, data for these patients are scarce.

15.3.3 Lyme Disease

Lyme disease is a spirochetal infection, which is transmitted by the bite of infected *Ixodes* spp. ticks. In most cases, it is caused by *Borrelia burgdorferi*. The disease is diffused especially in wooded areas. Cardiac involvement occurs during the early disseminated phase of the disease. *B. burgdorferi* can affect all layers of the heart, causing a transmural inflammation, with a predominance of macrophage and lymphocytes. Moreover, vasculitis of the small and large intramyocardial vessel can occur [15].

The cardiac manifestations are usually coincident with other symptoms of the disease (erythema, arthritis, or neurologic disease); however, in rare cases, there is an exclusive cardiac involvement. The principal manifestation of Lyme carditis is self-limited alteration of the conduction system and commonly varying degrees of atrioventricular block. Less frequently pericarditis, endocarditis, myocarditis, pericardial effusion, myocardial infarction, coronary artery aneurysm, QT interval prolongation, tachyarrhythmias, and congestive heart failure have been reported [15]. Lyme myopericarditis is often self-limiting and mild. However, occasionally patients can develop symptomatic myocarditis with cardiac dysfunction [15]. Lardieri et al. reported two cases of patients affected by DCM in which *B. burgdorferi* was grown in the culture of myocardial biopsies. Cardiac function returned to normal following treatment with penicillin, in addition to standard heart failure therapy [16].

The diagnosis of Lyme carditis is challenging and requires the confirmation of the association between historical, clinical, and laboratory data. The disease is diagnosed most easily when the cardiac involvement presents in association with a history of thick bite and classical Lyme manifestations (erythema migrans, arthritis), in the setting of positive serologic testing for *B. burgdorferi* antibodies [15]. Echocardiography may provide evidence of myocardial dysfunction. Cardiac MRI plays a supportive role, typically displaying non-specific epicardial contrast enhancement [17].

15.3.4 Treatment

Antibiotic therapy in the early stages of the disease prevents or attenuates later complications. Patients who have minor cardiac involvement (PR interval less than 300 ms) and no other symptoms should receive oral antibiotics, amoxicillin or doxycycline. Patients who have more severe cardiac involvement, such as second- or third-degree atrioventricular block or congestive heart failure, should be hospitalized and treated with intravenous ceftriaxone or high-dose penicillin G. Complete atrioventricular block usually resolves within 1 week, while minor conduction disturbances regress in 6 weeks [15].

15.4 Dilated Cardiomyopathy Associated with Neuromuscular Diseases: Co-working with Neurologists

Neuromuscular diseases encompass a broad spectrum of diagnoses with overlapping but distinct phenotypes [18], and most forms of cardiac involvement are detected from childhood to the second decade of life, but others can remain asymptomatic until later in life [18].

DCM occurs in a variety of inherited neuromuscular disorders and represents the interface between the cardiology and neurology specialties. Patients with DCM should undergo a comprehensive examination which includes a neuromuscular examination in order to detect potential neuromuscular disorders. Moreover, serum creatine kinase (CK) dosage is useful during the diagnostic work-up of DCM with potential skeletal muscle involvement (see Table 15.1).

- X-linked recessive muscular dystrophies include Duchenne muscular dystrophy (DMD) with a more severe phenotype and Becker muscular dystrophy (BMD) with milder and more variable phenotype. These are caused by mutations within the dystrophin gene, located on the X chromosome. Physical exam can reveal calf pseudohypertrophy, shortening of the Achilles tendons and hyporeflexia or areflexia in weak muscles, lumbar lordosis which compensates for gluteal weakness, and the classic Gower's sign (the use of the hands and arms to "walk" up the own body from a squatting position due to lack of hip and thigh muscle strength). The incidence of cardiomyopathy in DMD increases with age. Although it is estimated that 25% of boys have cardiomyopathy at 6 years of age and 59% by 10 years of age, cardiac involvement is nearly ubiquitous in older patients with DMD, as more than 80% of young men over 18 years of age demonstrate evidence of cardiac dysfunction [19, 20]. Cardiac involvement leads to a progressive decline in cardiac function with age, resulting in ventricular dysfunction that contributes to early death for heart failure. DMD causes a primary cardiomyopathy characterized by extensive fibrosis of postero-basal left ventricular wall, resulting in the characteristic electrocardiographic change of tall right precordial R waves and deep Q waves in leads I, aVL, and V5–6. Clinical cardiologist should be aware of this "red flag" which may orient to a dystrophin-related cardiomyopathy. Currently, clinical guidelines recommend the initial cardiac screening at the time of diagnosis of DMD, every 2 years until 10 years of age and then yearly thereafter. It seems that angiotensin converting enzyme inhibitors (ACEi) and beta-blockers may delay the onset and the progression of cardiac dysfunction and have to be recommended earlier in this disease and should become the mainstay of treatment of dystrophinopathic cardiomyopathy [21, 22].

- Emery-Dreifuss muscular dystrophy (EDMD) is a genetically heterogeneous disorder that can be inherited as an X-linked recessive, autosomal dominant or autosomal recessive disorder. The disease is generally characterized by progressive muscle wasting and weakness with typically early contractures of the elbows, Achilles tendons, and spine. DCM is seen in most patients with EDMD with common association of atrioventricular defects; however there is no correlation between the degree of neuromuscular involvement and the severity of cardiac abnormalities. Arrhythmogenic dilated cardiomyopathy and ventricular tachyarrhythmias are more common in autosomal dominant form (due to lamin A/C mutations).
- Limb-girdle muscular dystrophy (LGMD) is still used as a generic term to describe those patients with muscular dystrophy of girdle distribution. Indeed, it is characterized by proximal weakness affecting the pelvic and shoulder girdles. There is broad clinical heterogeneity among the various LGMDs, and cardiac involvement is very common in lamin A/C mutation, which presents arrhythmias and conduction abnormalities and sarcoglycan disease which frequently presents a DCM phenotype.
- Myotonic muscular dystrophies, type 1 and type 2, are characterized by myotonia, seen as an impaired relaxation after muscle contraction. Myotonic dystrophy is a multisystemic disease and can be associated with DCM [23–26]. Cardiac manifestations include also atrioventricular block with occasional progression to complete heat block, atrial fibrillation, ventricular tachyarrhythmias, and reduced left ventricular ejection fraction.

15.5 Primary Iron-Overload Cardiomyopathy: Co-working with the Hematologists

Iron-overload cardiomyopathy can result from a primary disorder of iron metabolism or from secondary causes of iron overload, such as hematologic disorders. Hereditary hemochromatosis is commonly due to mutations in the HFE gene, an autosomal recessive disorder in which there is increased intestinal iron absorption. Cardiac hemochromatosis is an important and potentially preventable cause of heart failure [27]. This is initially characterized by diastolic dysfunction and conduction disturbances and in later stages by DCM. When evaluating a new cardiomyopathy, screening for iron overload should include serum ferritin and transferrin saturation. Cardiac involvement in hemochromatosis can often be diagnosed on the basis of history, clinical examination, laboratory testing, and noninvasive imaging. Myocardial iron overload can be detected also by CMR.

Current treatment modalities to remove excess iron stores include therapeutic phlebotomy and iron-chelating agents; congestive heart failure should be treated with standard heart failure treatment regimens. Timely diagnosis and treatment can prevent and in some cases reverse left ventricular dysfunction.

15.6 Cardiomyopathy Related to Chemotherapeutic Agents: Co-working with Oncologists

Cancer patients receiving chemotherapy have an increased risk of developing cardiovascular complications. Cardiotoxicity is one of the most concerning of these complications and is defined as a left ventricular ejection fraction (LVEF) decline of ≥5 to <55% with heart failure symptoms or an asymptomatic decrease of LVEF ≥10 to <55% during cancer therapy [2, 28].

Two different patterns of cytotoxicity have been recognized:

- Type I refers to the effects of the drugs that determine acute myocyte injury, causing irreversible damage and depressed cardiac function on a dose-dependent basis. The most commonly accepted pathophysiological mechanism of cardiotoxicity is oxidative damage: these molecules form complexes with iron causing free radicals production [29]. Anthracyclines are the prototype for this category. The cardiac damage is dose-dependent; for this reason, in an attempt to reduce this injury, the initial dose, which is recommended not to be exceeded, is usually the one that has shown to cause less than 5% of heart failure cases. In comparison with other cardiomyopathies, anthracycline cardiotoxicity appears to have a substantially worse prognosis, with mortality rates up to 60% at 2 years. The hazard ratio for mortality has been reported as being over threefold that of idiopathic dilated cardiomyopathy [30]. For this reason, cardiac-sparing and cardioprotective strategies have been developed to reduce cardiac damage.
- Type II refers to a pattern of often reversible cardiomyopathy with no evidence of acute myocyte injury. This type of cytotoxicity is not dose-dependent. Cardiac damage does not appear to occur in all patients, is expressed in a broad range of severity, and is not associated with identifiable ultrastructural abnormalities. Trastuzumab, a monoclonal antibody, is an example of these agents and may cause a reversible myocyte dysfunction.

Patients undergoing chemotherapy should have careful clinical evaluation and assessment of cardiovascular risk factors and comorbidities before initiating the treatment.

After the treatment beginning, the most frequently used modality for detecting cardiotoxicity is the periodic measurement of left ventricular ejection fraction by using echocardiography. Global systolic longitudinal strain assessed by speckle tracking technology has been reported to accurately predict a subsequent decrease in ejection fraction [31]. The use of cardiac biomarkers, in particular troponins, during cardiotoxic chemotherapy, has emerged in the last decade and has proven to be a sensitive and specific tool for early identification and monitoring of anticancer drug-induced cardiac injury. Brain natriuretic peptide (BNP) may be useful, but its role in routine surveillance to define high-risk patients is not well established [28, 31].

The timing of cardiotoxicity surveillance, using echocardiography and biomarkers, needs to be personalized to the patients, considering their baseline cardiovascular risk and the specific cancer treatment protocol. Baseline echocardiography is recommended in all patients. Lifelong surveillance should be offered to patients treated with high doses of anthracycline and to survivors of childhood cancer [31].

15.6.1 Treatment

If left ventricular ejection fraction decreases >10% to a value below the lower limit of normal, ACEi and beta-blockers are recommended [31]. Moreover, when heart failure develops during chemotherapy, it is important to refer the patients to a cardio-oncology specialist and to have a close liaison with the oncology team to determine the necessity and duration of any interruption of cancer treatment [28, 31]. The time from the detection of cardiotoxicity, at the surveillance echocardiography, to the start of heart failure therapy is a crucial variable for recovery of cardiac dysfunction [32]. The historical dogma that anthracycline toxicity is irreversible is mainly due to the fact that the cardiac damage was identified late, while it has been shown that the large majority of patients with left ventricular dysfunction can improve with early therapy [2].

15.7 Alcoholic Cardiomyopathy

Alcoholic cardiomyopathy is a form of acquired dilated cardiomyopathy associated with a long history of heavy alcohol abuse (commonly defined as the consumption of over 80–90 g per day over a period of at least 5 years). The disease has a similar prevalence in men and women, although women seem to require a lower total lifetime dose of ethanol to develop symptoms.

Several mechanisms are implicated in mediating the adverse effects of ethanol: oxidative stress, apoptotic cell death, impaired mitochondrial bioenergetics/stress, derangements in fatty acid metabolism and transport, and accelerated protein catabolism [33]. Moreover, genetic factors may predispose to the disease. In a recent study, Ware et al. have shown that truncation variants in the gene encoding titin (TTNtv) represent an important genetic predisposition to alcoholic cardiomyopathy and that the combination of these variants and excess alcohol consumption is associated with worse left ventricular ejection fraction in patients affected by dilated cardiomyopathy [34].

Alcoholic cardiomyopathy is characterized by depressed cardiac output, reduced myocardial contractility, and dilatation of all the chambers of the heart. The effect of alcohol on left ventricular function is dose-dependent and progressive, causing, initially, a subclinical diastolic and/or systolic dysfunction, up to the development of low-output dilated cardiomyopathy, leading to episodes of congestive heart failure and even to sudden death [35]. Echocardiography is able to detect subclinical changes in cardiac function, which occur in the early stages of the disease, as abnormal Doppler transmitral flow pattern, indicating impaired left ventricle relaxation; changes in left ventricle volume before the changes in cardiac mass and impairment of diastolic filling may be a sensitive marker of the detrimental effect of alcohol on the heart [36].

Other clinical manifestations of alcoholic cardiomyopathy are arrhythmias. Indeed, chronic alcohol abuse produces multiple physiologic aberrancies in the heart, including ultrastructural changes, effects on the QT interval and heart rate variability, and proarrhythmic electrolyte abnormalities, creating a substrate for triggering nonfatal and fatal arrhythmias [35, 37].

The natural history of alcoholic cardiomyopathy compared with idiopathic dilated cardiomyopathy has been a highly controversial issue [38, 39]. The largest series of patients with alcoholic cardiomyopathy and the earliest to include significant numbers of patients receiving beta-blocker therapy, as well as angiotensin-converting enzyme inhibitor therapy, reported a better prognosis with alcoholic cardiomyopathy than with idiopathic dilated cardiomyopathy [40].

15.7.1 Treatment

Complete alcohol withdrawal is usually recommended to all patients with alcoholic cardiomyopathy [41]. Medical therapy is no different from that for other etiologies of heart failure. Moreover, any nutritional deficiencies should be corrected. The use of vitamin supplements is recommended in case of a deficiency, in particular B complex vitamins. Furthermore, it is necessary to correct the electrolyte disturbances, in order to avoid dangerous arrhythmias.

References

1. Japp AG, Gulati A, Cook SA, Cowie MR, Prasad SK. The diagnosis and evaluation of dilated cardiomyopathy. J Am Coll Cardiol. 2016;67:2996–3010.
2. Bozkurt B, Colvin M, Cook J, Cooper LT, Deswal A, Fonarow GC, et al. Current diagnostic and treatment strategies for specific dilated cardiomyopathies: a scientific statement from the American Heart Association. Circulation. 2016;134:e579–646.
3. Miller BH, Putman CE. The chest radiograph and sarcoidosis. Reevaluation of the chest radiograph in assessing activity of sarcoidosis: a preliminary communication. Sarcoidosis. 1985;2:85–90.
4. Birnie DH, Nery PB, Ha AC, Beanlands RSB. Cardiac sarcoidosis. J Am Coll Cardiol. 2016;68:411–21.

5. Birnie DH, Sauer WH, Bogun F, Cooper JM, Culver DA, Duvernoy CS, et al. HRS expert consensus statement on the diagnosis and management of arrhythmias associated with cardiac sarcoidosis. Heart Rhythm. 2014;11:1305–24.
6. Wijetunga M, Rockson S. Myocarditis in systemic lupus erythematosus. Am J Med. 2002;113:419–23.
7. Doherty NE, Siegel RJ. Cardiovascular manifestations of systemic lupus erythematosus. Am Heart J. 1985;110:1257–65.
8. Gordon C, Amissah-Arthur M-B, Gayed M, Brown S, Bruce IN, D'Cruz D, et al. The British Society for Rheumatology guideline for the management of systemic lupus erythematosus in adults: executive summary. Rheumatology. 2017;57:14–8.
9. Dhakal BP, Kim CH, Al-Kindi SG, Oliveira GH. Heart failure in systemic lupus erythematosus. Trends Cardiovasc Med. 2018;28:187–97.
10. Myung G, Forbess LJ, Ishimori ML, Chugh S, Wallace D, Weisman MH. Prevalence of resting-ECG abnormalities in systemic lupus erythematosus: a single-center experience. Clin Rheumatol. 2017;36:1311–6.
11. Pérez-Molina JA, Molina I. Chagas disease. Lancet. 2018;391:82–94.
12. Marin-Neto JA, Cunha-Neto E, Maciel BC, Simões MV. Pathogenesis of chronic Chagas heart disease. Circulation. 2007;115:1109–23.
13. de Andrade JP, Marin Neto JA, de Paola AAV, Vilas-Boas F, Oliveira GMM, Bacal F, et al. I Latin American guidelines for the diagnosis and treatment of Chagas' heart disease: executive summary. Arq Bras Cardiol. 2011;96:434–42.
14. Rassi A, Rassi A, Rassi SG. Predictors of mortality in chronic Chagas disease. Circulation. 2007;115:1101–9.
15. Fish AE, Pride YB, Pinto DS. Lyme carditis. Infect Dis Clin North Am. 2008;22:275–88.
16. Lardieri G, Salvi A, Camerini F, Ciñco M, Trevisan G. Isolation of Borrelia burgdorferi from myocardium. Lancet. 1993;342:490.
17. Munk PS, Ørn S, Larsen AI. Lyme carditis: persistent local delayed enhancement by cardiac magnetic resonance imaging. Int J Cardiol. 2007;115:2006–8.
18. Feingold B, Mahle WT, Auerbach S, Clemens P, Domenighetti AA, Jefferies JL, et al. Management of cardiac involvement associated with neuromuscular diseases: a scientific statement from the American Heart Association. Circulation. 2017;136:e200–31.
19. Nigro G, Comi LI, Politano L, Bain RJI. The incidence and evolution of cardiomyopathy in Duchenne muscular dystrophy. Int J Cardiol. 1990;26:271–7.
20. Bushby K, Finkel R, Birnkrant DJ, Case LE, Clemens PR, Cripe L, et al. Diagnosis and management of Duchenne muscular dystrophy, part 1: diagnosis, and pharmacological and psychosocial management. Lancet Neurol. 2010;9:77–93.
21. Fayssoil A. Angiotensin-converting enzyme inhibitors and beta-blockers in cardiac asymptomatic patients with Duchenne muscular dystrophy. Indian Heart J. 2010;62:273.
22. Viollet L, Thrush PT, Flanigan KM, Mendell JR, Allen HD. Effects of angiotensin-converting enzyme inhibitors and/or beta blockers on the cardiomyopathy in Duchenne muscular dystrophy. Am J Cardiol. 2012;110:98–102.
23. Jefferies JL, Eidem BW, Belmont JW, Craigen WJ, Ware SM, Fernbach SD, et al. Genetic predictors and remodeling of dilated cardiomyopathy in muscular dystrophy. Circulation. 2005;112:2799–804.
24. Sommerville RB, Vincenti MG, Winborn K, Casey A, Stitziel NO, Connolly AM, et al. Diagnosis and management of adult hereditary cardio-neuromuscular disorders: a model for the multidisciplinary care of complex genetic disorders. Trends Cardiovasc Med. 2017;27:51–8.
25. McNally EM, Sparano D. Mechanisms and management of the heart in myotonic dystrophy. Heart. 2011;97:1094–100.
26. Wahbi K, Babuty D, Probst V, Wissocque L, Labombarda F, Porcher R, et al. Incidence and predictors of sudden death, major conduction defects and sustained ventricular tachyarrhythmias in 1388 patients with myotonic dystrophy type 1. Eur Heart J. 2017;38:751–8.
27. Gulati V, Harikrishnan P, Palaniswamy C, Aronow WS, Jain D, Frishman WH. Cardiac involvement in hemochromatosis. Cardiol Rev. 2014;22:56–68.

28. Curigliano G, Cardinale D, Suter T, Plataniotis G, De azambuja E, Sandri MT, et al. Cardiovascular toxicity induced by chemotherapy, targeted agents and radiotherapy: ESMO clinical practice guidelines. Ann Oncol. 2012;23:vii155–66.
29. Zhang S, Liu X, Bawa-Khalfe T, Lu L-S, Lyu YL, Liu LF, et al. Identification of the molecular basis of doxorubicin-induced cardiotoxicity. Nat Med. 2012;18:1639–42.
30. Felker GM, Thompson RE, Hare JM, Hruban RH, Clemetson DE, Howard DL, et al. Underlying causes and long-term survival in patients with initially unexplained cardiomyopathy. N Engl J Med. 2000;342:1077–84.
31. Zamorano JL, Lancellotti P, Rodriguez Muñoz D, Aboyans V, Asteggiano R, Galderisi M, et al. 2016 European Society of Cardiology position paper on cancer treatments and cardiovascular toxicity. Eur Heart J. 2016;37:2768–801.
32. Cardinale D, Colombo A, Bacchiani G, Tedeschi I, Meroni CA, Veglia F, et al. Early detection of anthracycline cardiotoxicity and improvement with heart failure therapy. Circulation. 2015;131:1981–8.
33. Piano MR, Phillips SA. Alcoholic cardiomyopathy: pathophysiologic insights. Cardiovasc Toxicol. 2014;14:291–308.
34. Ware JS, Amor-salamanca A, Tayal U, Govind R, Serrano I, Pascual-figal DA, et al. Genetic etiology for alcohol-induced cardiac toxicity. J Am Coll Cardiol. 2018;71:2293–302.
35. Fernández-Solà J. Cardiovascular risks and benefits of moderate and heavy alcohol consumption. Nat Rev Cardiol. 2015;12:576–87.
36. Lazarević AM, Nakatani S, Nešković AN, Marinković J, Yasumura Y, Stojičić D, et al. Early changes in left ventricular function in chronic asymptomatic alcoholics: relation to the duration of heavy drinking. J Am Coll Cardiol. 2000;35:1599–606.
37. George A, Figueredo VM. Alcohol and arrhythmias: a comprehensive review. J Cardiovasc Med. 2010;11:221–8.
38. Fauchier L, Babuty D, Poret P, Casset-Senon D, Autret ML, Cosnay P, et al. Comparison of long-term outcome of alcoholic and idiopathic dilated cardiomyopathy. Eur Heart J. 2000;21:306–14.
39. Prazak P, Pfisterer M, Osswald S, Buser P, Burkart F. Differences of disease progression in congestive heart failure due to alcoholic as compared to idiopathic dilated cardiomyopathy. Eur Heart J. 1996;17:251–7.
40. Guzzo-Merello G, Segovia J, Dominguez F, Cobo-Marcos M, Gomez-Bueno M, Avellana P, et al. Natural history and prognostic factors in alcoholic cardiomyopathy. JACC Heart Fail. 2015;3:78–86.
41. Guzzo-Merello G, Cobo-Marcos M, Gallego-Delgado M, Garcia-Pavia P. Alcoholic cardiomyopathy. World J Cardiol. 2014;6:771–81.

Permissions

All chapters in this book were first published in DC, by Springer; hereby published with permission under the Creative Commons Attribution License or equivalent. Every chapter published in this book has been scrutinized by our experts. Their significance has been extensively debated. The topics covered herein carry significant findings which will fuel the growth of the discipline. They may even be implemented as practical applications or may be referred to as a beginning point for another development.

The contributors of this book come from diverse backgrounds, making this book a truly international effort. This book will bring forth new frontiers with its revolutionizing research information and detailed analysis of the nascent developments around the world.

We would like to thank all the contributing authors for lending their expertise to make the book truly unique. They have played a crucial role in the development of this book. Without their invaluable contributions this book wouldn't have been possible. They have made vital efforts to compile up to date information on the varied aspects of this subject to make this book a valuable addition to the collection of many professionals and students.

This book was conceptualized with the vision of imparting up-to-date information and advanced data in this field. To ensure the same, a matchless editorial board was set up. Every individual on the board went through rigorous rounds of assessment to prove their worth. After which they invested a large part of their time researching and compiling the most relevant data for our readers.

The editorial board has been involved in producing this book since its inception. They have spent rigorous hours researching and exploring the diverse topics which have resulted in the successful publishing of this book. They have passed on their knowledge of decades through this book. To expedite this challenging task, the publisher supported the team at every step. A small team of assistant editors was also appointed to further simplify the editing procedure and attain best results for the readers.

Apart from the editorial board, the designing team has also invested a significant amount of their time in understanding the subject and creating the most relevant covers. They scrutinized every image to scout for the most suitable representation of the subject and create an appropriate cover for the book.

The publishing team has been an ardent support to the editorial, designing and production team. Their endless efforts to recruit the best for this project, has resulted in the accomplishment of this book. They are a veteran in the field of academics and their pool of knowledge is as vast as their experience in printing. Their expertise and guidance has proved useful at every step. Their uncompromising quality standards have made this book an exceptional effort. Their encouragement from time to time has been an inspiration for everyone.

The publisher and the editorial board hope that this book will prove to be a valuable piece of knowledge for researchers, students, practitioners and scholars across the globe.

List of Contributors

Marco Merlo and Gianfranco Sinagra
Cardiovascular Department, Azienda Sanitaria Universitaria Integrata, Trieste, Italy

Chiara Daneluzzi and Antonio Cannatà
Cardiovascular Department, Azienda Sanitaria Universitaria Integrata, University of Trieste

Luisa Mestroni
Cardiovascular Institute and Adult Medical Genetics Program, University of Colorado Anschutz Medical Campus, Aurora, CO, USA

Paola Naso, Luca Falco, Aldostefano Porcari, Andrea Di Lenarda and Gerardina Lardieri
Cardiovascular Department, Azienda Sanitaria Universitaria Integrata, University of Trieste (ASUITS), Trieste, Italy

Valerio De Paris, Federico Biondi and Davide Stolfo
Cardiovascular Department, Azienda Sanitaria Universitaria Integrata, University of Trieste (ASUITS), Trieste, Italy

Marco Merlo and Gianfranco Sinagra
Cardiovascular Department, Azienda Sanitaria Universitaria Integrata, Trieste, Italy

Marco Merlo
Cardiovascular Department, Azienda Sanitaria Universitaria Integrata, Trieste, Italy

Marco Gobbo, Jessica Artico and Stefania Franco
Cardiovascular Department, Azienda Sanitaria Universitaria Integrata, University of Trieste (ASUITS), Trieste, Italy

Elena Abate
Cardiovascular Department, Azienda Sanitaria Universitaria Integrata, University of Trieste (ASUITS), Trieste, Italy
Klinik für Innere Medizin 3, Universitätsklinikum Halle (Saale), Halle (Saale), Germany

Matteo Dal Ferro and Marta Gigli
Cardiovascular Department, Azienda Sanitaria Universitaria Integrata, University of Trieste (ASUITS), Trieste, Italy

Giovanni Maria Severini
Medical Genetics Laboratory, Institute of Maternal and Child Health IRCCS Burlo Garofolo, Trieste, Italy

Luisa Mestroni
Cardiovascular Institute and Adult Medical Genetics Program, University of Colorado Anschutz Medical Campus, Aurora, CO, USA

Gianfranco Sinagra
Cardiovascular Department, Azienda Sanitaria Universitaria Integrata, Trieste, Italy

Marco Merlo and Gianfranco Sinagra
Cardiovascular Department, Azienda Sanitaria Universitaria Integrata, Trieste, Italy

Davide Stolfo, Thomas Caiffa and Alberto Pivetta
Cardiovascular Department, Azienda Sanitaria Universitaria Integrata, University of Trieste (ASUITS), Trieste, Italy

Bruno Pinamonti, Antonio De Luca and Renata Korcova
Cardiovascular Department, Azienda Sanitaria Universitaria Integrata, University of Trieste (ASUITS), Trieste, Italy

Elena Abate
Cardiovascular Department, Azienda Sanitaria Universitaria Integrata, University of Trieste (ASUITS), Trieste, Italy
Klinik für Innere Medizin 3, Universitätsklinikum Halle (Saale), Halle (Saale), Germany

Gherardo Finocchiaro
Cardiology Clinical and Academic Group, St George's, University of London, London, UK

Giancarlo Vitrella, Giorgio Faganello and Gaetano Morea
Cardiovascular Department, Azienda Sanitaria Universitaria Integrata di Trieste (ASUITS), Trieste, Italy

Lorenzo Pagnan, Manuel Belgrano and Maria Assunta Cova
Diagnostic and Interventional Radiology Department, Azienda Sanitaria Universitaria Integrata di Trieste (ASUITS), Trieste, Italy

Rossana Bussani and Furio Silvestri
Department of Pathology, Azienda Sanitaria Universitaria Integrata, University of Trieste (ASUITS), Trieste, Italy

Andrea Perkan and Piero Gentile
Cardiovascular Department, Azienda Sanitaria Universitaria Integrata, University of Trieste (ASUITS), Trieste, Italy

Gianfranco Sinagra
Cardiovascular Department, Azienda Sanitaria Universitaria Integrata, Trieste, Italy

Massimo Zecchin and Tullio Morgera
Cardiovascular Department, Azienda Sanitaria Universitaria Integrata, University of Trieste (ASUITS), Trieste, Italy

Daniele Muser
Cardiac Electrophysiology, Cardiovascular Medicine Division, Hospital of the University of Pennsylvania, Philadelphia, PA, USA

Cardiothoracic Department, University Hospital of Udine, Udine, Italy

Laura Vitali-Serdoz
Division of Electrophysiology, Department of Cardiology, Klinikum Coburg, Coburg, Germany

Alessandra Buiatti
Cardiovascular Department, Azienda Sanitaria Universitaria Integrata, University of Trieste (ASUITS), Trieste, Italy
Klinik und Poliklinik für Innere Medizin I–Kardiologie, Klinikum rechts der Isar–Technische Universität München, Munich, Germany

Pierluigi Lesizza, Aneta Aleksova and Benedetta Ortis
Cardiovascular Department, Azienda Sanitaria Universitaria Integrata, University of Trieste (ASUITS), Trieste, Italy

Antonio Paolo Beltrami
Pathology Department, School of Medicine, University of Udine, Udine, Italy

Mauro Giacca
Molecular Medicine Laboratory, International Centre for Genetic Engineering and Biotechnology (ICGEB), Trieste, Italy

Gianfranco Sinagra
Cardiovascular Department, Azienda Sanitaria Universitaria Integrata, Trieste, Italy

Antonio Cannatà, Davide Stolfo and Cosimo Carriere
Cardiovascular Department, Azienda Sanitaria Universitaria Integrata, University of Trieste (ASUITS), Trieste, Italy

Marco Merlo and Gianfranco Sinagra
Cardiovascular Department, Azienda Sanitaria Universitaria Integrata, Trieste, Italy

Alessandro Altinier, Alessia Paldino, Marta Gigli and Aniello Pappalardo
Cardiovascular Department, Azienda Sanitaria Universitaria Integrata, University of Trieste (ASUITS), Trieste, Italy

Gianfranco Sinagra
Cardiovascular Department, Azienda Sanitaria Universitaria Integrata, Trieste, Italy

Marco Merlo and Gianfranco Sinagra
Cardiovascular Department, Azienda Sanitaria Universitaria Integrata, Trieste, Italy

Giulia De Angelis, Antonio Cannatà and Laura Massa
Cardiovascular Department, Azienda Sanitaria Universitaria Integrata, University of Trieste (ASUITS), Trieste, Italy

Gianfranco Sinagra and Marco Merlo
Cardiovascular Department, Azienda Sanitaria Universitaria Integrata, Trieste, Italy

Enrico Fabris, Simona Romani, Francesco Negri, Davide Stolfo and Francesca Brun
Cardiovascular Department, Azienda Sanitaria Universitaria Integrata, University of Trieste (ASUITS), Trieste, Italy

Index

www.ingramcontent.com/pod-product-compliance
Lightning Source LLC
LaVergne TN
LVHW080804220926
848485LV00011B/147